BASIC ORTHOPAEDIC SCIENCES

BASIC ORTHOPAEDIC SCIENCES
The Stanmore Guide

Edited by

Manoj Ramachandran BSc(Hons) MBBS(Hons) MRCS(Eng) FRCS(Orth)
Paediatric and Young Adult Orthopaedic Fellow
Royal National Orthopaedic Hospital
Stanmore, UK

Associate Editors

Deborah M Eastwood MB FRCS
Consultant Orthopaedic Surgeon
Great Ormond Street Hospital for Children, London; and
Royal National Orthopaedic Hospital, Stanmore, UK

Dishan B Singh FRCS(Orth)
Consultant Orthopaedic Surgeon
Royal National Orthopaedic Hospital, Stanmore, UK

John AM Skinner MBBS FRCS(Eng) FRCS(Orth)
Consultant Orthopaedic Surgeon
Royal National Orthopaedic Hospital, Stanmore, UK

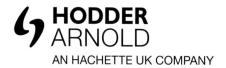
HODDER
ARNOLD
AN HACHETTE UK COMPANY

Hodder Arnold
First published in Great Britain in 2007 by
Hodder Arnold, an imprint of Hodder Education,
an Hachette UK company
338 Euston Road, London NW1 3BH

http://www.hoddereducation.com

Hachette UK's policy is to use papers that are natural, renewable and
recyclable products and made from wood grown in sustainable forests. The
logging and manufacturing processes are expected to conform to the
environmental regulations of the country of origin.

Whilst the advice and information in this book are believed to be true and
accurate at the date of going to press, neither the authors nor the publisher
can accept any legal responsibility or liability for any errors or omissions that
may be made. In particular (but without limiting the generality of the
preceding disclaimer) every effort has been made to check drug dosages;
however it is still possible that errors have been missed. Furthermore, dosage
schedules are constantly being revised and new side effects recognized. For
these reasons the reader is strongly urged to consult the drug companies'
printed instructions before administering any of the drugs recommended in
this book.

British Library Cataloguing in Publication Data
A catalogue record for this book is available from the British Library

Library of Congress Cataloging-in-Publication Data
A catalog record for this book is available from the Library of Congress

ISBN   978 0 340 885 024

2 3 4 5 6 7 8 9 10

Commissioning Editor:	Sarah Burrows
Project Editor:	Francesca Naish
Production Controller:	Joanna Walker
Cover Design:	Nichola Smith
Indexer:	Laurence Errington

Typeset in 9.5/12 pt Berling by Phoenix Photosetting, Chatham, Kent
Printed and bound in Spain by Graphycems

What do you think about this book? Or any other Hodder Arnold title?
Please visit our website: www.hoddereducation.com

For Joanna.
Everything I do is for you and you only.

Contents

Contributors

Pramod Achan FRCS(Orth)
Consultant Orthopaedic Surgeon
Royal London Hospital, London

Paul Allen MBBS FRCS
Consultant Orthopaedic Surgeon
Princess Alexandra Hospital, Harlow

William Aston BSc MRCS(Ed)
Specialist Registrar in Trauma and Orthopaedics
Royal National Orthopaedic Hospital, Stanmore

Rajiv Bajekal MCh(Orth) FRCS(Orth)
Consultant Orthopaedic Surgeon
Barnet General Hospital, London

Marcus Bankes BSc(Hons) MBBS(Hons) FRCS(Orth)
Consultant Orthopaedic Surgeon
Guy's and St Thomas' Hospital, London

Peter Bates BSc MRCS
Specialist Registrar in Trauma and Orthopaedics
Royal National Orthopaedic Hospital, Stanmore

Lisa Bellows BSc(Hons)
Orthotist
Great Ormond Street Children's Hospital, London

George Bentley ChM FRCS
Professor of Orthopaedics (retired) and locum
consultant
Royal National Orthopaedic Hospital, Stanmore

Rolfe Birch MChir FRCS
Professor of Orthopaedic Neurological Surgery
Royal National Orthopaedic Hospital, Stanmore

Gurdeep Biring BSc MBBS MRCS MSc (Ortho Eng) FRCS
(Orth)
Specialist Registrar in Trauma and Orthopaedics
Royal National Orthopaedic Hospital, Stanmore

Gordon Blunn BSc PhD
Head, Centre of Biomedical Engineering
Institute of Orthopaedics and Musculoskeletal
Science, Stanmore

Rick Brown MA FRCS(Orth)
Consultant Orthopaedic Surgeon
Cheltenham General Hospital, Cheltenham

Peter Calder FRCS(Orth)
Consultant Orthopaedic Surgeon
Royal National Orthopaedic Hospital, Stanmore

Stephen R Cannon FRCS
Consultant Orthopaedic Surgeon, Clinical Director
and Chair of the London Bone and Soft Tissue
Tumour Unit
Royal National Orthopaedic Hospital, Stanmore

Richard Carrington MBBS FRCS FRCS(Orth)
Consultant Orthopaedic Surgeon
Royal National Orthopaedic Hospital, Stanmore

Subhamoy Chatterjee MBBS MRCS(Ed) MSc (Distinction)
Specialist Registrar in Trauma and Orthopaedics
University College Hospital, London

Deborah M Eastwood MB FRCS
Consultant Orthopaedic Surgeon
Great Ormond Street Hospital for Children, London;
and
Royal National Orthopaedic Hospital, Stanmore

David Evans FRCS
Consultant Hand Surgeon and Clinical Director
The Hand Clinic, Windsor

Mark Falworth FRCS(Eng) FRCS (Orth)
Specialist Registrar in Trauma and Orthopaedics
Royal National Orthopaedic Hospital, Stanmore

Michael Fox BSc MRCS
Specialist Registrar in Trauma and Orthopaedics
Royal National Orthopaedic Hospital, Stanmore

Fares Haddad BSc MCh(Orth) FRCS(Orth) Dip Sports Med
Consultant Orthopaedic Surgeon
University College and Middlesex Hospitals, London

Alister Hart MA FRCS(Orth)
Specialist Registrar in Trauma and Orthopaedics
Royal National Orthopaedic Hospital, Stanmore

Aresh Hashemi-Nejad MBBS FRCS FRCS(Orth)
Consultant Orthopaedic Surgeon
Royal National Orthopaedic Hospital, Stanmore

Caroline Hing BSc MBBS MSc MD FRCS(Orth)
Specialist Registrar in Trauma and Orthopaedics
Royal National Orthopaedic Hospital, Stanmore

Brian Hsu MBBS
Registrar in Trauma and Orthopaedics
Royal North Shore Hospital, Sydney, Australia

Vikas Khanduja MBBS FRCS(G) MSc FRCS(Orth)
Specialist Registrar in Trauma and Orthopaedics
Royal National Orthopaedic Hospital, Stanmore

Simon Lambert BSc FRCS(Ed) FRCS (Orth)
Consultant Orthopaedic Surgeon
Royal National Orthopaedic Hospital, Stanmore

David Little MMBS FRACS(Orth) PhD
Head, Orthopaedic Research and Biotechnology and
Consultant Orthopaedic Surgeon
The Children's Hospital at Westmead, Sydney,
Australia

Rohit Madhav MBBS FRCSEd(Orth)
Consultant Orthopaedic Surgeon
University College and Middlesex Hospitals, London

Linda Marks FRCP
Consultation in Rehabilitation Medicine
Royal National Orthopaedic Hospital, Stanmore

Nimalan Maruthainar FRCSEd(Orth)
Consultant Orthopaedic Surgeon
Royal Free Hospital, London

Jay Meswania
Technical Manager, Centre of Biomedical
Engineering
Institute of Orthopaedics and Musculoskeletal
Science, Stanmore

Fergal Monsell MSc FRCS(Orth)
Consultant Orthopaedic Surgeon
Bristol Children's Hospital, Bristol

Mark Mullins MA FRCS(Orth)
Consultant Orthopaedic Surgeon
Royal London Hospital, London

Amir Ali Narvani BSc MBBS(Hons) MRCS MSc(Sports
Med)(Hons)
Specialist Registrar in Trauma and Orthopaedics
Barnet General Hospital, London

Natasha Rahman BSc(Hons) MBBS MRCS
Specialist Registrar in Trauma and Orthopaedics
Royal London Hospital, London

Manoj Ramachandran
Paediatric and Young Adult Fellow
Royal National Orthopaedic Hospital, Stanmore

Navin Ramachandran BSc(Hons) MBBS(Hons) MRCP
Specialist Registrar in Diagnostic Radiology and
Honorary Lecturer
St George's Hospital and the University of London,
London

Vijai Ranawat BSc(Hons) MBBS MRCS
Specialist Registrar in Trauma and Orthopaedics
Royal National Orthopaedic Hospital, Stanmore

Asif Saifuddin BSc(Hons) MBChB MRCP FRCR
Consultant Musculoskeletal Radiologist
Royal National Orthopaedic Hospital, Stanmore

Nicholas Saw FRCS(Orth)
Consultant Orthopaedic Surgeon
The Princess Alexandra Hospital NHS Trust,
Harlow, Essex

Dishan B Singh FRCS(Orth)
Consultant Orthopaedic Surgeon
Royal National Orthopaedic Hospital, Stanmore

John AM Skinner MBBS FRCS(Eng) FRCS(Orth)
Consultant Orthopaedic Surgeon
Royal National Orthopaedic Hospital, Stanmore

Cheh Chin Tai MA FRCS(Orth)
Specialist Registrar in Trauma and Orthopaedics
Whittington Hospital, London

Tim Waters BSc MRCS
Specialist Registrar in Trauma and Orthopaedics
Royal National Orthopaedic Hospital, Stanmore

Alan White MB BCh FRCS FRCS(Orth)
Consultant Orthopaedic Surgeon
Southend Hospital, Southend

Andrew Williams MBBS FRCS FRCS(Orth)
Consultant Orthopaedic Surgeon
Chelsea and Westminster Hospital, London

Lester Wilson FRCS(Eng) FRCS(Orth)
Consultant Spinal Surgeon
Royal National Orthopaedic Hospital, Stanmore

Foreword

Knowledge of basic science is an essential platform on which to build an understanding of orthopaedics. It is necessary for day-to-day clinical work, research, publications and examinations. This book has been developed to cover the major areas of basic science required by orthopaedic surgeons and all those associated with musculoskeletal function and dysfunction.

Although it would be impossible to cover every facet of basic science, the sections are wide-ranging, from statistics to biomechanics and from pharmacology to gait analysis. Sections on all the musculoskeletal tissues have been included, together with sections on the functions of all the joints. Relevant areas of biomaterials, friction and lubrication, together with the basic tools of research, including statistics, have also been included in a form that provides the essence of knowledge required of the trainee.

The majority of the chapters have a junior and senior author. Each senior author has an expertise in the area covered, while the junior author has provided the focus required for postgraduate orthopaedic examinations. Each section is well organized and easy to read and contains a wealth of information essential to the reader. The viva questions are useful in assessing the reader's understanding of the section with an added essential reading section for the examination candidate.

Basic Orthopaedic Sciences: The Stanmore Guide has been ably edited by Manoj Ramachandran, Paediatric and Young Adult Fellow on the Stanmore Rotation, who is to be congratulated in bringing together such a disparate group of topics, along with the contributors for making many difficult topics so understandable.

I am sure this book will become a necessary addition to any library for those requiring information on orthopaedic basic sciences in a concise and readable form.

George SE Dowd MD MCh(Orth) FRCS
Co-Director of Training, Royal National
Orthopaedic Hospital Rotation and Consultant
Orthopaedic Surgeon
Royal Free Hospital and Wellington Knee Unit,
London; and
Training Programme Director, Royal National
Orthopaedic Hospital, Stanmore

Preface

How many times have you heard a colleague say, "I once knew everything about articular cartilage/hip biomechanics/statistics (*substitute any orthopaedic basic science topic here*) but I seem to have forgotten the exact details. Anyway, you're the one sitting the exam, not me!" Oh, how trainees love to hear those dulcet tones of encouragement…

I like to think that learning orthopaedic basic sciences is somewhat similar to learning anatomy at medical school. It is certainly better to have learnt once than not at all. Equally, it is better to have understood concepts than to have committed facts to rote memory. Having spouted all these wise words though, I still feel that there is an awful lot to learn in orthopaedic basic sciences. The aim of this book is to tease out the pertinent points that are relevant both to exam situations and day-to-day clinical practice. Although originally conceived with postgraduate orthopaedic exams in mind, the final text has evolved into a primer in basic sciences for all health professionals with an interest in orthopaedics, mainly as a result of the input from all the contributors.

This first edition has drawn from and expanded on the popular "Stanmore Basic Sciences course" run at the Royal National Orthopaedic Hospital in Middlesex, UK. The book's scope and focus were determined by feedback from candidates on the course and from field-testing at its various stages of development (which makes it sound much more impressive than it really was!). Ideas such as bold highlighting of key words and concepts, and the use of only five key references for further reading, were added along the way. Diagrams have been kept simple for ease of reproduction as and when required. Although the book is not exhaustive, and indeed does not claim to be, a working knowledge of the text should serve the readers well in their journey through the quagmire that is basic sciences.

Finally, a personal note. I wanted to put together a text that doesn't insult the reader by aiming too low and omitting key information. Equally, aiming too high (as some books do) would be disastrous. I've settled for a happy medium. I urge you, the reader, having read this book, to rest safe in the knowledge that you are at the higher end of the orthopaedic basic science Gaussian curve. And from this vantage position, from where you can attack any exam-related or basic science query, I urge you to send me feedback so I can improve upon this edition and perhaps even invite you onto the panel of authors on the next one.

Now all you have to do is start by learning how exactly a Gaussian curve is defined…

Manoj Ramachandran
manojorthopod@gmail.com
London 2006

Acknowledgements

I'd like to start by thanking all the authors for putting up with my constant nagging about deadlines. I hope you all think it was worth the effort. The senior reviewers did a great job too. I must single out Dishan Singh as the book's catalyst during its embryonic stages. The conversations we had back in 2002 are the reason why this book even came into being. In addition, Deborah Eastwood worked tirelessly (as always!) in the latter stages of the book's development to ensure that deadlines were met and people were chased up.

I'd also like to thank and congratulate the team at Hodder Arnold for making this book happen. Finally, I must thank everyone in my personal life for putting up with me during my multiple projects. My deepest gratitude though goes to my wife, Joanna.

1

Statistics

MANOJ RAMACHANDRAN, DAVID LITTLE AND FARES HADDAD

INTRODUCTION

A working knowledge of statistics is essential for any healthcare professional working within the sphere of orthopaedics. At its most basic, statistics involves the handling of data, best thought of in three ways:

- **Data collection**, e.g. surveys, studies.
- **Data presentation**, e.g. measurement of central tendency and variation.
- **Data interpretation**, e.g. hypothesis testing, confidence intervals.

In reality, experienced statisticians working in conjunction with orthopaedic surgeons commonly perform data-handling with access to computerized statistical packages. Orthopaedic surgeons should know how to critique data in print and how to design, implement and analyse the results of a study.

DATA TYPE

Types of data are summarized in Table 1.1.

DATA PRESENTATION

Plotting of data allows determination of central tendency and spread (or variability). The

Table 1.1 Types of data analysed in statistics

	Description	Discrete/ continuous?	Qualitative/ quantitative?	Parametric/ non-parametric?
Nominal	*Categories without order, e.g. eye colour, marital status*	*Discrete*	*Qualitative*	*Non-parametric*
Ordinal	*Ordered categories, e.g. Ficat grades*	*Discrete*	*Qualitative*	*Non-parametric*
Integer	*Number of counts, e.g. papers published*	*Discrete*	*Quantitative*	*Parametric or non-parametric*
Ratio	*Zero at origin, value independent of units, e.g. age, distance*	*Continuous*	*Quantitative*	*Parametric or non-parametric*
Interval	*Distances between units are of known size, e.g. hours spent revising*	*Continuous*	*Quantitative*	*Parametric or non-parametric*

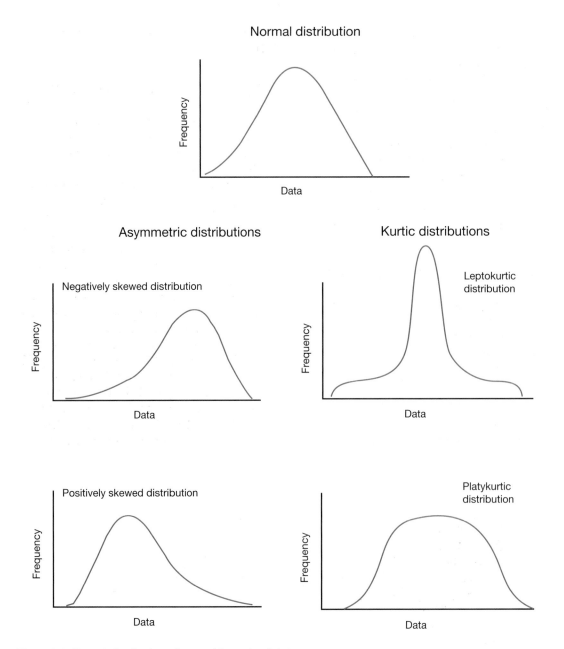

Figure 1.1 *Normal distribution, skew and kurtosis of data.*

familiar symmetrical bell-shaped curve of a **normal** (or **Gaussian**) **distribution** (Figure 1.1), which allows for the use of the mean as a measure of central tendency and of the more powerful parametric tests, is a rare event in orthopaedics.

Bell-shaped curves, when asymmetrical, are not distributed normally. A **skewed distribution** is asymmetrical and has a tail, which is either positive or negative. If data distribution is skewed, then the median or mode has to be used to measure central tendency. If there is doubt about the normality of a distribution, then it is best to assume that any given distribution is not normal and, therefore, data should be tested for normality (see later).

Kurtosis is a measure of the relative peaked-ness or flatness of a distribution compared with a normal distribution. Positive kurtosis (**leptokurtosis**) indicates a relatively peaked distribution, while negative kurtosis (**platykurtosis**) indicates a relatively flat distribution.

Transformation is the method by which non-normal data can be normalized in order to allow parametric testing. Biological variables that follow a logarithmic (or square, square-root or reciprocal) distribution may be converted to a normal distribution and the data then retested to see whether they are skewed.

MEASURES OF CENTRAL TENDENCY

- **Mean:** the average of the data, measured by dividing the sum of all the observations by the number of observations.
- **Median:** the central value of the data; used for ordinal data.
- **Mode:** the data value with the most frequency; used for nominal data.

For **perfectly normally distributed** data, the **mean, median and mode are the same**. This

does not hold true for skewed data (Figure 1.2).

MEASURES OF SPREAD/VARIABILITY

- **Range:** the lowest and highest values of the data. The range does not give much information about the spread of the data about the mean.
- **Percentiles:** groupings of data into brackets of 1 per cent, 10 per cent or, more commonly, 25 per cent (known as quartiles).
- **Variance:** the measure of the spread where the mean is the measure of the central tendency. Variance is the corrected sum of squares about the mean $[\sigma (x - \text{mean})^2 / (n - 1)]$.
- **Standard deviation (σ):** the square root of the variance (the use of the square root gives the same dimension as the data). For reasonably symmetrical bell-shaped data, one standard deviation (SD) contains roughly 68 per cent of the data, two SD contains roughly 95 per cent of the data and three SD contains around 99.7 per cent of the data (Figure 1.3). **A normal distribution is defined uniquely by two parameters, the**

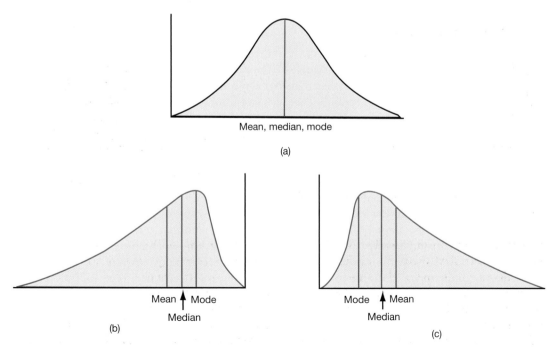

Figure 1.2 *Mean, median and modes for different data spreads.*

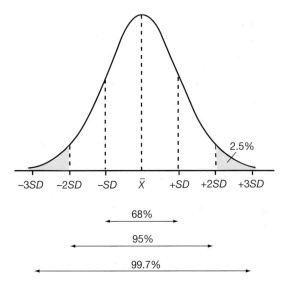

Figure 1.3 *Standard deviations (SD) of normally distributed data.*

mean and the SD of the population. Other features of a normal distribution include that it is **symmetrical** (mean = mode = median) and that the data are **continuous**.

- **Coefficient of variation**: defined as (SD/mean) × 100. Indicates how big the SD is in comparison with the mean: if SD is high, then the data are highly variable.
- **Standard error of the mean**: defined as the SD divided by the square root of the sample size. Used in relation to a sample rather than the population as a whole. The formula does not assume a normal distribution. It measures how closely the sample mean approximates the population mean.
- **Confidence intervals**: ranges on either side of a sample mean giving a rapid visual impression of significance. Confidence intervals (CI) are equal to the values between the confidence limits (CL) and are a set number of standard errors of estimate of the mean (SEM) from the mean on either side. For a large sample, 95% CIs are approximately two SEMs either side of the mean. Confidence intervals are preferred to P values (see below) because:
  - CIs relate to the sample size;
  - a range of values is provided;
  - CIs provide a rapid visual impression of significance;
  - CIs have the same units as the variable.

DATA INTERPRETATION

All good studies test hypotheses. When statistics are used to examine data concerning hypotheses, the key concept is that of the **null hypothesis**, where a primary assumption is made that any difference seen occurred purely by chance. The collected data are then tested to disprove the null hypothesis; if the result is statistically significant, then the hypothesis is rejected on the basis that it is wrong. The difference, therefore, must be real and did not occur by chance.

It is possible to calculate the probability that any difference seen did occur by chance. Orthopaedic surgeons are usually willing to accept a 5 per cent probability that the difference seen was due to chance ($P = 0.05$). If P is less than 0.05, then this suggests that the probability of the difference seen being due to chance is less than 5 per cent (for $P < 0.001$, the probability is less than 0.1 per cent).

ERRORS

Errors may arise when accepting or rejecting the null hypothesis. A **type I (α) error** occurs when a difference is found but in reality there is not a difference (i.e. a false-positive result, and therefore the null hypothesis is rejected incorrectly). This is one of those 5 per cent of cases where the difference occurred by chance. A good analogy is convicting an innocent person of a crime. We can protect against type I errors by reducing significance levels, although this increases the risk of a type II error occurring. Note that the risk of a type I error decreases as the acceptable P value is lowered, but then bigger study samples are needed in order to protect against a type II error.

A **type II (β) error** occurs when no difference is found but in reality a difference does exist (i.e. a false-negative result, and therefore the null hypothesis is accepted incorrectly). A good analogy here is failing to convict a person who is guilty of a crime. Type II errors are usually the result of a small sample size; therefore, it is important to perform a power analysis before undertaking a study. We can protect against type II errors with statistical power. Note that type I and type II errors are related inversely. Type II errors are common in orthopaedic studies.

A **type III (γ) error** occurs rarely when the researcher correctly rejects the null hypothesis but incorrectly attributes the cause. In other words, the researcher misinterprets cause and effect. Type III error is also used facetiously to refer to the mistake of switching the definitions of type I and type II errors.

POWER ANALYSIS

A statistical power analysis is a method of determining the number of subjects needed in a study in order to have a reasonable chance of showing a difference if one exists. The statistical power is the probability of demonstrating a true effect or statistically significant difference and is defined by $1 - \beta$ expressed as a percentage. The statistical power is therefore the probability that the test will correctly reject the null hypothesis. Power analysis must be performed before a study commences; without power analysis, it is difficult to know whether any lack of statistical significance is due to the lack of a real difference or due to a small sample size. When reviewing a study that lacks a statement about power, a post-hoc power analysis can be useful in estimating the probability of type II error.

Factors affecting power analyses

- size of the difference between the means (the larger the difference, the easier it is to detect a difference and the greater the power);
- spread of the data (the larger the spread, the less likely a difference will be detected);
- acceptable level of significance (i.e. the *P* value that is set);
- sample size (power increases with increasing sample size);

- variability in observations (the larger the variability, the lower the power);
- experimental design (e.g. within subjects versus between subjects);
- type of data (parametric versus non-parametric).

If the power of an experiment is low, then there is a good chance that the experiment will be inconclusive or give a type II error; thus, it is important to consider power in the design of experiments. As a general rule, if the clinically relevant difference approximates one SD of the measured variable, then 17 (or about 20) subjects are required in each group.

STUDY DESIGN

The first decision is whether the study is to be observational or experimental. In an **observational study**, the investigator observes rather than alters events. A review of the prevalence of pulmonary emboli after total hip replacement is an example of an observational or descriptive study. In an **experimental study**, the investigator applies a manoeuvre and then observes the outcome. For example, a surgeon may conduct a randomized trial comparing the effects of warfarin and heparin on the prevalence of deep venous thromboses in patients managed with total hip replacement. The investigator must also decide on the timeline of the study:

Study timelines

- **Retrospective study:** the outcome of interest has already occurred and the patient or cohort (group of patients) is followed forward in time from a point in the past.
- **Prospective study:** follows the patient or cohort forward in time; stronger than a retrospective study.
- **Cross-sectional study:** examines patients or events at one point in time without follow-up; used, for example, when looking at the prevalence of a condition or describing the distribution of variables.

The next step is the generation of a null hypothesis. Following this, a statistician is usually required to perform a power analysis in order to calculate the sample size. Value judgements are made regarding the risks of type I and type II errors acceptable based on the clinical and financial consequences of such a result. Typically, the type I (α) error is set at 0.05 and the type II (β) is set at 0.20, i.e. a power of 80 per cent. Calculation of the sample size also requires knowledge of the effect size (i.e. the difference expected between the means) and an estimation of the variance.

When performing multiple tests, there is an increased risk of a type I error and so the acceptable P value may have to be decreased. An example of correcting for this is the **Bonferroni correction**, which states simply that if one is testing n independent hypotheses, then one should use a significance level of $0.05/n$. For example, if there are two independent hypotheses, then a result would be declared significant only if P is less than 0.025. Note that although tests are rarely independent, the Bonferroni correction is a very conservative procedure that is unlikely to reject the null hypothesis. Other corrections are available, e.g. Tukey's least significant difference procedure.

SIGNIFICANCE TESTING

It is important to note that there may be a difference between clinical and statistical significance. To test for **statistical significance**, think about the following:

- What **type** of data have been used in the study?
- What is the **sample size**? (The larger the sample size, the easier it is to test, as parametric or non-parametric tests may be used.)
- Are the groups **distributed normally**?
- Do the data need to be **transformed** so that we can make a normality assumption?
- Are the groups interdependent? (Use a paired test.)
- Is a **single**- or **two-tailed** P value necessary? (If the direction – positive or negative – of the difference between the sample means is known, then only a one-tailed P value is necessary.)

Always remember that the magnitude of the difference between the data sets under consideration determines clinical significance. For example, a 5 per cent change in callus size is unlikely to be relevant, but a 25 per cent change may be relevant. The P value does not relate to clinical significance but merely tells us how certain we are that the difference we are considering is real.

Next, the type of test to be used is considered. Tests can be parametric or non-parametric. **Parametric tests** assume that data were sampled from a particular form of distribution, such as a normal distribution; **non-parametric tests** make no such assumption.

Features of parametric tests

- Assumes the data were sampled from a normal population.
- Observations must be independent.
- Populations must have the same variance.
- Can use absolute difference between data points.
- Increased power for a given sample size (n).
- Rarely exists in orthopaedics.

Features of non-parametric tests

- No assumptions are made about the origins of the data.
- No limitations on types of data.
- Rank order of values.
- Less likely to be significant.
- Decreased power for a given n.
- Cannot relate back to any parametric properties of the data.

It is best to use non-parametric tests if the outcome is a rank or score and the population is clearly not Gaussian, or if some of the values are off the scale (too high or low to measure). If unsure, there are statistical tests to determining whether the distribution of any measured data differs significantly from a

Table 1.2 Statistical tests for use in certain situations

	Normal distribution (from Gaussian population)	Not distributed normally, (e.g. rank, score, measurement)	Nominal data (binomial outcome)
Describing one group	Mean, SD	Median, interquartile range	Proportion
Two treatments in different groups	Unpaired t-test	Mann–Whitney U test (rank test)	Chi-squared test (Fisher's for small samples)
Two treatments in same or matched group(s)	Paired t-test	Wilcoxon signed rank test	McNemar's test
More than two treatments in different groups	ANOVA	Kruksal–Wallis test	Chi-squared test
More than two treatments in same or matched group(s)	Repeated measures ANOVA	Friedman test	Cochrane Q test
Quantify association between two variables	Pearson correlation	Spearman correlation	Contingency coefficients
Predict value from another measured variable	Simple linear or non-linear regression	Non-parametric regression	Simple logistic regression
Predict value from several measured or binomial variables	Multiple linear or nonlinear regression		Multiple logistic regression

ANOVA, analysis of one-way variance; SD, standard deviation.

Gaussian distribution, e.g. the Kolmogorov–Smirnoff and Shapiro–Wilk tests.

Table 1.2 indicates which tests to use in which situation.

It is worth knowing a little about the following tests:

PAIRED T-TEST

This should be used when there is a pair of observations on a single subject, e.g. blood pressure before and after application of a tourniquet. If there are multiple observations, then analysis of one-way variance (ANOVA) should be used. Note that the t-test is also known as Student's t-test (it was developed by WS Gosset, writing under the pseudonym 'Student').

UNPAIRED T-TEST

This can be used to compare two random samples provided they both follow a normal distribution. Samples can be of differing size but should be independent, i.e. there must be no chance that a subject could appear in both of the groups being compared.

ANALYSIS OF ONE-WAY VARIANCE

ANOVA determines the probability that two or more samples were drawn from the same parent population. ANOVA can be subclassified by secondary or grouping variables (two-way ANOVA), e.g. blood pressure before and after two different antihypertensive drugs. If some of the measurements were made in the same subjects, then the data can be corrected for repeated measures. Note that comparison of two samples with one-way ANOVA is very similar to performing an unpaired t-test.

CHI-SQUARED TEST

The chi-squared (χ^2) test can be used for qualitative data. It is used only on actual numbers of occurrences (i.e. frequencies), but not proportions, percentages, means or other derived statistics. The test compares distribution of a categorical variable in a sample with the distribution of a categorical variable in another sample. It assesses whether the observed data fit the expected pattern using the equation $\chi^2 = \sigma (O - E)^2/E$, where O is observed data and E is expected data. The test is unreliable if any of the expected values is less than five (in which case, use **Fisher's exact test** instead). If the number of subjects is small (less than 30), **Yates' continuity correction** has to be made in order to avoid individual values having an overly significant effect on the end result. Note that McNemar's test is a variant of the χ^2 test and is used for paired nominal data.

CORRELATION AND REGRESSION

Correlation measures the degree of association between two parameters, with the correlation coefficient (r) being anywhere between -1 and $+1$. The latter is sometimes called **Pearson's correlation coefficient** after its originator and is a measure of linear (i.e. parametric) association. If one parameter increases as the other does, then the correlation coefficient is positive (and vice versa). The data are always represented on a **scatter plot**. If a curved line is needed to express the relationship, then more complicated measures of correlation must be used, specifically **Spearman's rank for non-parametric data**.

Once correlation is established, regression is the line drawn over the scatter plot using a regression equation $y = a + bx$, with the **regression coefficient** being the direction coefficient of the regression line. Regression shows how one variable changes on average with another and can be used to find out what one variable is likely to be when the other is known. Regression relationships may be linear, multiple or logistic. The regression function r^2 indicates what amount of variance in the dependent variable is related to variance in the independent variable. For example, if knee pain correlates with walking distance by $r^2 = 0.6$, then 60 per cent of the variation in walking distance can be explained by variation in knee

pain. The remaining 40 per cent of variability is not explained.

DATA COLLECTION

In orthopaedics, there has been a drive to categorize different types of study according to the levels of evidence that they provide (Table 1.3). In general, the increasing levels of evidence are as follows:

EXPERT OPINIONS

Expert opinions are essentially what an expert in the field has to say on a given subject.

CASE SERIES

With case series, the outcomes of a group are reported, but there is no comparison group. Case series are very weak in terms of causation. They should act as a stimulus for more powerful studies.

CASE–CONTROL STUDIES

Case–control studies are retrospective studies where cases are gathered with a certain outcome and then compared with controls (either historical or prospective) that did not have the same outcome in order to look back at the effects of interventions or treatments. These studies are quick and cheap to perform and, if constructed carefully, can yield clinically relevant information, e.g. odds ratios (see below). Unfortunately, case–control studies are full of methodological biases.

COHORT STUDIES

In a cohort study, two groups, one of which has undergone an intervention or treatment, are followed up over time in order to compare outcomes such as onset of disease or adverse events. These studies are useful for identifying incidence and for establishing relative risk. Problems with cohort studies include diagnostic access bias (due to preselection), expense, and decreased validity due to loss to follow-up.

Table 1.3 Levels of evidence in orthopaedics

Level	Therapeutic studies (investigating results of treatment)	Prognostic studies (investigating outcome of disease)	Diagnostic studies (investigating a diagnostic test)	Economic and decision analyses (developing an economic or decision model)
I	RCT (a) Significant difference (b) No significant difference, but narrow CI Systematic reviews of level I RCTs (studies homogeneous)	Prospective study Systematic review of level I studies	Testing of previously developed diagnostic criteria in series of consecutive patients (with universally applied reference gold standard) Systematic review of level I studies	Clinically sensible costs and alternatives; values obtained from many studies; multi-way sensitivity analyses Systematic review of level I studies
II	Prospective cohort study Poor-quality RCT (e.g. 80% follow-up) Systematic review (a) Level II studies (b) Non-homogeneous level I studies	Retrospective study Study of untreated controls from a previous RCT Systematic review of level II studies	Development of diagnostic criteria on basis of consecutive patients (with universally applied reference gold standard) Systematic review of level II studies	Clinically sensible costs and alternatives; values obtained from limited studies; multi-way sensitivity analyses Systematic review of level II studies
III	Case–control study Retrospective cohort study Systematic review of level III studies		Study of non-consecutive patients (no consistently applied reference gold standard) Systematic review of level III studies	Limited alternatives and costs; poor estimates Systematic review of level III studies
IV	Case series (no, or historical, control group)	Case series	Case–control study Poor reference standard	No sensitivity analyses
V	Expert opinion	Expert opinion	Expert opinion	Expert opinion

CI, confidence interval; RCT, randomized controlled trial.

RANDOMIZED CONTROLLED TRIALS

Randomized controlled trials (RCTs) are the gold standard. Groups of patients are randomized to either receive or not receive an intervention or treatment, and the outcomes are compared in a prospective manner. The aim of the study and the hypothesis to be tested are stated clearly. Important features of RCTs, other than power analysis, include the following:

- **Randomization:** this ensures that all prognostic variables, both known and unknown, will probably be distributed equally among the treatment groups. This avoids bias in treatment assignment. Types of randomization include the following:
  - **Simple:** treatment allocations are assigned by computer-generated tables. This method may not be appropriate in small or multicentre trials. Note that dates of birth and days of the week are not

appropriate methods of randomization.

- **Stratified:** if there are prognostic variables that are extremely important, then stratification ensures equal distribution between treatment groups. The computer program also takes into account previously identified confounding factors. Generally, only two or three variables are stratified. Stratification is practical only in large trials and should be performed by centre in multicentre trials.
- **Block:** treatment is allocated by blocks of set size. This ensures that an equal number of patients is assigned to each treatment. For example, if the block size is six, then three receive treatment A and three receive treatment B.

- **Generalizability:** it is important to know to what or whom the results of the study apply (e.g. patients, surgeons) and also what the clinical implication of the results will be.
- **Sample selection:** inclusion and exclusion criteria should be decided upon and stated clearly in advance.
- **Outcome selection:** measures of outcome should be valid, reproducible and responsive to change. The choice of outcome should be clinically relevant. Note that objective outcomes, although measured more easily than subjective outcomes, may not always be the best choice. It is also worth considering primary and secondary outcome measures. Analysis is best made on an intention-to-treat basis, i.e. if a subject drops out during the study or changes treatment, that subject should still be included in the analyses. Another way of looking at this is to analyse according to the treatment that the subject was assigned to rather than the treatment that the subject actually underwent. The opposite of intention-to-treat analysis is analysis **per protocol** or **on study**.
- **Bias:** this refers to a flaw in impartiality that introduces systematic error into the methodology and results of a study. Bias can be reduced in a number of ways, including randomization, masking (previously known as blinding), and meticulous attention to the study protocol. Types of bias include the following:

- **Experimenter bias:** during either selection or treatment (can be reduced by randomization).
- **Observational/experimental bias:** errors in the measurement or classification of disease (can be reduced by masking). An example of observational bias is the use of hip and knee scoring systems, where errors may occur if adjacent joints are also diseased.
- **Patient bias.**
- **Publication bias.**
- **Confounding factors:** these are independent variables that interfere with the drawing of statistically valid conclusions from a study. These factors may not be distributed equally between groups and so introduce a form of bias known as confounding bias. Confounding bias can be reduced by matching (e.g. by age) or stratification.
- **Masking/blinding:** this protects against bias. Blinding can be single (only the patient is blinded) or double (both the patient and the investigator are blinded).
- **Ethics:** consent from an ethics committee (usually local or regional) is required for RCTs.
- **Publication:** it is important to know where the study is to be published, which generally depends on the audience at which it is aimed.
- **Sequential analysis:** two modalities are compared, power is determined, analysis is performed at predetermined points, and the trial is stopped when statistical significance is reached.
- **Equivalence study:** this is a RCT in which two treatments are expected to have the same outcome. The research hypothesis is that there is a difference between the two groups (known as the alternative hypothesis, as opposed to the null hypothesis). Studies such as this are used, for example, to compare prophylactic methods for preventing deep vein thromboses.

META-ANALYSES AND SYSTEMATIC REVIEWS

Meta-analyses are becoming increasingly popular with the advent of evidence-based medicine

(EBM). The aim is to find the relevant evidence from several studies in an unbiased manner and to appraise each paper, including all randomized trials, for methodological quality. The results are then reported as a common estimate with its confidence interval. Meta-analyses are at the top of the evidence hierarchy, but they may vary in their methodologies, may be heterogeneous in their results, may paint an overly rosy picture because of publication bias (i.e. reporting positive more often than negative results) and may duplicate data.

Systematic reviews are different from meta-analyses, in that no common estimate or confidence intervals are given. The Cochrane Collaboration organizes and publishes highly detailed systematic reviews in its database and maintains a register of all published RCTs. The Cochrane Collaboration also maintains a prospective register of RCTs as they commence.

TESTS AND OUTCOMES

It is worth knowing a little about screening and epidemiology for examination situations and everyday practice. Wilson and Jungner expanded on the criteria for a screening test in a World Health Organization (WHO) document in 1968. This paper is in Spanish, but the essentials have been distilled below (use the mnemonic 'IATROGENIC' to remember the main points):

Screening criteria

- The condition should be an **Important** health problem with known **Incidence**.
- There is an **Accepted** and effective treatment.
- **Treatment** and diagnostic facilities should be available.
- **Recognizable** latent and early symptomatic stage(s) should be present, and consideration should be given to whether early pick-up at the latent stage leads to intervention and to whether intervention improves outcome.

- **Opinions** on who to treat are agreed.
- There is **Guaranteed** safety, sensitivity and specificity of the test.
- **Examination** and/or treatment are acceptable to the patient.
- The **Natural** history of the condition should be known.
- Tests are **Inexpensive** and simple to perform.
- The screening programme should be **Cost-effective**, with a policy drawn up on whom to treat, and it should be **Continuously** rolled out and repeated at intervals.

Epidemiology is the study of the frequency and cause of disease in human populations. The following definitions are worth remembering:

INCIDENCE

Incidence is the rate of occurrence of new disease in a population previously free of disease. The rate is found by dividing the number of new cases in the study period by the number of individuals at risk at the beginning of the study period.

PREVALENCE

Prevalence is the frequency of a disease at a given time. The frequency is found by dividing the number of patients with the disease by the sum of the number of the patients with the disease and the number of patients at risk.

SENSITIVITY

Sensitivity is the ability of a test to exclude false negatives (FN), i.e. the ability of a test to pick up all cases of a disease. The sensitivity is found by dividing the number of true positives (TP) by the sum of all the patients with the condition $[TP/(TP + FN)]$, i.e. true positive/disease positive (Table 1.4).

SPECIFICITY

The specificity is the ability of a test to exclude false positives, i.e. to exclude the disease.

Table 1.4 Standard contingency table

	Disease positive	Disease negative
Test positive	True positive (TP)	False positive (FP)
Test negative	False negative (FN)	True negative (TN)

Table 1.5 Calculating odds ratios

	Success	Failure	Totals
Control	a	b	a + b
Treatment	c	d	c + d

Specificity is found by dividing the number of true negatives by the sum of all the patients without the condition [TN/(TN + FP)], i.e. true negative/disease negative.

POSITIVE PREDICTIVE VALUE

The positive predictive value (PPV) is the probability that a subject who tests positive is truly positive, i.e. the PPV indicates the significance of a positive test. The PPV is found by dividing all positive test results in patients with the disease by the total number of positive test results [TP/(TP + FP)], i.e. true positive/test positive.

NEGATIVE PREDICTIVE VALUE

The negative predictive value (NPV) is the probability that a subject who tests negative is truly negative, i.e. the NPV indicates the significance of a negative test. The NPV is found by dividing all negative test results in patients without the condition by the total number of negative test results [TN/(TN + FN)], i.e. true negative/test negative.

ACCURACY

The accuracy gives an idea of how often a test is correct [(TP + TN)/(TP + TN + FP + FN)].

ODDS RATIO

The odds ratio (OR) is often used in case–control studies. The OR is the ratio of the odds that an event will occur in one group to the odds that the event will occur in the other group. If we consider Table 1.5:

- Success rate in the control group $(CSR) = a/(a + b)$.
- Success rate in the treatment group $(TSR) = c/(c + d)$.
- $OR = (c/d)/(a/b) = cb/ad$.
- Relative risk reduction $= (TSR - CSR)/CSR$.

VALIDITY

The validity is the extent to which a test or outcome measure actually measures what it purports to measure. Tests have to be **precise** (consistency of repeated measures) and **accurate** (represent what they mean to represent). The different types of validity include:

- **Construct validity:** the extent to which a measure corresponds to theoretical concepts or constructs concerning the phenomenon of interest.
- **Content validity:** the extent to which a measure represents the domain of interest.
- **Criterion or concurrent validity:** correlating scores on a new instrument or test with external criteria known or believed to measure the attribute.

RESPONSIVENESS TO CHANGE

The test has to be able to reflect the positive or negative effects of any interventions. This has to be tested in a clinical setting.

RELIABILITY

The reliability assesses the random error of a measure. It is important to consider reliability within the same assessor (**intra-observer**) and with different assessors (**interobserver**). Clinical disagreement is ubiquitous in medicine, e.g. classification systems have come under a great deal of scrutiny. If two clinicians do not agree, then the classification cannot be accurate. In general, most systems show at best slight to moderate agreement. Sources of disagreement may arise from the following:

- **The examiner:**
  - Understanding of classification
  - Prior expectation
  - Level of expertise and experience
- **The classification:**
  - Vague
  - Complex
  - Inaccurate
- **The tool:**
  - Inaccurate
  - Imprecise

When measuring agreement, one must be aware that, as a result of the law of averages, there is bound to be agreement by chance. **Kappa analysis** involves adjusting the observed proportion of agreement in relation to the proportion of agreement expected by chance. Kappa analysis is used for categorical data. A value of 1.0 indicates complete agreement, a value of 0 indicates that the agreement can be explained purely by chance, and a negative value suggests systematic disagreement. **Cronbach's alpha** is used for multiple variables. Note that kappa analysis can be weighted or unweighted. **Weighted kappa statistics** allow for the measuring of observer agreement in rank scales, taking into account the agreement by chance and bringing the magnitude of disagreement into calculation. Further criteria that have been used in kappa analysis include the Landis and Koch (1977) and Svenholm criteria. The former uses the following subclassification: 0–0.2, slight agreement; 0.2–0.4, fair agreement; 0.4–0.6, moderate agreement; 0.6–0.8, substantial agreement; 0.8–1.0, almost perfect agreement.

Note that **interclass correlation coefficients** are used when testing reliability of continuous data.

SURVIVAL ANALYSIS

Survival analysis is a study in which outcome of an intervention is plotted over time, which allows for variable dates of entry and for patients to be followed up for different lengths of time. Data can be analysed continuously (**actuarial method**) or at times of failure (**Kaplan–Meier product-limit method**), or a combination of both can be used (**life-table analysis**); the latter is preferred in orthopaedics, as the presentation of both a complete life table and a survival curve allow the probability of failure to be calculated. It is easy to abuse survival analysis; due care must be given to the definition of failure, the treatment of loss to follow-up and death, and the cohort effect.

In order to construct a life table for joint replacements, the first step is to define an endpoint or outcome. There may be several endpoints, such as success, failure, death (often used in survivorship of cancer) or revision (most often used in joint replacements).

For joint replacements, the number of joints being followed and the number of failures are determined for each year after operation. For each time period, the number of patients at risk, the number of failures and the number of patients withdrawn are recorded. The latter includes patients who have died, patients who have reached the end of the trial and patients lost to follow-up. Patients who complete the trial and deaths are treated as successful withdrawals. Successful withdrawals are also known as **censored data** or **non-endpoints**; they do not count as failures and affect only the number of patients at risk. Losses to follow-up can be treated as unsuccessful or successful withdrawals, but this must be clarified in the methodology.

The number of individuals at risk during each year is calculated as the number of patients at the beginning of the year less half the number of withdrawals. The **percentage failure rate for each year** is determined from the number at risk and the number of failures (by dividing the number of failures during the interval by the number of patients at risk); from this, the percentage success rate is calculated. **Cumulative estimate of survival** is calculated as (100% – cumulative probability of failure). The **annual survival rate** is calculated by cumulating the success rate for all previous years and the year in question.

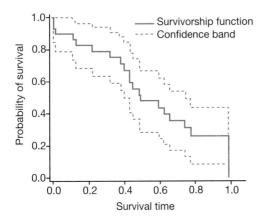

Figure 1.4 *Example of Kaplan–Meier survival analysis curve.*

In life-table analysis the survival rates are calculated annually, while in Kaplan–Meier analyses the rates are recalculated each time a failure occurs (Figure 1.4).

Calculations are performed at regular intervals according to the method used, and graphs are drawn with steps at each time point or failure. The **survivorship curve** is the cumulative estimate of survival plotted with 95 per cent CLs (or CIs). Upward blips or solid circles are used to represent censored data on graphs. When reporting survival analysis, one must include 95 per cent CIs, best- and worst-case scenarios and, most importantly, the number of patients left at longer follow-up. Typically, very small numbers remain at the latest time interval, and these data are the least reliable. One must not extrapolate the results beyond the defined time periods, and only specific hard endpoints must be used.

FURTHER READING

Bland, JM. *An Introduction to Medical Statistics.* Oxford: Oxford University Press, 2000.

Greenhalgh, T. *How to Read a Paper: The Basics of Evidence Based Medicine.* London: BMJ Publishing Group, 1997.

Griffin, D, Audige, L. Common statistical methods in orthopaedic clinical studies. *Clin Orthop Relat Res* 2003;**413**:70–9.

Kocher, MS, Zurakowski, D. Clinical epidemiology and biostatistics: a primer for orthopaedic surgeons. *J Bone Joint Surg Am* 2004;**86**:607–20.

Murray, DW, Carr, AJ, Bulstrode, C. Survival analysis of joint replacements. *J Bone Joint Surg Br* 1993;**75**:697–704.

2

Genetics

PETER CALDER AND ARESH HASHEMI-NEJAD

INTRODUCTION

Our understanding of genetics has advanced greatly since 1953, when Watson and Crick first deduced the structure of **deoxyribonucleic acid (DNA)**. Conditions once grouped by phenotype have been shown to have similar genotypes. Knowledge of the genes responsible for specific diseases can lead to more accurate classifications and prognosis and, possibly, improved treatment techniques.

A basic knowledge of disease inheritance and genetic disorders is required by the orthopaedic surgeon. Learn to draw a family pedigree of single-gene inheritance and know the gene mutations of the more common conditions.

CHROMOSOMAL STRUCTURE AND FUNCTION

Chromosomes are structures found within the cell nucleus. The karyotype of a normal human somatic cell is 46 chromosomes (the diploid number). This includes 22 autosomal pairs and two sex chromosomes (Figure 2.1).

Chromosomes are composed of **DNA**, **ribonucleic acid (RNA)**, **polysaccharides**, and **histone** and **non-histone proteins**. Normally chromosomes cannot be seen under a light microscope, but during cell division they become condensed, allowing visualization at 1000× magnification. Chromosomes are thin thread-like structures that have a **short p arm** and a **long q arm** separated by a constriction known as the **centromere** (Figure 2.1). The chromosomes have three basic shapes depending on the centromere location. **Metacentric** chromosomes have p and q arms of approximately equal length, e.g. chromosome 1. **Submetacentric** chromosomes have p and q arms of differing lengths, e.g. chromosome 6. In **acrocentric** chromosomes, the centromere is near one end and, therefore, there is a very small p arm and a correspondingly long q arm, e.g. chromosome 13.

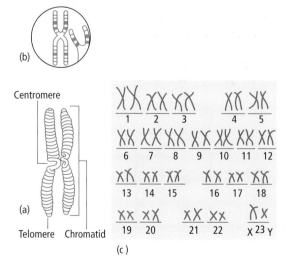

Figure 2.1 *Diagram of 23 paired human chromosomes.* *(a) Structure of a chromosome. (b,c) Male karyotype.*

DEOXYRIBONUCLEIC ACID

DNA sequences are arranged in a specific order to form genes. About 100 000 genes make up the human genome. DNA is a polymer of **deoxyribonucleotides** composed of a **nitrogenous base**, a **sugar** and a **phosphate group**. The bases contain the genetic information and are derived from **purines** or **pyrimidines**. The **purine bases** are **adenine** and **guanine**; the **pyrimidine bases** are **thymine** and **cytosine**. Watson and Crick deduced the double-helical structure of DNA with paired bases in the centre. Hydrogen bonds between the bases hold the two chains together. Adenine is always paired with thymine, and guanine with cytosine (Figure 2.2).

Growth and division of somatic cells is via the process of **mitosis**. Replication of DNA involves unwinding of the double helix, allowing a complementary DNA daughter strand to be formed using the original strand as a template. This is a semi-conservative process, as each new helix contains one of the original chromosomal strands.

Genes code for protein synthesis. During the process of **transcription**, templates are produced from the DNA in the form of messenger **ribonucleic acid (mRNA)**. The mRNA exits the nucleus into the cellular cytoplasm. By combining with other RNA molecules, such as transfer RNA (tRNA) and ribosomal RNA (rRNA), **protein synthesis (translation)** takes place at the **ribosomes**. Proteins have many different biological functions: mechanical tissue strength seen in skeletal tissues is due to the presence of collagen; muscle contraction occurs with the interaction of actin and myosin protein filaments; proteins act as transport molecules and enzymes during biological reactions; and the immune system relies on complex proteins in the form of antibodies.

INHERITANCE

In normal somatic cells, females have two X chromosomes and males have one X and one Y chromosome. During the process of **meiosis**, the chromosomes separate to form a **haploid** number, including one copy of each **autosome** and a single sex chromosome. A child inherits one half of his or her autosomal pair and one sex chromosome from each parent. The mother can contribute only an X chromosome, but the father can contribute either an X or a Y sex chromosome.

CHROMOSOMAL ABNORMALITIES

Chromosomal abnormalities can involve whole chromosomes or result from structural changes of one or more chromosomes.

Examples of chromosomal abnormalities

- **Whole-chromosome abnormalities:**
  - monosomy, e.g. Turner syndrome;
  - trisomy, e.g. Down syndrome, Klinefelter syndrome.
- **Structural abnormalities:** point mutations, deletions, inversions, translocations.

WHOLE-CHROMOSOME ABNORMALITIES

Whole-chromosome anomalies include the loss and/or gain of a whole chromosome, referred to as **aneuploidy**. This can affect the autosomes or

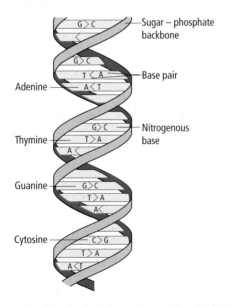

Figure 2.2 *Structure of deoxyribonucleic acid (DNA).*

the sex chromosomes. In general terms, the loss of a chromosome has a greater effect on an individual than the loss of a gene due to the loss of more genetic information.

Monosomy

Monosomy, the loss of one chromosome, occurs less often than an increase in number of chromosomes. Survival does not occur with the loss of one half of an autosome, but it is possible to lose one X chromosome. This is documented as XO and is known as **Turner syndrome**. The incidence is approximately 1 in 2000 live births, although Turner syndrome is more commonly seen in aborted fetuses. The syndrome is exclusively found in females.

Clinically, Turner syndrome is seen as a short female with skeletal abnormalities, including cubitus valgus, medial tibial exostosis and a short fourth metacarpal/metatarsal. Other malformations include craniofacial, renal-tract and cardiovascular abnormalities. The condition is inherited. The paternal X chromosome is more likely to be missing, usually as a sporadic event.

Trisomy

In **trisomy**, the cells have an **extra chromosome**. The most common trisomy compatible with life is trisomy 21, or **Down syndrome**. The incidence of Down syndrome is around 1 in 660 live births, with an increased risk in mothers over the age of 35 years. The aetiology in 94 per cent of cases is the **failure of separation of the autosomal pair during meiosis**. This produces a gamete with two homologous chromosomes, which, when joined with a normal gamete during fertilization, produces trisomy. In 3.5 per cent of case, chromosomal rearrangement occurs following **translocation** of one of the autosomes. The remaining 2.5 per cent of cases occur due to **mosaicism**, in which some of the body cells have a normal complement of 46 chromosomes but others have 47 chromosomes. Mosaicism occurs following defects in mitosis during formation of the zygote.

Orthopaedic manifestations in Down syndrome include atlantoaxial instability in 12–20 per cent, joint laxity with recurrent dislocation of the patella, and increased risk of slipped upper femoral epiphysis.

The addition of an extra X sex chromosome is seen in **Kleinfelter's syndrome** (XXY). The incidence of this syndrome is 1 in 1000 male births. Clinically, this results in a tall, thin male with infertility and hypogonadism.

STRUCTURAL ABNORMALITIES

Changes in the structure of the chromosomes may involve one or both copies of a gene. The **genotype** is the inherited genetic code that produces the physical appearance known as the **phenotype**. Disorders occur at specific alleles on one or both individual autosomes. An **allele** is defined as one or two alternative forms of a gene that can have the same locus on homologous chromosomes and are responsible for alternative traits. If both alleles are similarly involved, then there is a homozygous trait; if the alleles differ, then there is a heterozygous trait.

The alteration in chromosomal structure may occur at specific nucleotide bases, known as **point mutations**, or may involve larger parts of the chromosome. Examples include **deletions**, where part of the chromosome is removed, with a consequent loss of genetic material; **inversions** of part of the chromosome by 180 degrees, which results in misreading of the genetic code as the DNA is out of the correct sequence; and **translocations** of genetic material from one chromosome to another.

SINGLE-GENE INHERITANCE

Gene defects may be inherited by autosomal chromosomal transmission or may be linked to X chromosomes. Defects can be either dominant or recessive. The **penetrance** of a genetic disorder relates to the probability that the phenotype will be expressed.

The **severity** of the phenotypic expression may alter between individuals with the same genotype; this is known as **variable expressivity**. An example is Marfan syndrome, an autosomal dominant condition that results in a defect in collagen formation. Abnormalities may occur in the cardiovascular, optic and skeletal systems. Patients with Marfan syndrome may express all of the symptoms (severe involvement) or have very few symptoms (milder form).

Incomplete penetrance is defined as inheritance of the mutant gene without expression of the phenotype of the disorder. This is in contrast to **variable expressivity**, in which the patient always expresses some of the symptoms.

Examples of single-gene inheritance

- **Autosomal dominant:** achondroplasia, osteogenesis imperfecta, neurofibromatosis.
- **Autosomal recessive:** mucopolysaccharidoses (except Hunter syndrome), sickle cell anaemia.
- **X-linked dominant:** hypophosphataemic rickets.
- **X-linked recessive:** Duchenne's muscular dystrophy, haemophilia A.

AUTOSOMAL DOMINANT INHERITANCE

Affected individuals are heterozygous for the mutation. Homozygous individuals of the allele usually are more severely affected and usually do not survive to term. There is a 50 per cent chance of inheritance from one heterozygous parent:

	A (Mutant gene)	n (Normal gene)
n	An – affected	nn – normal
n	An – affected	nn – normal

Males and females are affected equally. Examples of autosomal dominant conditions include achondroplasia, osteogenesis imperfecta (OI) and neurofibromatosis type 1 (NF1).

Achondroplasia

This is the most common form of **short-limb** or **disproportionate rhizomelic dwarfism**. It is inherited as complete penetrance. Eighty-seven per cent of cases are as a result of a new mutation. The gene is encoded on chromosome 4, locus p16.3. The mutation affects the gene for **fibroblast growth factor receptor 3 (FGFR3)**. Hypochondroplasia has a milder

phenotype than achondroplasia and is caused by mutation of other regions of the *FGFR3* gene.

Osteogenesis imperfecta

This is a generalized disease of connective tissue due to a quantitative or qualitative **defect of type I collagen**. It has marked clinical and genetic heterogeneity. Sillence in 1981 classified the condition into types I–IV, with subgroups A and B in types I and IV, where B represents dentinogenesis imperfecta. Initially, inheritance of types I and IV was thought to be autosomal dominant, and that of types II and III autosomal recessive. However, it is now accepted to be an autosomal dominant condition, with cases from unaffected parents being due to mosaicism rather than recessive genes.

Type I collagen is the major extracellular protein in bone, skin and tendons. It is a heterotrimer made of two $\alpha 1$ chains (tropocollagen) and one $\alpha 2$ chain in a triple helix structure. The pro-$\alpha 1$ chain is encoded by the *COL1A1* gene on chromosome 17 and the pro-$\alpha 2$ chain is encoded by the *COL1A2* gene on chromosome 7.

In the **common type 1 OI**, the clinical features include osteopenia, mild bone fragility, grey/blue sclera and ligament laxity. The *COL1A1* mutant allele results in failure of production of the pro-$\alpha 1$ chain due to a premature stop codon. The mRNA remains within the nucleus, resulting in only 50 per cent production of normal $\alpha 1$ chain. Other epidemiological and genetic factors affect the disease process, as there is a spectrum of severity.

In **more severe types of OI**, there are mutations of either the *COL1A1* or the *COL1A2* gene, resulting in a mixture of normal and abnormal collagen chains. The $\alpha 1$ chains are long molecules consisting of 338 repeating triplet amino-acid sequences, usually glycine, proline and hydroxyproline. The most common mutation is the substitution of the small glycine molecule with a larger amino acid. This results in 50 per cent of abnormal $\alpha 1$ and $\alpha 2$ chains being formed. These abnormal chains bind to form an abnormal collagen molecule that interferes with the extracellular matrix formation by impairing the function of the normal $\alpha 1$ chains.

Neurofibromatosis type 1

NF1 is inherited as complete penetrance, but it has a high variable expressivity. Fifty per cent of patients have a fresh gene mutation. The gene is encoded on chromosome 17, locus q11.2. The gene encodes the protein neuro-fibromin which acts as a tumour suppressor.

AUTOSOMAL RECESSIVE INHERITANCE

Affected individuals are homozygous for the genetic mutation. Heterozygous individuals are known as carriers. There is a 25 per cent chance of producing an affected individual from two parental carriers:

	A (mutant gene)	n (normal gene)
A	AA – affected	An – carrier
n	An – carrier	nn – normal

Males and females are affected equally. Most autosomal recessive conditions produce errors of metabolism due to the deficiency of specific enzymes. This can result in an accumulation of substrate or product, or both. Examples of autosomal recessive disorders include mucopolysaccharidoses and sickle cell anaemia.

Mucopolysaccharidoses

Type I Hurler mucopolysaccharidosis

Skeletal changes include diaphyseal broadening of short misshapen bones. Flaring of the rib cage and widening of the medial end of the clavicle are also present. Anterior wedging of the vertebral bodies produces a kyphosis and a thoracolumbar gibbus. There is odontoid hypoplasia and a J-shaped sella turcica.

Type IV Morquio A and B mucopolysaccharidosis

Skeletal changes include marked platyspondyly, with ovoid shaped vertebrae and odontoid hypoplasia, flaring of the rib cage, flattening of the femoral heads, genu valgum and joint laxity. There is a deficiency of N-acetyl galactosamine-6-sulphatase in type A; the gene

has been mapped to chromosome 16 q24.3. In type B, there is a deficiency of beta-galactosidase; the gene has been mapped to chromosome 3 p21.33.

Sickle cell anaemia

Sickling of red cells occurs as a result of an inherited autosomal recessive single-gene mutation, leading to substitution of glutamine for valine at position 6 of the beta-globin chain of haemoglobin.

X-LINKED DOMINANT INHERITANCE

Either sex can be affected. The phenotype is dominant when a heterozygous female expresses the phenotype:

Affected male	X	X
X^{AD} (affected dominant)	$X^{AD}X$	$X^{AD}X$
Y	XY	XY

From the above table, all daughters will inherit the affected gene from an affected male, but no sons will be affected.

Affected female	X^{AD} (affected dominant)	X
X	$X^{AD}X$	XX
Y	$X^{AD}Y$	XY

From the above table 50 per cent of sons and 50 per cent of daughters risk inheriting the mutated gene from an affected mother.

An example of an X-linked dominant disorder is **hypophosphataemic rickets**. Males express the disease fully, but females have variable expressivity in the heterozygous genotype.

X-LINKED RECESSIVE INHERITANCE

The phenotype is recessive when expressed by a homozygous female. All males are affected, as they possess only one X chromosome. Heterozygous females are carriers.

Female carrier	X^{AR} (affected recessive)	X
X	$X^{AR}X$	XX
Y	$X^{AR}Y$	XY

From the above table, there is a 25 per cent chance of producing a normal male and equally

Table 2.1 Musculoskeletal disorders and their genetic defects

Musculoskeletal disorder	Genetic mutation
Achondroplasia/hypochondroplasia	Fibroblast growth factor (FGF) receptor 3
Diastrophic dysplasia	Sulphate transporter
Duchenne's muscular dystrophy	Dystrophin
Jansen metaphyseal chondrodysplasia	PTH/PTHrP receptor
Marfan syndrome	Fibrillin
Multiple epiphyseal dysplasia	Cartilage oligomeric matrix protein (COMP) or type IX collagen (COL9A2)
Multiple hereditary exostoses	EXT1, EXT2 genes
Osteogenesis imperfecta	Type I collagen
Pseudo achondroplasia	COMP
Schmid metaphyseal dysplasia	Type X collagen
Spondyloepiphyseal dysplasia	Type II collagen
Thanatophoric dysplasia	FGF receptor 3
X-linked hypophosphataemic rickets	PEX (cellular endopeptidase)

a normal female. In addition there is a 25 per cent risk of producing an affected male and equally a female carrier.

Carrier female and affected male	X^{AR} (affected recessive)	X
X^{AR} (Affected recessive)	$X^{AR} X^{AR}$	$X^{AR} X$
Y	$X^{AR} Y$	XY

The affected male transmits the affected gene through all his daughters. If the female is also a carrier, then there is a 25 per cent risk of producing an affected female, an affected male, a female carrier or a normal male.

Examples of X-linked recessive disorders include Duchenne's muscular dystrophy, a deficiency of the protein dystrophin, and haemophilia A, which produces a deficiency in clotting factor VIII.

Many of the gene defects for common musculoskeletal disorders have now been characterized (Table 2.1).

MULTIFACTORIAL INHERITANCE

Many orthopaedic conditions are derived from multiple gene defects and environmental factors. Examples include developmental dysplasia of the hip, talipes equinovarus and neural tube defects. These conditions demonstrate familial inheritance but do not behave like single-gene disorders. The risk of the condition being inherited in subsequent relatives increases compared with the population but decreases in subsequent-degree relatives. An example is talipes equinovarus, which has an incidence of 1 in 1000 births. In first-degree relatives of an affected parent, there is a 25 times increased risk of the condition; this risk decreases in second-degree relatives to a five times higher risk.

GENETIC COUNSELLING

The aim of genetic counselling is to provide information to allow informed decisions to be made on the risk of inheritable disease being transmitted in future pregnancies. Parents need to be made aware that the risk documented for any condition – one in four for autosomal recessive conditions, one in two for autosomal dominant conditions – refers to each specific pregnancy, i.e. if one child is affected, the next pregnancy cannot be guaranteed to produce a normal child as one of the other possible outcomes for the original pregnancy. Subsequent pregnancies carry the original risk of inheritance. Prenatal diagnosis can be achieved by various methods, including amniocentesis, chorionic villous biopsy and fetal imaging techniques such as ultrasound.

Viva questions

1 What are chromosomes composed of? What is the basic structure of DNA?

2 What chromosomal abnormalities are you aware of?

3 Draw an inheritance table for an autosomal dominant condition of your choice.

4 Do you know of any X-linked dominant conditions? What is the risk of future offspring developing the condition?

5 Osteogenesis imperfecta (OI) is an example of single-gene inheritance. What are the different types of OI? What are the clinical manifestations?

FURTHER READING

Cole, WG. Genes and orthopaedics. *J Bone Joint Surg Br* 1999;**8**:190–2.

Cole, WG. Advances in osteogenesis imperfecta. *Clin Orthop Relat Res* 2002;**401**:6–16.

Dietz, FR, Mathews, KD. Update on the genetic bases of disorders with orthopaedic manifestations. *J Bone Joint Surg Am* 1996;**78**:1583–98.

Econs, MJ. New insights into the pathogenesis of inherited phosphate wasting disorders. *Bone* 1999;**25**:131–5.

Horton, WA. Fibroblast growth factor receptor 3 and the human chondrodysplasias. *Curr Opin Pediatr* 1997;**9**:437–42.

3
Skeletal embryology and limb growth

RICK BROWN AND DEBORAH EASTWOOD

INTRODUCTION

Some of the major challenges in paediatric orthopaedics relate to congenital or acquired limb deformities. Before the pathological conditions can be considered, it is essential to have a comprehensive understanding of both limb development in utero and the pivotal role of the physis in growth.

NORMAL EMBRYONIC LIMB DEVELOPMENT

The embryo develops in both a proximal-to-distal direction and a rostral-to-caudal direction. The upper-limb buds appear at 4 weeks of age, followed by the lower-limb buds a few days later. A **limb bud** comprises **mesoderm** covered by a thin surface of **ectoderm**.

The mesoderm forms limb mesenchyme with separate areas forming the **somite** and the **lateral mesodermal plate**. The lateral mesoderm forms the bone and connective tissue, while the somatic mesoderm forms the muscle. The **Homeobox (HOX)** gene controls mass and local growth in the distal direction of the condensing mesenchyme. The **zone of proliferating activity** (ZPA) in the ectoderm, whose activity is mediated by the **sonic hedgehog (Shh)** genes, directs development in the anterior-to-posterior direction, producing the **apical ectodermal ridge**

(AER) at the tip of the limb bud from which the digits form (Figure 3.1).

As embryonic development progresses, first the mesenchyme condenses and then chondrocytes differentiate within the mesenchyme (**chondrification**). This chondrocyte formation and cartilage differentiation first occurs in the diaphyseal region of the humerus and the femur. These new chondrocytes start to produce a matrix of glycosaminoglycans. The cartilaginous mesenchyme (the **cartilage anlage**) then undergoes resorption and cavitation between future segments in a process of **segmentation**, leading to the formation of the primitive joint. This will later be followed by development of the intra-articular structures. For example, a discoid meniscus results if the meniscus fails to

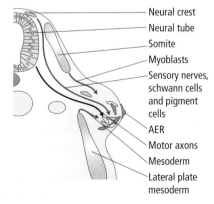

Figure 3.1 *Diagram of a limb bud, showing site of the apical ectodermal ridge (AER).*

Neural crest
Neural tube
Somite
Myoblasts
Sensory nerves, schwann cells and pigment cells
AER
Motor axons
Mesoderm
Lateral plate mesoderm

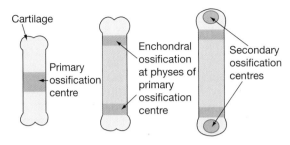

Cartilage

Primary ossification centre

Enchondral ossification at physes of primary ossification centre

Secondary ossification centres

Figure 3.2 *Diagrammatic representation of an early fetal bone with a primary ossification centre alone, a midterm fetal bone showing the site of enchondral ossification, and a late fetal bone with addition of the secondary ossification centres.*

differentiate fully at this stage; this happens in less than 1 per cent of knees and occurs most commonly on the lateral side.

Simultaneously with joint formation, the **primary ossification centre** (Figure 3.2) develops with hypertrophy of the mid-diaphyseal chondrocytes and invasion by blood vessels, which form a primitive nutrient artery system. Initially, **intramembranous ossification** occurs circumferentially from the periosteum around this primary ossification centre. However, in the epiphyseal regions, the cartilage cells become hypertrophic, and after vascular invasion the process of **enchondral ossification** commences. By the twelfth week, ossification centres are present in all long bones.

At around the ninth week, the limbs rotate. The upper and lower limbs rotate through 90 degrees laterally and medially, respectively. This results in a lateral thumb and a medial hallux.

Towards the end of fetal development, the earliest **secondary ossification centre** (Figure 3.2) develops at the distal femur. By this time, a separate system of blood vessels has grown into the epiphysis. Initially, these vascularized chondrocytes within the epiphyseal cartilage hypertrophy to form a central mass. This mass forms a spherical physis over its entire surface, which later reshapes into a hemispherical physeal outer surface and a discoid non-physeal surface towards the metaphysis.

The distal femoral secondary ossification centre should be present after 36 weeks; failure to see this centre on the radiograph of a neonate implies prematurity or a skeletal

abnormality. Other secondary centres appear throughout early childhood, including the capital femoral epiphysis that ossifies sometime after 3 months and should be seen before age 1 year. The sequential development of these centres acts as a monitor of skeletal age.

In childhood, the hemispherical physis of the secondary ossification centre becomes less active, with production of few new chondrocytes. It thins until it is replaced by subchondral bone and articular cartilage. As skeletal maturity is reached, the physis is resorbed, allowing the metaphyseal and epiphyseal blood systems to merge.

ABNORMAL LIMB DEVELOPMENT IN UTERO

If the normal sequence of events described above is disturbed during the first trimester of pregnancy, congenital limb deformities can occur. Although the precipitating cause of the majority of such deformities is unknown, for some specific problems the pathology is understood. An example of this occurred with the use of the drug thalidomide. This drug had an antiangiogenic effect that interrupted the development of the vascularization of the ossification centres, leading to a clinical picture of phocomelia.

The International Society of Hand Surgeons (Swanson 1976) has classified congenital limb anomalies into seven general groups related to the underlying pathology (Table 3.1).

Table 3.1 Swanson's classification of congenital limb deformities

Group	Example
Failure of formation	*Fibular deficiency*
Failure of separation	*Tarsal coalitions*
Hypoplasia	*Hypoplastic digit*
Overgrowth	*Macrodactyly*
Duplication	*Polydactyly*
Constriction ring syndromes	*Amniotic bands*
Dysplasias or syndromes	*Achondroplasia*

Both upper and lower congenital limb deformities can also be divided anatomically into longitudinal and transverse types. In **longitudinal deformities**, an abnormality is produced along one side of the whole limb, although the abnormality may be more marked in the distal rather than the proximal segment. The deficiency may be on either the pre-axial or the post-axial side of the limb. In a **transverse limb deformity**, proximal to the level of the insult there is normal growth. Distal to the insult, growth and development are affected variably.

In the lower limb, a defect in the cartilage anlage may lead to a **proximal focal femoral deficiency** (PFFD). The precise aetiology of the defect is unknown, and the clinical picture involves varying degrees of acetabular dysplasia and femoral hypoplasia. There is always a coxa vara, and a pseudarthrosis may be present from birth or soon after. Atkins classified PFFD according to the shapes of the femoral head and acetabulum, while Gillespie and Torode categorized the condition according to the presence and quality (i.e. stability) of the hip and knee joints because of the influence of joint stability on the success of leg-lengthening treatment.

In a post-axial lower-limb deficiency such as **fibular deficiency** (or **hemimelia**), either there is a complete absence of the fibula or the fibula is short. The lateral rays of the foot may also be deficient, and segmentation of the tarsal bones may have failed, leading to a tarsal coalition. This in turn leads to the development of a ball-and-socket ankle joint. In the proximal segment of the limb, some femoral shortening will be apparent with a valgus, externally rotated unstable knee secondary to hypoplasia of the lateral femoral condyle and absent cruciate ligaments.

Absence of part of the tibia in the form of a **tibial deficiency** (or **hemimelia**) (a pre-axial deficiency) occurs less commonly but with a genetic predisposition. There are associated medial ray toe deformities and indeed pre-axial upper limb deformities. Jones classified the condition according to the radiographic appearance of the tibia in infancy.

In the upper limb, the longitudinal defor-mities are again pre-axial (radial) or post-axial

(ulna) deficiencies. A radial deficiency is relatively common and usually associated with other congenital disorders, e.g. VACTERL (vertebral, cardiac anomalies, anal atresia, tracheo-oesophageal fistula, renal disorders, limb anomalies) syndrome. **Radio-ulnar synostosis** is a more common disorder due to a failure of separation in which the child has a loss of supination and pronation.

A number of conditions have been described as **packaging disorders**, in which limbs that have been formed normally in the first trimester are moulded into abnormal positions in the third trimester. These include **plagiocephaly**, **torticollis**, **infantile skeletal skew** and **calcaneovalgus feet**. In general, these are all self-correcting conditions that the surgeon needs only to review.

Moulding is also believed to play a role in some forms of developmental hip dysplasia, congenital talipes equinovarus and forefoot adductus. Moulding may explain the predilection for development hip dysplasia to affect the left side. In utero, the left side of the fetus most commonly lies against the mother's spine, producing an adduction force on the left hip.

NORMAL LIMB GROWTH IN CHILDHOOD

A bone grows longitudinally by **enchondral ossification** at the physis, while circumferential growth occurs at the zone of Ranvier at the level of the physis and by **appositional ossification** in the osteogenic layer of the periosteum along the diaphysis. The **zone of Ranvier** contains osteoblasts, fibroblasts and chondrocytes. The **perichondial ring of LaCroix** is a strong fibrous structure that secures the epiphysis to the metaphysis. In addition, enchondral ossification at the hemispherical physis of the secondary ossification centre provides both growth in limb length and contouring of the articular surface.

The physis comprises a highly ordered layered structure of chondrocytes in an extracellular matrix. The chondrocytes are arranged in the longitudinal axis of the bone

Epiphyseal blood vessels

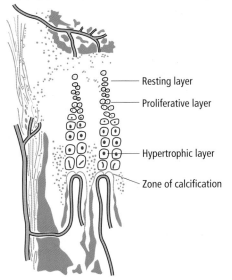

Resting layer

Proliferative layer

Hypertrophic layer

Zone of calcification

Metaphysis with blood vessels

Figure 3.3 *Layers of a physis.*

into four layers (Figure 3.3); the nomenclature of these layers varies from book to book, but the function of each layer does not.

Layers of the physis

- resting (reserve or germinal);
- proliferative;
- hypertrophic;
- calcification.

Each chondrocyte progresses through a sequence of changes as it moves from layer to layer. In the **resting** and **proliferative** layers, the cells are relatively small and surrounded by a mechanically strong thick layer of matrix. In the **resting** layer, germinal cells of stem-cell origin are found. These cells exist in an area of low oxygen tension and respond to circulating hormones. The cells contribute to the growth of both the physis and the secondary ossification centre.

As the cells **proliferate**, they appear as thin discs and palisade, and in the extracellular matrix longitudinal orientation of the collagen fibres occurs. This is an area of high oxygen tension. With **hypertrophy** of the chondrocytes (to five to ten times their original size), there is physically less space for the extracellular matrix and its strengthening effect, and this is therefore the weakest layer of the physis.

In the **zone of provisional calcification**, the metaphyseal vascular invasion allows calcification of the matrix to occur, and programmed cell death of the chondrocytes is initiated. With the vascular invasion come osteoblasts and osteoclasts, allowing the formation of the primary bone and its subsequent remodelling.

There are a number of key physes relevant to orthopaedic practice. In the arm, 80 per cent of humeral growth occurs at the proximal physis, while 75 per cent of the growth of the radius occurs distally. The sequence of appearance of the distal humeral physis is important in understanding paediatric elbow injuries (Figure 3.4). The first is the **C**apitellum (2 years), followed approximately every 2 years by the **R**adial head, medial (**I**nternal) epicondyle, **T**rochlear, **O**lecranon and **L**ateral (external) epicondyle (use the mnemonic **CRITOL** to remember the order). Thus, no secondary centres are visible in an infant, making interpretation of the transphyseal fracture difficult. In a transphyseal fracture, the relationship of the radius to the ulna is preserved, unlike a dislocation around the elbow or a displaced intraphyseal fracture.

Two-thirds of lower-limb growth occurs around the knee, with 70 per cent attributable to the distal femoral physis. For the last 4–6 years of skeletal growth, one can estimate that the distal femur grows at 9 mm/year and the proximal tibia at 6 mm/year. The proximal femur and distal tibia account for only a few millimetres (3–4 mm) each per year.

The apophysis of the ilium closes sequentially from lateral to medial. This Risser sign acts as a guide to maturity of the spine and the likelihood of a further deterioration of a scoliosis curve.

Like all other physes, the acetabulum responds to the forces applied across it, which allows the extensive remodelling required after both closed and open reductions for developmental hip dysplasia. After the age of

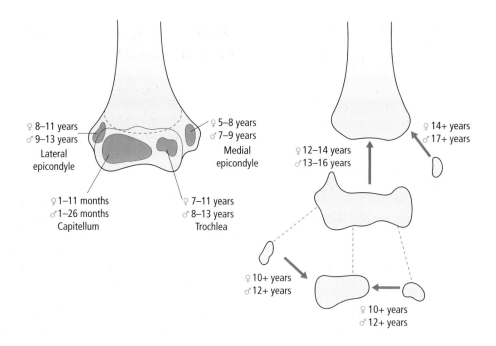

Figure 3.4 *Distal humeral secondary ossification centres: (a) age of appearance, (b) age of fusion.*

8 years, the triradiate cartilage begins to close. Thus, a reshaping innominate osteotomy, such as the Pemberton osteotomy, must be performed before closure of this physis. A fracture of the acetabulum in a young child that involves the triradiate cartilage may lead to growth arrest and secondary acetabular dysplasia.

In the infant foot, most bones comprise a cartilaginous mass with a circumferential physis and have great potential for remoulding. This, along with the visco-elastic properties of tendons and ligaments, is the basis for the high success rate of early conservative treatments such as that of Ponseti.

TRAUMA TO THE NORMAL GROWTH PLATE

Physeal injuries account for 15–30 per cent of all childhood fractures. However, nearly a third occur in the phalanges, and growth arrest occurs in less than 10 per cent. The energy of a fracture process passes like a lightning bolt through the hypertrophic layer of the physis. In an undulating physis such as the distal femur, however, the fracture line does not pass cleanly through a single layer of the physis, and thus there is a significantly higher risk of the reserve cell layer being damaged and resulting in a growth arrest.

Salter and Harris (1963) devised the most commonly used classification of physeal fractures. Type I is rare and is most commonly seen in infants or as a form of a pathological fracture. An acute unstable slipped upper femoral epiphysis has been considered as a form of type I Salter and Harris fracture. Type II fractures are most common, with a Thurston–Holland metaphyseal fragment. Growth deformity is thought to be rare, except in high-risk sites such as the distal femur. The epiphyseal type III fracture is usually intra-articular and requires anatomic reduction for joint congruity. Both type IV and V injuries have a high risk for developing growth arrest and joint incongruity. Mercer Rang modified this classification system by the addition of a Salter–Harris type VI fracture involving an injury to the perichondrial ring.

Growth disturbances can result from a bridge of bone forming across the physeal cartilage. The **bars** can be **peripheral**, **central** or **linear**. If large enough, a central bridge may lead to a limb-length discrepancy, while a more peripheral bar may produce an angular deformity. A physis may become less active following a single injury or as a result of repetitive injury or irradiation, but these factors may well have a lesser deforming effect on growth. Both computed tomography (CT) and magnetic resonance imaging (MRI) techniques can be used to map the size and location of a bony bridge in order to plan management.

A bony bridge with a surface area of more than 40 per cent of the entire growth plate is not resectable. If a lesser percentage is involved and significant growth remains, resection can be performed by a Lagenskiöld technique involving removal of the bony bridge through a metaphyseal window and tunnel to the area of damage. The defect in the physis is then filled with an interposition graft, often of fat taken locally, which prevents recurrence of the bony bridge or bar. A physeal bar that is starting to cause an unacceptable angular deformity may be best managed by surgical closure of the remaining physis. If complete closure of a physis has occurred, then in order to prevent leg-length discrepancy complete closure of the contralateral physis should be considered in a patient of appropriate age (usually within 3–4 years of skeletal maturity).

It is advised to follow up high-risk physeal injuries for a long enough period to exclude growth arrest. This is when the metaphysis has satisfactorily grown away from the physis, which may be confirmed by the presence of parallel Harris growth arrest lines.

The physis responds in a predictable manner to applied stresses and strains. Remodelling will occur at the physis due to forces acting in the plane of motion of the joint according to **Wolff's law**, which states that **bone remodels according to the applied stresses**. Similarly, in non-traumatic conditions such as Blount's disease, the medial physis of the proximal tibia experiences a large compressive force, slowing physeal activity according to the **Heuter–Volkmann principle**, leading to further collapse into tibia vara.

ABNORMAL GROWTH PROCESSES AROUND THE PHYSIS

CONGENITAL CONDITIONS

These problems occur in utero and have been discussed previously in this chapter.

METABOLIC CONDITIONS

In all forms of rickets, there is a failure of calcification of the chondrocytes in the provisional zone of calcification of the physis. There is normal matrix, but it fails to calcify. This is followed by disorderly invasion by blood vessels. Radiographically, this results in a widened, thickened physis and a hazy appearance of the metaphysis, with flaring and cupping due to persistence of cartilage in the metaphysis.

INFECTION

Most paediatric orthopaedic infections are spread by the haematogenous route. The rich metaphyseal blood supply explains the preponderance of osteomyelitis occurring in metaphyseal sites in children. In infancy, most presentations of septic arthritis of the hip and shoulder are secondary to metaphyseal infection that has discharged into the joint. Rarely, an epiphyseal osteomyelitis may present in a neonate due to the temporary presence of transphyseal vessels.

ENDOCRINE CONDITIONS

A slip of the upper femoral epiphysis is believed to have a complex multifactorial aetiology, with hormones such as thyroxine and oestrogen thought to play a role. A slip after menarche is very rare, suggesting that an alteration in the peripubertal sex hormonal status is important. Several theories have suggested that the fibrous ring has a period of relative weakness in early adolescence, while the mean body mass index (BMI) of patients has been shown to be higher, resulting in a greater load across the weaker physis. Other factors may act either by altering the mineral content of the extracellular matrix or by altering the hypertrophic changes in the hypertrophic zone. The increased incidence among people of Afro-Caribbean and Pacific Island descent may suggest a genetic component.

In hypothyroidism, enchondral bone formation at the physis is delayed. This produces reduced overall limb growth with an irregular and fragmented epiphysis, which may be difficult to distinguish from multiple epiphyseal dysplasia (MED) and Perthes' disease.

DEVELOPMENTAL CONDITIONS

Skeletal dysplasias are a diverse group of developmental disorders of bone and/or cartilage that result in altered limb growth and are often due to a defect in the growth plate. The Rubin classification divides these conditions according to the location of the defect and whether there is increased or decreased activity (Table 3.2, Figure 3.5).

Table 3.2 Rubin's classification of skeletal dysplasias

Epiphysis	Hyperplasia	Trevor's disease
	Hypoplasia	SED, MED, pseudo achondroplasia
Physis	Hyperplasia	Enchondromatosis
	Hypoplasia	Achondroplasia
Metaphysis	Hyperplasia	Hereditary multiple exostoses
	Hypoplasia	Osteopetrosis
Diaphysis	Hyperplasia	Diaphyseal dysplasia
	Hypoplasia	Osteogenesis imperfecta

MED, multiple epiphyseal dysplasia; SED, spondyloepiphyseal dysplasia.

The most common dysplasia is achondroplasia, which is a disorder of reduced enchondral ossification in the proliferative zone of the physis. Intramembranous and appositional ossification are minimally affected.

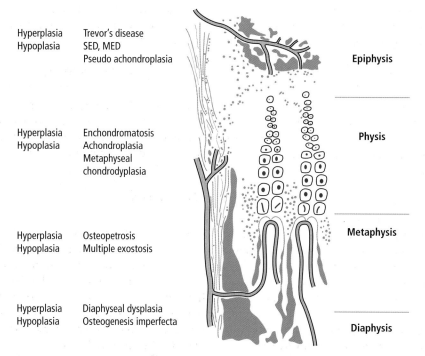

Hyperplasia	Trevor's disease
Hypoplasia	SED, MED
	Pseudo achondroplasia

Epiphysis

Hyperplasia	Enchondromatosis
Hypoplasia	Achondroplasia
	Metaphyseal
	chondrodyplasia

Physis

Hyperplasia	Osteopetrosis
Hypoplasia	Multiple exostosis

Metaphysis

Hyperplasia	Diaphyseal dysplasia
Hypoplasia	Osteogenesis imperfecta

Diaphysis

Figure 3.5 *Physis showing level of phenotypic defects leading to skeletal dysplasias.*
MED, multiple epiphyseal dysplasia; SED, spondyloepiphyseal dysplasia.

Thus, there is reduced growth of the long bones but sparing of the flat skull bones, which gives the characteristic appearance of macrocephaly, frontal bossing and rhizomelic limb shortening. The genetic defect, resulting in a single amino-acid substitution, alters the production of the fibroblast growth factor receptor 3 (FGFR-3), which is believed to be important for physeal function.

Epiphyseal hypoplasia can result in conditions with small, deformed or weakened epiphyses, such as in spondyloepiphyseal dysplasia (SED), MED and pseudo achondroplasia. However, it is now known that these conditions with similar epiphyseal radiographic changes are due to very different genetic defects. SED is due to a defect in the *COL2 A1* gene coding for the type II collagen found in the epiphysis. Both the more severe form of MED and pseudo achondroplasia result from defects in the gene coding for the cartilage oligomeric matrix protein (COMP).

Defects in the *COL2 A1* gene have also been found in adult patients with early onset of primary osteoarthritis, suggesting that this may be at the extreme end of the spectrum of a hypoplastic epiphyseal dysplasia.

Osteogenesis imperfecta has been described as a diaphyseal hypoplasia, where defective collagen production results in weakened, soft, deformed bones. In the most common form (Sillence type 1), only 50 per cent of the normal collagen is produced; in the other forms, there is both a qualitative and a quantitative reduction in the amount of normal collagen. Despite possessing a weak bone matrix, these patients are able to heal bone well.

Hyperplasia and overactivity of the epiphysis occur in the rare condition Trevor's disease (dysplasia epiphysealis hemimelica), in which an epiphyseal osteochondroma is produced. These occur mostly in the ankle and knee joint. The term 'hemimelica' is used because the lesions are located on only one side of the bone or limb.

Ollier's disease is multiple enchondromatosis characterized by lesions filled with hyaline cartilage that are continuous with the growth plate but extend into the metaphysis and diaphysis. Therefore, the disease is classified as a hyperplasia of the physis. A variant with multiple enchondromata and vascular malformations is known as Maffucci syndrome, which is associated with a high risk of malignant transformation.

The most common tumour-like skeletal dysplasia is hereditary multiple exostoses (diaphyseal aclasis). Patients with this condition have multiple osteochondromata that grow from the metaphysis in a diaphyseal direction. It is considered to be a metaphyseal hyperplasia. As in the other tumour-like dysplasias, the lesions cease growing after physeal closure.

TUMOURS

In addition to the tumour-like dysplasias, tumours can affect the growing bone in many ways. The most common childhood cancer is acute lymphocytic leukaemia, which results in characteristic transverse lines in the metaphysis.

When differentiating between a benign and malignant appearance of a lesion, a general rule is that benign lesions such as a unicameral bone cysts do not cross the physis. Any tumour that crosses a physis should be suspected to be malignant.

ENVIRONMENTAL ASPECTS

The cells in the physis, especially in the proliferative layer, are very sensitive to irradiation. Growth disturbance and deformity can occur after treatment for childhood cancers.

CONCLUSION

The activity of the physis is central to the understanding of paediatric orthopaedics. Development of the physis starts in utero, however, where, along with the developing limb, it can be affected by a variety of insults that may be detectable antenatally on ultrasound scan or may become apparent only with further growth in infancy and childhood. After birth, the physis again may be affected by injury and disease.

Viva questions

1 When does the limb bud of the embryo first appear?

2 What is a secondary ossification centre?

3 Draw a sketch of a physis.

4 Through which layer of the physis do fractures occur?

5 How is the physis affected by rickets?

FURTHER READING

Gillespie, R, Torode, IP. Classification and management of congenital abnormalities of the femur. *J Bone Joint Surg Br* 1983;**65**:557–68.

Jones, DH, Barnes, J, Lloyd-Roberts, G. Congenital aplasia and dysplasia of the tibia with intact fibula: classification and management. *J Bone Joint Surg Br* 1978;**60**:31–9.

Rivas, R, Shapiro, F. Structural stages in the development of the long bones and epiphyses. *J Bone Joint Surg Am* 2002;**84**:85–100.

Rubin, P. *Dynamic Classification of Bone Dysplasias*. Chicago, IL: Year Book Medical Publishers, 1964.

Salter, RB, Harris, WR. Injuries involving the epiphyseal plate. *J Bone Joint Surg Am* 1963;**45**:587–622.

Swanson, AB. The classification of congenital limb malformations. *J Hand Surg Am* 1976;**1**:8–22.

4

Orthopaedic pharmacology

MANOJ RAMACHANDRAN AND NATASHA RAHMAN

INTRODUCTION

Orthopaedic surgeons should have a sound working knowledge of the indications for, and the actions and adverse effects of, any therapeutic drug that they prescribe on a regular basis. This chapter provides an overview of the common classes of drugs encountered by orthopaedic surgeons. Antibiotics are discussed in Chapter 5.

ANALGESIC AND ANTI-INFLAMMATORY DRUGS

The choice and route of analgesic drug administration depends on the nature and duration of the pain. A **progressive approach** is used, starting with **simple analgesics** such as paracetamol and non-steroidal anti-inflammatory drugs (NSAIDs), supplemented first by **weak opioid analgesics** and later by **strong opioids**. As a general rule, severe acute pain (e.g. trauma, postoperative pain) is treated with strong opioid drugs given by injection. Mild inflammatory pain (e.g. rheumatoid arthritis) is treated with NSAIDs supplemented by weak opioids given orally. Severe chronic pain (e.g. severe rheumatoid arthritis, back pain) is treated with strong opioids given orally, subcutaneously or epidurally. In addition, patient-controlled analgesic systems may be used.

There are four main classes of analgesic drug:

- opioid analgesics;
- NSAIDs;
- centrally acting non-opioid drugs, e.g. paracetamol, amitriptyline, carbamazepine;
- local anaesthetics.

OPIOID ANALGESICS

Examples

- **Strong:** morphine, diamorphine, fentanyl, pethidine, buprenorphine.
- **Weak:** codeine, dihydrocodeine, dextropropoxyphene.

Essentials

Opioid analgesics **mimic endogenous opioid peptides** by causing a prolonged activation of **opioid receptors**, usually mu (μ) receptors. Opioid receptors are distributed widely throughout the central nervous system and are concentrated most highly in areas involved in nociception, such as the **dorsal horn of the spinal cord** and the **thalamus**. Opioid analgesics function via opioid receptors to facilitate opening of potassium channels (causing hyperpolarization) and calcium channels (inhibiting transmitter release) at the neuronal level, acting via G-proteins linked to adenylate cyclase. The clinical effects of these drugs are **analgesia**, **sedation** and **euphoria**.

Adverse effects

- **Respiratory depression:** this can be reversed with naloxone (short-acting) or naltrexone (long-acting), although reversal is more difficult with overdoses of partial μ agonists, such as dextropropoxyphene (found in co-proxamol) and buprenorphine.
- **Nausea and vomiting:** due to stimulation of the chemoreceptor trigger zone. Strong opioids must be given with an antiemetic.
- **Constipation:** laxatives are usually required with strong opioids.
- **Tolerance** and **dependence** to strong opioids in addicts.
- **Postural hypotension:** due to depression of the vasomotor centre and release of histamine.
- **Biliary spasm, constriction of the sphincter of Oddi:** particularly with morphine.
- **Pruritus:** due to histamine release.
- **Bronchoconstriction:** due to histamine release.

Miscellaneous facts

- Diamorphine (also known as heroin) is more lipid-soluble than morphine and so has a faster onset of action than morphine.
- Fentanyl can be given transdermally for chronic pain.
- Buprenorphine is an effective analgesic when given sublingually but is associated with prolonged vomiting.

NON-STEROIDAL ANTI-INFLAMMATORY DRUGS

Examples

- **Salicylic acid derivatives:** aspirin.
- **Propionic acid derivatives:** ibuprofen, naproxen (low incidence of side-effects, first-line treatment in inflammatory arthropathies).
- **Miscellaneous:** diclofenac, indometacin.
- **Selective cyclo-oxygenase 2 (COX-2) inhibitors:** celecoxib, rofecoxib (fewer gastrointestinal side effects, but increased risk of cardiovascular morbidity and mortality –

therefore used with caution).
- **Oxicams:** piroxicam (long half-life, but associated with high incidence of gastrointestinal bleeding in elderly people).
- **Pyrazolones:** azapropazone (potent, but high incidence of side effects).

Essentials

Although NSAIDS are a chemically diverse group, they all **inhibit cyclo-oxygenase (COX)**, resulting in **inhibition of prostaglandin synthesis** (Figure 4.1). COX exists as a constitutive isoform (COX-1) in most tissues, where it has a housekeeping function, but at sites of inflammation, COX-2 (a second isoform) is stimulated by cytokines. NSAIDs exert their anti-inflammatory actions via inhibition of COX-2. The inhibition of COX-1 by NSAIDs results in gastrointestinal damage (**dyspepsia, nausea, gastritis**) as a result of loss of the gastroprotective effects of prostaglandins E2 (PGE_2) and I2 (PGI_2), which inhibit gastric acid secretion, increase blood flow through the gastric mucosa and have a cytoprotective action.

Aspirin is an **irreversible inactivator of COX**, acting by acetylating a serine residue of the constitutive form of the enzyme. Other NSAIDs are reversible non-selective competitive inhibitors of COX. COX-2 inhibitors are more selective in their action. NSAIDS are **analgesics** (via inhibition of prostaglandins, which sensitize nociceptive nerve endings to inflammatory

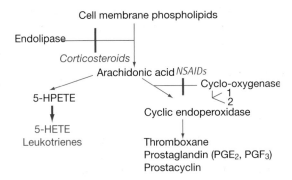

Figure 4.1 *Mechanism of action of non-steroidal anti-inflammatory drugs (NSAIDs) and corticosteroids.* 5-HETE, 5-hydroxyeicosatetraenoic acid; 5-HPETE, 5-hydroperoxyeicosatetraenoic acid; PGE_2, prostaglandin E2; PGF_3, prostaglandin F3.

mediators such as histamine and bradykinin), **anti-inflammatory agents** (via inhibition of prostaglandins, leading to less vasodilation and oedema) and **antipyretics** (by inhibition of the endogenous pyrogen interleukin 1 (IL1), which acts via prostaglandins to elevate the hypothalamic set point for temperature control in fever).

Adverse effects

- **Gastrointestinal:** see above.
- **Renal:** prostaglandins are involved in the control of renal blood flow and sodium and water excretion, particularly in patients with conditions associated with increased vasoconstrictor catecholamines and angiotensin II release, such as congestive cardiac failure and cirrhosis. Inhibiting renal prostaglandin synthesis can result in sodium retention, reduced blood flow and subsequent reversible renal insufficiency.
- **Pulmonary:** bronchospasm in aspirin-sensitive asthmatic patients (the triad of aspirin sensitivity, asthma and nasal polyposis is known as Samter syndrome).
- **Minor effects:** rash, urticaria, photosensitivity reactions.

Miscellaneous facts

Aspirin is increasingly being thought of as a cardiovascular drug rather than an NSAID due to its antiplatelet effects (inhibition of platelet aggregation). Aspirin also has beneficial effects in the prevention of colorectal cancer and in delaying the onset of Alzheimer's disease.

PARACETAMOL (ACETAMINOPHEN)

Essentials

Paracetamol is generally considered to be a **weak inhibitor of the synthesis of prostaglandins**. Its mechanism of action may be via the production of reactive metabolites by the peroxidase function of COX-2, which could deplete glutathione, a cofactor of enzymes such as PGE synthase. COX-3, an isoenzyme of COX-1 found in the central nervous system,

has been suggested to be the site of action of paracetamol, but this selective interaction is unlikely to be clinically relevant. The central action of paracetamol may also be due to activation of descending serotonergic pathways.

Paracetamol has analgesic and antipyretic actions but only weak anti-inflammatory effects. It is well absorbed orally and does not cause gastric irritation.

Adverse effects

- **Analgesic-associated nephropathy:** may occur following long-term high doses of paracetamol.
- **Hepatotoxicity in overdose:** potentially fatal liver damage can occur by saturation of the normal conjugating enzymes causing the drug to be converted by mixed-function oxidases to N-acetyl-p-benzoquinone imine. If this metabolite is not inactivated by conjugation with glutathione (using N-acetylcysteine or methionine), it reacts with cell proteins, causing hepatocyte necrosis.

LOCAL ANAESTHETICS

Examples

- **Esters:** cocaine, procaine.
- **Amides:** lignocaine, bupivacaine, prilocaine.

Essentials

Local anaesthetics **block action potential initiation and propagation** in neurons by physically plugging the transmembrane pore of sodium channels. Local anaesthetics are **ampiphilic** molecules with a hydrophobic aromatic group linked by an ester or amide bond to a basic amine group. Their activity is strongly pH-dependent, being increased at alkaline pH when the proportion of ionized molecules is low, which allows them to penetrate the nerve sheath and axonal membrane as the unionized form is more membrane-permeant. Local anaesthetics block conduction in the following order: small myelinated axons, unmyelinated axons, large myelinated axons. Therefore, nociceptive and sympathetic transmission in Aδ and C fibres is blocked first. Local anaesthetics may be given topically, by direct infiltration, intravenously, as nerve blocks, or by spinal or epidural administration.

Esters are rapidly hydrolysed by plasma cholinesterases, and amides are metabolized in the liver.

Adverse effects

- **Central nervous system effects:** agitation, confusion, tremors progressing to convulsions, respiratory depression.
- **Cardiovascular effects:** myocardial depression and vasodilation, leading to a drop in blood pressure.
- **Hypersensitivity reactions.**

GLUCOCORTICOIDS

Examples

- **Mildly potent (class I):** hydrocortisone.
- **Moderately potent (class II):** triamcinolone.
- **Potent (class III):** methylprednisolone.
- **Very potent (class IV):** betamethasone dipropionate.

Essentials

Glucocorticoids have **anti-inflammatory** and **immunosuppressive** effects. They act on all phases of the inflammatory response, from the early changes of acute inflammation to the later proliferative changes of chronic inflammation. Glucocorticoids interact with intracellular receptors, forming **steroid–receptor complexes** that **modify gene transcription** at the DNA level, resulting in either **induction or inhibition of protein synthesis**. Examples include inhibition of transcription of the genes for COX-2, phospholipase A2 (PLA_2; an endolipase) and cytokines such as the interleukins, and increased synthesis of lipocortin 1, which exerts its anti-inflammatory actions by inhibiting endolipases (Figure 4.1). Glucocorticoids also directly **depress monocyte/macrophage function, decrease circulating T-cell levels**, and directly **inhibit lymphocyte transport** to the site of antigenic stimulation and antibody production.

Glucocorticoids can be given orally, topically or parenterally. They are bound to corticosteroid-binding globulin in the blood and enter cells by diffusion, eventually being metabolized in the liver.

Adverse effects

The adverse effects of glucocorticoids are best remembered using the mnemonic 'I WAS HOPPING MAD':

- **Infection** (including reactivation of nascent infections, e.g. tuberculosis).
- **Wasting** of muscles (due to protein loss).
- **Adrenal insufficiency.**
- **Sugar disturbances** (hyperglycaemia, diabetes).
- **Hypotension.**
- **Osteoporosis** (due to increase in bone catabolism; one mechanism is the inhibition of vitamin D_3-mediated induction of the osteocalcin gene in osteoblasts).
- **Peptic ulcer.**
- **Pancreatitis.**
- **Proximal myopathy** (due to protein loss).
- **Incidental** (moon facies, 'orange-on-stick' appearance due to central obesity, easy bruising, hirsutism).
- **Necrosis** of the femoral head.
- **Glaucoma**, cataracts.
- **'MAD'** (psychological changes, e.g. euphoria, depression, psychosis, emotional lability).

ANTICOAGULANTS

Anticoagulants are used in the prophylaxis and treatment of thromboembolism. There are several classes of these drugs:

- **Vitamin K antagonists:** warfarin.
- **Inhibitors of thrombin:**
  - unfractionated heparin;
  - low-molecular-weight heparins (LMWH), e.g. enoxaparin, dalteparin;
  - fondaparinux;
  - oral thrombin inhibitors, e.g. melagatran.

WARFARIN

Essentials

Warfarin is a coumarin derivative with a structure similar to vitamin K. Warfarin is active orally. It **blocks vitamin K-dependent γ-carboxylation of glutamate residues** on factors II, VII, IX and X, resulting in the production of modified factors known as **PIVKA** (proteins in vitamin K absence). These modified factors cannot bind calcium and therefore become inactive in coagulation. Warfarin takes **2–3 days to achieve its full anticoagulant effect**, as the inactive factors slowly replace those originally present. The effects of warfarin are monitored with the prothrombin time, which is expressed as an international normalized ratio (INR). Warfarin has a **long half-life** (around 40 h), and it takes as long as 5 days for the INR to return to normal after cessation of treatment. Warfarin is metabolized by hepatic microsomal enzymes to inactive 7-hydroxywarfarin.

Adverse effects

- **Haemorrhage:** in overdosage (reverse acutely with clotting factor concentrates or fresh frozen plasma; if severe, consider intravenous vitamin K).
- **Drug interactions:** drugs that induce (e.g. barbiturates, carbamazepine) or inhibit (e.g. ethanol, metronidazole) hepatic microsomal enzymes may have an effect on the action of warfarin, either leading to haemorrhage on their withdrawal or to potentiation of its action.
- **Teratogenicity**.

INHIBITORS OF THROMBIN

Essentials

Heparin is a **naturally occurring glycosaminoglycan** of varying molecular weight (5000–15 000). It is given by injection (subcutaneous or intravenous) and is **short-acting**. Heparin forms a 1 : 1 complex with anti-thrombin III (Figure 4.2), a protease inhibitor that **inactivates thrombin** (factor II) when bound to heparin. The heparin–anti-thrombin II complex also inactivates factor Xa (among others). When heparin is given intravenously, its effects need to be monitored with the activated partial thromboplastin time (APTT). Heparin has a short duration of action (4–6 h).

LMWH–anti-thrombin III complex inhibits factor Xa only, resulting in less bleeding. LMWHs have **longer half-lives** and therefore require only **single daily dosing**. They are given by subcutaneous injection. Prophylactic doses do not require monitoring.

Adverse effects

- **Haemorrhage:** less with LMWHs than with heparin. Bleeding with heparin can normally

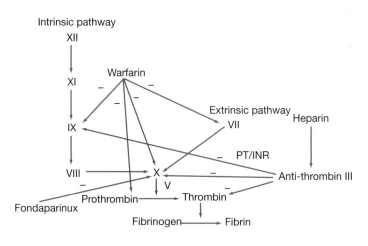

Figure 4.2 *Sites of action of anticoagulants on the coagulation cascade.*
INR, international normalized ratio; PT, prothrombin time.

be controlled by stopping its administration, but in severe cases protamine sulphate (a basic peptide that combines with the acidic heparin) may be required.

- **Allergic reactions**.
- **Heparin-induced thrombocytopenia** (HIT).
- **Osteoporosis**: when used long-term.
- **Thrombosis**: rare.

Miscellaneous facts

- **Fondaparinux** is a pentasaccharide that precisely inhibits factor Xa and has been shown to **reduce venous thromboembolism** more effectively than LMWHs in hip and knee arthroplasty and fractures of the hip. It is given at least 6 h after surgery and at least 12 h after removal of the spinal/epidural catheter in order to avoid the risk of surgical or neuraxial bleeding.
- **Melagatran** is a newer **direct oral thrombin inhibitor** with a number of important advantages over warfarin, including a wide therapeutic and safety window, the lack of need for monitoring, and no reported interactions with other drugs.

DRUGS ACTING ON BONE METABOLISM

BONE REMODELLING

Remodelling of bone occurs continuously throughout life (see Chapter 13). To summarize, the cycle commences with osteoclast recruitment by cytokines, e.g. interleukin 6 (IL-6). The osteoclasts adhere to areas of trabecular bone and dig pits by secreting hydrogen ions and proteolytic enzymes (Figure 4.3).

This action leads to liberation of factors that are embedded in bone, such as insulin-like growth factor 1 (IGF-1). These in turn recruit and activate osteoblasts, which have been primed to develop from precursor cells by parathyroid hormone (PTH) and 1, 25-dihydroxycholecalciferol (calcitriol). Osteoblasts invade the pits and synthesize and secrete osteoid, the organic matrix of bone. The osteoid is then mineralized, i.e. complex calcium phosphate crystals (hydroxyapatites) are deposited. Osteoblasts and their precursors

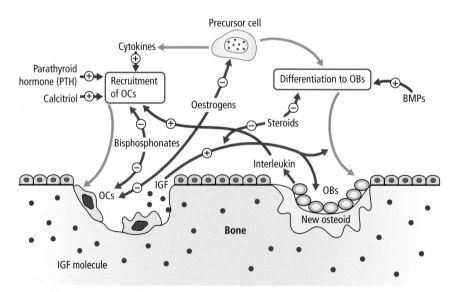

Figure 4.3 *Bone remodelling cycle and the site of action of cytokines and drugs. Note that oestrogens are thought to exert their anti-osteoporotic effects by up-regulating transforming growth factor beta (TGF-β), which results in apoptosis of osteoclasts (OC) and osteoblasts (OB). BMP, bone morphogenic protein; IGF, insulin-like growth factor.*

secrete IGF-1 (which becomes embedded in the osteoid) and other cytokines, such as IL-6, which in turn recruit osteoclasts (a return to the start of the cycle). Bone metabolism and mineralization therefore involves the action of PTH, the vitamin D family, cytokines and calcitonin.

BISPHOSPHONATES

Essentials

This class of drug is characterized by a **P—C—P backbone resistant to phosphatases** (Figure 4.4), in contrast to pyrophosphate, which has a P—O—P backbone. No known enzymes can metabolize the P—C—P backbone of bisphosphonates, resulting in considerable longevity of these drugs once administered.

Bisphosphonates act by **directly stabilizing the hydroxyapatite crystal**, making it more resistant to resorption. **Aminobisphosphonates** such as pamidronate and alendronate have more **specific osteoclastic activity** than early bisphosphonates such as etidronate. Aminobisphosphonates also **directly inhibit the action of osteoclasts** (via the mevalonate pathway, inhibiting farnesyl pyrophosphate (FPP) synthase), preventing prenylation (formation of brush border) and functioning of signalling proteins required for osteoclast formation.

Bisphosphonates are given orally (poorly absorbed) or parenterally. Around 50 per cent of a dose accumulates at sites of bone mineralization, where it remains until the bone is absorbed.

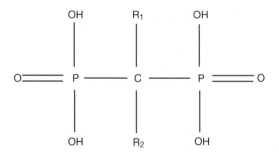

Figure 4.4 *Chemical structure of bisphosphonates.*

Bisphosphonates are used clinically to treat postmenopausal and glucocorticoid-induced osteoporosis, Paget's disease of bone and malignant hypercalcaemia. They are also used in paediatric orthopaedics for the treatment of decreased bone mineral density and pain in conditions such as osteogenesis imperfecta and fibrous dysplasia.

Adverse effects

- Oral intake must be on an empty stomach, which can cause **gastric pain** and **oesophagitis**.
- Rarer reported adverse effects include **transient leucopenia** and ophthalmic changes, such as **scleritis**.

VITAMIN D DERIVATIVES

Essentials

Vitamin D analogues are commonly used in the treatment of metabolic bone disease. There are several vitamin D derivatives available for clinical use (Table 4.1). All vitamin D derivatives can be given orally and are well absorbed from the intestine. Vitamin D derivatives are fat-soluble, and bile salts are essential for absorption.

Adverse effects

- Excessive intake leads to **hypercalcaemia**.
- Increased requirements for vitamin D if on certain anticonvulsive medication, e.g. **phenytoin**.

CALCITONIN

Essentials

The mechanism of action of calcitonin is discussed in Chapter 13. Calcitonin is available for clinical use in natural (porcine – calcitonin) and synthetic (salmon – salcalcitonin) forms. Porcine calcitonin may contain traces of thyroid hormones and can lead to antibody production.

Calcitonin is given by subcutaneous or intramuscular injection or intranasally. It is used clinically to treat **Paget's disease of bone** (for

Table 4.1 Vitamin D derivatives and their clinical uses

Compound	Alternative name	Comments
Vitamin D3	*Cholecalciferol*	*Formed in skin from dehydrocholesterol by ultraviolet radiation*
Vitamin D2	*Ergocalciferol (calciferol)*	*Formed in plants by ultraviolet radiation; used clinically to treat rickets, osteomalacia and vitamin D deficiency due to malabsorption and liver disease*
25-OH-Vitamin D3	*Calcifediol*	*Main storage form of vitamin D*
1,25-OH-Vitamin D3	*Calcitriol*	*Most potent metabolite in regulating plasma calcium; used clinically to treat renal osteodystrophy (due to decreased calcitriol generation)*
1α-OH-cholecalciferol	*Alfacalcidol*	*Synthetic derivative of vitamin D3; undergoes hepatic 25-hydroxylation to calcitriol; used clinically to treat renal osteodystrophy (due to decreased calcitriol generation)*

pain relief and to reduce neurological complications), **malignant hypercalcaemia**, and as part of the therapy for **postmenopausal and glucocorticoid-induced osteoporosis**. Note that bisphosphonates are often the first-line drugs for these conditions.

Adverse effects

- **Nausea and vomiting**.
- **Facial flushing**.
- **Tingling sensation** in the hands.
- **Unpleasant taste** in the mouth.
- Increased risk of **stress fractures**, e.g. in the distal tibia, as the bone formed may be abnormal.

MISCELLANEOUS DRUGS

PARATHYROID HORMONE

PTH (teriparatide) is an anabolic agent used in the treatment of osteoporosis. The 1–34 portion of the 84-amino-acid peptide PTH can be given by subcutaneous daily injection. The anabolic effect of PTH results in increased bone formation and improved micro-architecture. PTH also activates bone lining cells and osteoblasts, particularly if intermittent

stimulation is used (with continuous stimulation by teriparatide, osteoclasts are stimulated more). Teriparatide works mainly on the periosteal surface of bone, but it also causes endosteal resorption, increasing the diameter of bone and its bending and torsional strength by increasing the second and polar moments of inertia. There are concerns regarding an increased incidence of osteosarcoma in rats (although high doses were used in these animal trials), blunting of the effects of co-administered bisphosphonates and high expense. Minor adverse effects include leg cramps and dizziness.

STRONTIUM

Strontium was originally detected in lead mines in the 1700s near Strontian in Scotland. It is a group 2, period 5 element in the periodic table, with atomic number 38. Strontium is similar to calcium, and thus dual-energy X-ray absorption (DEXA) scans following treatment with strontium look excellent. Strontium is given orally daily in ranelate form, which links two strontium atoms. Its effects are increased bone formation (anabolic effect) and decreased bone resorption (anti-catabolic effect). Strontium has shown early promise as a treatment for osteoporosis.

Viva questions

1 What are the different methods of achieving pain relief after joint arthroplasty?

2 What thromboprophylaxis regimen would you use for total hip arthroplasty?

3 What are the indications for the use of bisphosphonates in orthopaedics?

4 What classes of drug can be used to treat osteoporosis?

5 How do local anaesthetics work?

FURTHER READING

Bhattacharyya, T, Smith, RM. Cardiovascular risks of coxibs: the orthopaedic perspective. *J Bone Joint Surg Am* 2005;**87**:245–6.

Ekman, EF, Koman, LA. Acute pain following musculoskeletal injuries and orthopaedic surgery. Mechanisms and management. *J Bone Joint Surg Am* 2004;**86**:1316–27.

Mader, JT, Wang, J, Calhoun, JH. Antibiotic therapy for musculoskeletal infections. *J Bone Joint Surg Am* 2001;**83**:1878–90.

Morris, CD, Einhorn, TA. Bisphosphonates in orthopaedic surgery. *J Bone Joint Surg Am* 2005;**87**:1609–18.

Warwick, D. New concepts in orthopaedic thromboprophylaxis. *J Bone Joint Surg Br* 2004;**86**:788–92.

5

Inflammation and infection

VIKAS KHANDUJA AND MANOJ RAMACHANDRAN

INTRODUCTION

Inflammation and infection are large topics to cover in terms of the essentials required for day-to-day orthopaedic practice. Details of the virulence of microorganisms and the host response produced following an infection are beyond the scope of this chapter. However, a working knowledge of the common microorganisms causing infection in bones and joints, the common antibiotics used, and the mechanisms of action of the latter is essential. An in-depth knowledge of acute osteomyelitis and septic arthritis is invaluable and is thus covered in this chapter. Finally, a brief discussion on methicillin-resistant *Staphylococcus aureus* (MRSA) and tuberculosis (TB) is also required.

OVERVIEW OF INFLAMMATION

The five cardinal features of acute inflammation are **rubor** (erythema), **calor** (heat), **dolor** (pain), **tumor** (swelling) and **functio laesa** (loss of function). Acute inflammation follows a specific sequence. The initial phase is **vasoconstriction**, followed immediately by **vasodilation** and **increased vascular permeability**.

Further events include **leukocytic margination** and **emigration** (neutrophils, followed by monocytes) and **phagocytosis**, involving both intracellular degradation of ingested particles (oxygen-dependent and oxygen-independent mechanisms) and extracellular release of leukocyte products, e.g. lysosomal enzymes. When bacteria invade the musculoskeletal system, the initial response is an acute inflammatory reaction. This results in polymorphonuclear cells attacking and phagocytosing bacteria.

There are three possible outcomes to acute inflammation: complete **resolution**, healing by **scarring**, and progression to **chronic inflammation**. Chronic inflammation can occur due to a variety of causes, including **persistent infection** by intracellular microbes (e.g. tubercle bacilli, viral infections) that are of low toxicity but evoke an immunological reaction, **prolonged exposure** to non-degradable but potentially toxic substances (e.g. lung silicosis, asbestosis), and **immune** (particularly autoimmune) **reactions**.

The key cells in chronic inflammation are **mononuclear cells** (principally macrophages, lymphocytes and plasma cells), **fibroblasts** and **eosinophils** (in immune reactions). **Macrophages** are the central figures, their activation in inflammation being triggered by lymphokines (e.g. gamma-interferon) produced by immune-activated T-cells or non-immune factors such as exotoxin. The secretory products of macrophages induce characteristic chronic inflammatory changes, such as **tissue destruction** (proteases and oxygen-derived free radicals), **neovascularization** (growth factors), **fibroblast proliferation** (growth factors) and **connective tissue accumulation** (interleukin 1 [IL-1], tumour necrosis factor alpha [TNF-α]).

Lymphocytes have a reciprocal relationship with macrophages in chronic inflammation. Activated lymphocytes produce lymphokines, and these (particularly gamma-interferon) are major stimulators of macrophages. Activated macrophages produce monokines, which in turn influence B- and T-cell function.

BACTERIOLOGY

Microorganisms that can cause infection include bacteria, viruses, parasites and fungi. Of these, bacteria are the most common source of infection in bones and joints. Bacteria are **prokaryotic cells**, as they do not have a nucleus. The genetic material is aggregated in an area of the cytoplasm called the **nucleoid**. Bacteria do not possess a cytoplasmic compartment containing mitochondria and lysosomes. A consistent feature of all prokaryotes but not eukaryotes is the presence of a **cell wall**, which allows bacteria to resist osmotic stress. This cell wall differs in complexity between species, and bacteria are usually divided into two major groups – Gram-positive and Gram-negative bacteria – which reflect their cell-wall structure.

Bacteria are designated **Gram-positive** or **Gram-negative** depending on whether the cell membrane of the bacterium retains crystal-violet indium dye after an alcohol rinse. Gram-positive bacteria retain the dye and, hence, appear bluish under a light microscope. Gram-negative bacteria do not retain the dye, but they do retain the safranin O counter-stain and, hence, appear pink under a light microscope.

Bacteria can be classified further into **cocci** and **bacilli** depending on their shape. Cocci are round and bacilli are small rods. Examples of the common bacteria and their classification are given in Table 5.1.

SEPTIC ARTHRITIS AND OSTEOMYELITIS

DEFINITION

Septic arthritis is a condition characterized by **infection of the synovium and the joint space**. The infection causes an intense inflammatory reaction and release of proteolytic enzymes, leading to rapid destruction of the articular cartilage.

Osteomyelitis is an **acute or chronic inflammatory process of the bone** and its structures secondary to infection.

Table 5.1 Examples of common bacteria and their classification

Gram-positive cocci	Gram-negative cocci	Gram-positive bacilli	Gram-negative bacilli
Staphylococcus aureus, S. epidermidis	Branhamella catarrhalis	Clostridium tetani, C. perfringens	Pseudomonas aeruginosa
Enterococcus *spp.*	Neisseria gonorrhoea, N. meningitides	Bacillus anthracis	Eikenella corrodens
Streptococcus *spp.*		Actinomyces *spp.*	Haemophilus influenzae
		Corynebacterium *spp.*	Escherichia coli
		Nocardia asteroides	Salmonella typhi
		Listeria monocytogenes	Klebsiella pneumoniae
			Bacteroides fragilis

AETIOLOGY AND PATHOGENESIS

Septic arthritis and osteomyelitis are **common in children** but can also occur in adults, usually secondary to an immunocompromised state or an underlying medical condition such as diabetes. Septic arthritis and osteomyelitis can occur from **primary seeding of the synovial membrane**, secondarily from **infection in the adjacent metaphyseal bone**, or directly from **infection in the adjoining epiphysis**. In the shoulder, elbow, hip and ankle joints, the capsule overlaps a portion of the adjoining metaphysis. If the focus of osteomyelitis breaks through the metaphyseal bone, it can directly infect the joint and lead to concurrent septic arthritis.

Destruction of the articular cartilage begins quickly and is secondary to proteolytic enzymes released from synovial cells. IL-1 triggers the release of proteases from chondrocytes and synoviocytes in response to polymorphonuclear leukocytes and bacteria. Degradation results in the **loss of proteoglycans** from the articular cartilage by 5 days and **loss of collagen** by 9 days.

Impairment of the intracapsular vascular supply secondary to elevation of the intracapsular pressure and thrombosis of the vessels also play a role in the destruction of articular cartilage. The common sites of involvement in children are the hip and knee, but in the adult about 85 per cent of cases are mono-articular, the knee being the most common joint involved.

CLINICAL PRESENTATION

Typically, the disease has an **acute onset** and the child is irritable and febrile. If the infection involves the lower limb, the child usually has a **limp** and **refuses to bear weight**. Clinical examination of the involved joint reveals **resistance to passive motion** of the attempted joint and **severe pain on attempted motion**. In subcutaneous joints, increased **warmth**, **erythema**, soft-tissue **swelling** and **effusion** may be present. The joints are usually held in a position of maximal comfort; if the hip is involved, the child holds it in a position of flexion, abduction and external rotation. Neonates with septic arthritis may exhibit only irritability, lethargy, difficulty in feeding, and pseudo-paralysis of the affected limb. In osteomyelitis, tenderness is most acute over the involved area of bone, which is usually metaphyseal.

INVESTIGATIONS

Initial laboratory tests include a full blood count, acute-phase reactants, including erythrocyte sedimentation rate (ESR) and C-reactive protein (CRP), and blood cultures. The **white cell count** is usually greater than $12\,000/mm^3$, with 40–60 per cent polymorphonuclear leukocytes. **ESR** is usually elevated to more than 50 mm, and **blood cultures** are positive in about 30–50 per cent of cases. **CRP** is elevated and returns to normal fairly quickly after treatment.

Ultrasound of the affected joint, especially the hip, can detect an effusion and can be an aid in aspiration. **Radiographs** may show subluxation or dislocation of the joint and soft-tissue swelling around the affected joint. Radiographs can also reveal subtle changes such as joint-space widening in septic arthritis and metaphyseal rarefaction in early osteomyelitis. **Bone scans** may show a decreased-uptake 'cold scan' early in the disease process and an increased-uptake 'hot scan' later on.

Joint aspiration with immediate **Gram stain** and **microscopy** followed by **culture** and **sensitivity** remains the mainstay for diagnosis for septic arthritis. On direct examination, the aspirate may demonstrate **gross pus**. A **white cell count** of more than $50\,000/mm^3$ with 75 per cent of polymorphonuclear leukocytosis is usually seen. Gram stains are positive in only 30–50 per cent of the cases, and cultures of the aspirate are positive in about 50–80 per cent of cases. **Synovial protein levels** that are more than 40 mg/dL and are less than serum protein levels are consistent with septic arthritis. **Lactate levels** are typically elevated in the joint fluid in patients with septic arthritis. The **glucose level** in the aspirate is lower than that in the serum.

The diagnosis of osteomyelitis is usually made by a combination of clinical findings, radiographs, bone scanning and magnetic resonance imaging (MRI) scans, along with the aspiration of pus from the involved area and positive blood cultures. In chronic osteomyelitis, radiographic signs of necrotic bone (**sequestrum**) and periosteal new bone formation (**involucrum**) are evident.

TREATMENT

Septic arthritis is an emergency, and treatment should be expedited to prevent any permanent damage to the articular cartilage. Appropriate management involves **prompt diagnosis** followed by **surgical drainage** and **irrigation of the involved joint** with appropriate constitutional support, including hydration and antibiotics. A **drain** should be left in place following irrigation until the volume of the drainage decreases. If surgery is not followed by rapid recovery, **re-exploration** should be considered.

Intravenous antibiotics should be commenced immediately after aspiration of the involved joints. **Broad-spectrum** antibiotics are commenced initially based on the organisms suspected and subsequently changed to **specific** antibiotics, depending upon culture and sensitivity. The organisms responsible in various

Table 5.2 Organisms responsible for septic arthritis and osteomyelitis by age

Age group	Organisms
Infants (<1 year)	Group B streptococci
	Staphylococcus aureus
	Escherichia coli
Children (1–16 years)	S. aureus
	Streptococcus pyogenes
	Haemophilus influenzae
Adults (<16 years)	Staphylococcus epidermidis
	S. aureus
	Pseudomonas aeruginosa
	Serratia marcescens
	E. coli

age groups are summarized in Table 5.2. Intravenous antibiotics are usually given for 2 weeks and then **converted to oral antibiotics** for a total of 4–6 weeks, depending on the clinical response.

The approach to management of acute osteomyelitis is similar but may involve open drainage of pus if, for example, a subperiosteal abscess forms. If osteomyelitis becomes **chronic**, the management principles involve **drainage** and **debridement** of all necrotic tissue, with **preservation of the involucrum**, **obliteration of dead spaces** (e.g. with vascularized bone graft or vacuum-assisted closure), **adequate soft-tissue coverage** (e.g. with local or free flaps) and **preservation of skeletal stability**.

ANTIBIOTICS

Antibiotics are used for **prophylaxis**, to **eradicate infections**, and for **initial care** in open fractures and wounds. A comprehensive list of the antibiotics commonly used for musculoskeletal infections along with their groups, subgroups and mechanism of action is shown in Table 5.3. Table 5.4 summarizes the spectrum of activity and the common complications of these antibiotics.

ANTIBIOTIC DELIVERY

Antibiotics can be delivered in a variety of ways:

- **Oral**.
- **Intramuscular**.
- **Intravenous** and **home intravenous therapy** (via Hickman line).
- **Antibiotic beads and spacers**: aminoglycosides are impregnated in polymethylmethacrylate (PMMA) cement and used to treat infected total joint arthroplasty and osteomyelitis. The antibiotic used in this form is stable during the process of PMMA polymerization. Elution of antibiotic from PMMA is for a maximum of 6–8 weeks. This form delivers a very high local concentration of the antibiotic.
- **Osmotic pump**: delivers high concentration of antibiotic locally. Useful for osteomyelitis.

Table 5.3 Antibiotics commonly used in orthopaedics

Antibiotic group	Subgroup	Examples	Mechanism of action
Penicillins	Natural	Penicillin G (IV) Penicillin V (oral)	Bactericidal: inhibit bacterial peptidoglycan synthesis by binding to penicillin-binding proteins on bacterial cell membranes; also known as beta-lactam antibiotics
	Penicillinase-resistant	Flucloxacillin	
	Aminopenicillins	Ampicillin Co-amoxiclav Amoxicillin	
	Antipseudomonal	Piperacillin Ticarcillin Mezlocillin	
Cephalosporins	First generation	Cefradine Cefalexin	Bactericidal: inhibit bacterial cell-wall synthesis; also known as beta-lactams
	Second generation	Cefuroxime Cefaclor	
	Third generation	Ceftriaxone Ceftazidime	
	Fourth generation	Cefepime Cefpirome	
Carbapenems		Imipenem	Bactericidal: inhibits cell-wall synthesis
Monobactams		Aztreonam	Bactericidal: inhibit cell-wall synthesis; limited spectrum of activity, mainly against Gram-negative anaerobes
Aminoglycosides		Gentamicin Neomycin Tobramycin Amikacin	Bactericidal: inhibit bacterial protein synthesis by binding to cytoplasmic rRNA (30S subunit)
Macrolides		Erythromycin Clarithromycin Azithromycin	Inhibit dissociation of peptidyl tRNA from ribosomes during translocation by binding to the 50S subunit
Quinolones		Ciprofloxacin Ofloxacin Norfloxacin	Inhibit DNA gyrase, an enzyme that compresses DNA into super-coils
Glycopeptides		Vancomycin Teicoplanin	Inhibit cell-membrane synthesis by interfering with insertion of glycan subunits in cell wall
Tetracyclines		Tetracycline Doxycycline Minocycline	Bacteriostatic: inhibit bacterial protein synthesis by binding to cytoplasmic rRNA (30S subunit)
Others		Rifampicin	Bactericidal: prevents RNA transcription by inhibiting DNA-dependent RNA polymerase

DNA, deoxyribonucleic acid; IV, intravenous; rRNA, ribosomal ribonucleic acid; tRNA, transfer ribonucleic acid.

Table 5.4 Antibiotic spectrum of activity and complications

Antibiotic	Spectrum of activity	Complications
Penicillin	Mainly against Gram-positive cocci, Clostridium spp., Anthrax spp.; inactivated by bacterial beta-lactamases	Hypersensitivity reactions, haemolytic anaemia, CNS toxicity, colitis
Flucloxacillin	Staphylococcus spp.	As for penicillin, plus cholestatic jaundice, hepatitis
Co-amoxiclav (amoxicillin + beta-lactamase inhibitor clavulanic acid)	Staphylococcus aureus, Escherichia coli, Haemophilus influenzae, Bacteroides spp., Klebsiella spp.	As for penicillin, hepatitis, cholestatic jaundice, skin reactions
Piperacillin	Pseudomonas aeruginosa, Gram-negative bacilli	As for penicillin
Cephalosporins	First-generation cephalosporins very active against Gram-positive bacteria; fourth-generation cephalosporins active against Gram-negative bacteria; activity against Gram-positive bacteria decreases from first to fourth generations	Haemolytic anaemia, colitis, allergic skin reactions, disturbances in liver enzymes
Imipenem	Administered with cilastatin to prevent renal metabolism; active against aerobes and anaerobes and Gram-positive and Gram-negative bacteria	CNS toxicity, grand mal seizures, colitis
Gentamicin	Mainly against aerobic Gram-negative bacteria, Pseudomonas aeruginosa, Enterobacteriaceae spp.	Ototoxicity, nephrotoxicity, neuromuscular blockade
Erythromycin	Active against Streptococcus spp., Listeria monocytogenes, Moraxella catarrhalis, Mycoplasma pneumoniae, Legionella pneumophilia, Chlamydia pneumoniae	Can cause gastrointestinal reactions, e.g. nausea, vomiting, abdominal cramps
Ciprofloxacin	Mainly against Gram-negative bacteria	Gastrointestinal disturbances, tendonitis, increased risk of Achilles tendon rupture
Vancomycin	Excellent activity against S. aureus, Staphylococcus epidermidis, Enterococcus spp., MRSA	'Red-man syndrome' – flushing of head, neck and upper torso associated with hypotension; nephrotoxicity, ototoxicity, neutropenia, thrombocytopenia
Tetracycline	Mainly against Gram-positive bacteria	Colitis, staining of bone and teeth in children, hepatotoxicity in pregnancy

CNS, central nervous system; MRSA, methicillin-resistant Staphylococcus aureus.

ANTIBIOTIC RESISTANCE

There are two types of microbiological resistance: innate (or intrinsic) and extrinsic.

Innate or intrinsic antibiotic resistance

This implies that the bacterial cell inherently has properties that do not allow the antibiotic to act on it. Examples of innate or intrinsic resistance include:

- enzyme production that destroys the antibiotic;
- changes in cell-wall permeability;
- alterations in structural target (e.g. 30S and 50S ribosomes);
- mutations in efflux mechanisms;
- bypass of metabolic pathway;
- resistance via a combination of the above or multiple mechanisms.

Extrinsic antibiotic resistance

This implies that an organism acquires resistance to an antibiotic to which it was previously sensitive. This can take place due to a chance mutation in the genetic material of the cell or the acquisition of drug-resistant genes from other drug-resistant cells. This resistance is usually mediated via **plasmids**, small circles of double-stranded DNA. Plasmids carry genes for specialized functions and also carry one or more genes for antimicrobial resistance.

METHICILLIN–RESISTANT STAPHYLOCOCCUS AUREUS

DEFINITION AND PREVALENCE

MRSA is a Gram-positive coccus and a **major nosocomial pathogen**. The prevalence of MRSA is reported to be around 1.6 per cent within orthopaedic departments, compared with 0.3 per cent within general hospital settings. MRSA is a cause for significant concern due to its associated high morbidity and mortality and the financial implications if total joint arthroplasties are infected.

GENETICS

The staphylococci acquire their methicillin resistance due to the presence of an **acquired penicillin-binding protein**, PBP2a. This protein is encoded by the gene *mecA*, which is carried on the staphylococcal chromosome. The levels of resistance of the bacteria depend on the production of PBP2a.

COLONIZATION AND RISK FACTORS

Most MRSA infections are acquired by proximity and contact with other colonized patients. It is postulated that up to 25 per cent of hospital personnel are carriers of MRSA. Other important risk factors implicated in the acquisition of MRSA are:

- old age;
- previous hospitalization or surgery;
- prolonged hospitalization;
- open skin lesions;
- chronic medical illness;
- presence of invasive in-dwelling device;
- prolonged antibiotic therapy;
- exposure to another colonized or infected patient.

PREVENTION AND PROPHYLAXIS

The main areas of focus for prevention are **effective screening** to pick up high-risk patients and staff and appropriate **isolation** and **treatment of carriers**. Once these patients have been identified, they should be treated with **nasal mupirocin**; bathing in **antiseptic detergent**, such as 4% chlorhexidine or 2% triclosan, should be encouraged.

Education of nursing and medical staff on hand hygiene is essential. Alcohol-based hand rubs have been shown to be effective against hospital-acquired MRSA infection. However, compliance remains a major problem, with compliance rates of below 50 per cent being reported, despite publication of guidelines on regular hand hygiene.

MANAGEMENT

Once infection is established, management involves administering **intravenous glycopeptides**, which have become the mainstay of treatment. Vancomycin and teicoplanin are the drugs of choice. The advantage of teicoplanin over vancomycin is that the former has better bone penetration, is better tolerated, and can be administered as a bolus dose and, therefore, given on an outpatient basis.

Staphylococcal resistance to glycopeptides has been reported and is a cause for concern. There are also concerns about emergence of strains of *Staphylococcus aureus* with reduced sensitivity to vancomycin. Fortunately, the discovery of **oxazolidinones**, which inhibit an early step in protein synthesis, seems to have solved the problem of glycopeptide resistance. Linezolid, which was the first in this class of antibiotics to be used, has excellent tissue penetration, has 100 per cent bioavailability and can be given orally. **Linezolid** is recommended when conventional glycopeptides have failed or are not tolerated. The major adverse effect of linezolid is bone-marrow suppression with prolonged use.

TUBERCULOSIS

TB is a **chronic granulomatous condition** commonly caused by *Mycobacterium tuberculosis*. The incidence in developed countries is much lower than in developing countries. However, TB is on the rise again, partly due to the human immunodeficiency virus (HIV) epidemic. In addition, multiple drug-resistant strains of *M. tuberculosis* appear regularly.

PATHOGENESIS

Mycobacteria are **obligate aerobic acid-fast rods**. The infection usually **begins in the lung** and the subpleural region along with the draining lymphatics. The mediastinal lymph nodes are also involved. This is known as the primary (Gohn) complex. This primary infection can undergo complete resolution and remain quiescent, or it can spread systemically. Local spread into the lung can lead to **bronchopneumonia,** and haematogenous spread can lead to **miliary TB**, which involves the lung, bones, joints and spine; this is known as **secondary TB**.

CLINICAL PRESENTATION

Patients with pulmonary TB present with low-grade fever, productive chronic cough, weight loss and generalized weakness. Although skeletal involvement usually follows pulmonary involvement, only half of the patients with skeletal involvement have pulmonary disease. Skeletal involvement commonly includes the spine (**tuberculous spondylitis**), the fingers (**tuberculous dactylitis**), the appendicular skeleton (where **metaphyseal lytic lesions** with little or no sclerosis are found) and, rarely, the hip and knee joints (presenting as **mono-arthritis**). The important features of tuberculous mono-arthritis include florid synovitis, preservation of joint space and periarticular osteopenia.

DIAGNOSIS

The diagnosis is difficult to establish and requires a minimum of three large-volume **early-morning sputum** samples. The presence of **acid-fast bacteria under Ziehl–Neelsen stain** confirms the diagnosis. The bacteria appear as red acid-fast organisms under the stain. If microscopy is negative, the specimen is subjected to culture on **Lowenstein–Jensen medium** for a period of 6 weeks at 35–37°C; growth of bacteria in this medium confirms diagnosis. If both microscopy and culture are negative, then the gold standard for diagnosis remains **biopsy**. Histological sections reveal a **classic granuloma** with **caseating central necrosis**. The development of DNA probes, polymerase chain reaction (PCR) assays and liquid media has allowed more sensitive and rapid diagnosis, but these tests are not always specific.

SKIN TESTS

The basis of skin tests is a **delayed hypersensitivity reaction**. The two commonly employed tests are the Heaf test and the Mantoux test. Both tests involve exposing the patient's skin to purified protein derivative. A positive response includes the formation of papules on the skin after a designated number of hours. A positive response implies an active infection or previous BCG (Bacillus Calmette–Guèrin) vaccination.

TREATMENT

A combination regime of **first-line chemotherapeutic agents** such as ethambutol, rifampicin, pyrazinamide and isoniazid for a prolonged period (6–9 months) remains the mainstay of treatment. TB is usually treated for an extensive time period, as the organism grows slowly and there is a possibility of it becoming dormant. By using two or more antibiotics, the chance of developing resistance during this extended time is minimized.

Viva questions

1 Classify bacteria and give some examples of Gram-positive bacteria.

2 How do penicillins act? What are the different classes of penicillins? How do the classes differ?

3 How do bacteria develop resistance?

4 Describe the pathogenesis of septic arthritis.

5 What is MRSA, and how is it acquired?

FURTHER READING

De Boeck, H. Osteomyelitis and septic arthritis in children. *Acta Orthop Belg* 2005;**71**:505–15.

Lazzarini, L, Mader, JT, Calhoun, JH. Osteomyelitis in long bones *J Bone Joint Surg Am* 2004;**86**:2305–18.

Mader, JT, Wang, J, Calhoun, JH. Antibiotic therapy for musculoskeletal infections. *J Bone Joint Surg Am* 2001;**83**:1878–90.

Tuli, SM. General principles of osteoarticular tuberculosis. *Clin Orthop Relat Res* 2002;**398**:11–19.

Wong, KC, Leung, KS. Transmission and prevention of occupational infections in orthopaedic surgeons. *J Bone Joint Surg Am* 2004;**86**:1065–76.

6

Imaging techniques

MANOJ RAMACHANDRAN, NAVIN RAMACHANDRAN AND ASIF SAIFUDDIN

INTRODUCTION

Following the discovery of X-rays in 1895 by Wilhelm Konrad Röentgen, the initial application of radiography lay in the demonstration of fractures and radio-opaque foreign bodies. Subsequently, the specialties of orthopaedics and radiology have emerged and developed in parallel. A broad understanding of the techniques employed in radiology as applied to orthopaedics is required for the practising orthopaedic surgeon.

PLAIN RADIOGRAPHY

WHAT IS IT?

X-rays are a form of **high-energy radiation** belonging to the electromagnetic spectrum (Figure 6.1). They pass through the body, undergoing **differential absorption** by tissues.

In radiography, X-rays subsequently fall on to **fluorescent film–screen combinations** resulting in the formation of black silver crystals, a process known as film blackening. These film–screen combinations can be processed to give a radiographic image.

Tissues containing elements with a high atomic number, e.g. calcium in bone, absorb a high proportion of X-rays (**high beam attenuation**), resulting in less crystal formation on the film and, therefore, a white **radiodense** appearance. Tissues where little absorption of X-rays occurs, e.g. fat and air (**low beam attenuation**), give a black **radiolucent** appearance, as more crystals are formed on the film. Soft tissues, such as muscle, with **intermediate beam attenuation**, appear grey.

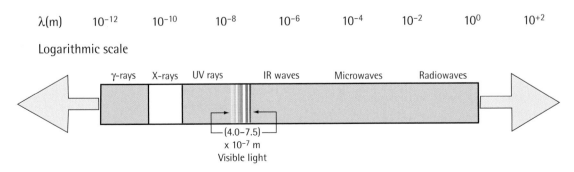

Figure 6.1 *Electromagnetic spectrum. IR, infrared; UV, ultraviolet.*

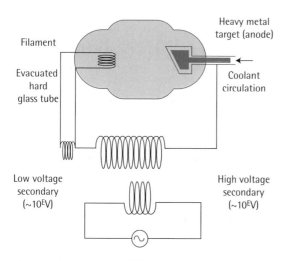

Figure 6.2 Production of X-rays.

HOW DOES IT WORK?

X-ray generation is achieved by **heating** a **fine filament** (the negative cathode, usually made of tungsten) to incandescence in a vacuum at a temperature of around 2200°C. This results in the emission of electrons, a process known as **thermionic emission** (Figure 6.2).

These free negatively charged electrons leave the surface of their atoms and are drawn towards the positive anode, a smooth metal fragment usually made of tungsten. The electrons hit the anode at about half the speed of light on an area known as the **focal spot**. Here, the free electrons may interact with any of the following:

- **Outer electrons of the target nucleus**, generating heat, which can lead to tube overheating. In order to reduce the generation of excess heat, the rotating anode disc was developed.
- **Inner electrons**, knocking them out of their orbit, with subsequent X-ray production.
- **Nucleus**, causing the free electron to slow down and change direction, resulting in the emission of X-rays from **braking radiation** (*bremsstrahlung*). This constitutes 80 per cent of the X-rays generated in the X-ray tube.

The quantity of X-rays produced is proportional to the number of electrons flowing from the cathode to the anode (measured in

milliamperes, mA). The quality, or penetrating property, of the X-ray beam is dependent on the energy of the electrons striking the target (which is determined by the kilovoltage, kV); the higher the kilovoltage, the more penetrating the X-ray photon.

As X-rays pass through matter, they can be **transmitted**, **absorbed** or **scattered**, resulting in attenuation. After passing through the patient, they fall on to an X-ray cassette, composed of the following:

- Carbon fibre or aluminium **front**, which acts as a filter to minimize beam attenuation, remove low-energy X-rays that are not diagnostically useful, and reduce the patient exposure required.
- Lead sheet **back** to decrease the backscatter of radiation.
- **Film**, consisting of a polyester base coated with fine photographic emulsion (silver iodobromide) sensitive to X-rays.
- Two **intensifying screens** on each side of the film – a polyester base coated with a dense layer of phosphor crystals (e.g. rare earths such as lanthanum or gadolinium) that absorbs X-rays and converts them into visible light, which in turn exposes the film.

Processing of the X-ray cassette involves **development** by alkaline immersion, **fixation** by acid immersion, **washing** and **drying**.

WHAT IS IT USED FOR?

Plain radiographs are often the **first-line investigation** in the assessment of musculoskeletal disorders. They also have wide applications in both elective and trauma surgery.

WHAT ARE ITS ADVANTAGES?

- Good for **assessing bone** due to its high calcium content and intrinsic X-ray contrast.
- **Cheap** and **easily obtained** in a clinical setting.

WHAT ARE ITS DISADVANTAGES?

- **Not sensitive to subtle bony destruction** or abnormalities.

- **Difficult to interpret in areas of complex anatomy** or where overlying structures obscure bone.
- **Form of ionizing radiation** and so appropriate precautions to reduce the overall dose must be taken, e.g.
  - request X-rays only when there is a clinical indication;
  - maximize the distance between the patient and the X-ray source;
  - use fast films and minimize exposure time (the latter also reduces blurring from patient movement);
  - use gonadal shields on patients where appropriate, and lead aprons, lead gloves and thyroid shields for staff in a theatre setting;
  - all staff should be trained in radiation protection, and staff exposure to radiation should be monitored.

ADDITIONAL TECHNIQUES AND ADVANCES

Digital imaging

- There is greater flexibility for image enhancement, storage, manipulation and retrieval, e.g. picture archiving and communication systems (PACS).
- As a phosphor-based storage plate is used, which is more sensitive than the rare earths used in film–screens, the overall radiation dose to the patient is reduced.
- Digital images do not have the high spatial resolution of radiographic film–screen combinations, although the quality is rising.
- Costs were once high but are now falling as the use of digital imaging becomes more widespread.

Fluoroscopy

- Imaging can be performed in real time, allowing dynamic assessment, e.g. arthrography, myelography.
- Digital subtraction techniques can be used to increase the contrast of the area of interest.

Conventional tomography (body–section radiography)

- This has now been replaced by computed tomography (CT).
- Brings bony structures of interest into focus by moving the X-ray tube as the exposure takes place, thus blurring adjacent structures and focusing in on area of interest.
- Radiation dose is even higher than that of a CT scan.

ULTRASOUND

WHAT IS IT?

Ultrasound uses high-frequency (3–50 MHz) sound waves generated by a transducer. These waves are reflected and refracted at tissue interfaces. Reflected waves return to the transducer, where they are converted into electrical signals in order to produce images.

HOW DOES IT WORK?

The ultrasound waves are produced by a transducer made of piezoelectric crystal. Piezoelectric crystals change shape when a voltage is applied across them and generate a voltage when their shape is altered.

A **DC voltage** is applied to the crystal and then reversed (or an AC current is used), leading to **expansion** and **contraction** of the surfaces and producing a **compression wave**, the sound wave. When coupled to the skin using lubricating gel, sound waves are **transmitted into the body** and **reflected back**. When the waves arrive back at the transducer, they distort the shape of the piezoelectric crystal, generating a voltage. The more sound waves that are reflected, the greater the voltage produced and the brighter the reflecting structure appears on the image (i.e. more reflective structures look brighter). The depth to echo-producing structures can be calculated by timing the period elapsed from sound-wave emission to detection. This depth information is combined with the reflectivity data to produce the final image.

The higher the frequency of the wave, the higher the spatial resolution; the attenuation within tissue is also higher, thus limiting visualization to superficial structures. **Doppler** can be used in addition to qualitatively and quantitatively observe **vascularity** and **blood flow**.

WHAT IS IT USED FOR?

- **Assessing tendons** (which normally have an echogenic fibrillar structure in the longitudinal plane and are ovoid in cross-section), both statically and dynamically, e.g. the rotator cuff and tendons around the foot and ankle.
- **Assessing masses** to see whether they are cystic or solid. Cystic masses are compressible and have a **hypoechoic** appearance (as they are weakly reflective), with associated posterior acoustic enhancement. Solid masses, which are strongly reflective (**hyperechoic**), may produce acoustic shadowing, i.e. reducing the intensity of echoes from regions behind them.
- **Confirming joint effusions**, especially in deep joints such as the hip and shoulder, with the advantage that **guided aspiration** and **therapeutic injections** can be performed.
- **Screening** and **evaluation** of developmental dysplasia of the hip.

WHAT ARE ITS ADVANTAGES?

- **No ionizing radiation** is involved, and so ultrasound is highly acceptable to patients.
- Ultrasound machines are **small, inexpensive** and **portable**.

- **Dynamic scanning** of active and passive movements can be performed.
- **No side effects** are known at the intensities used in clinical practice.
- Ultrasound is **pain-free** and **non-invasive**.

WHAT ARE ITS DISADVANTAGES?

- Ultrasound is highly **operator-dependent**, both for acquisition and interpretation, and has a long learning curve.
- The field of **view is often limited**.
- It may be **difficult to characterize** the imaged tissue.
- Ultrasound **cannot penetrate cortical bone**.

WHAT DO THOSE ADDITIONAL LETTERS STAND FOR?

A-mode scanning is **amplitude** mode, B-mode is **brightness** mode and M-mode is **time–motion** mode. B-mode is used most commonly in clinical practice, producing the two-dimensional images that orthopaedic surgeons are most familiar with. A-mode produces one-dimensional images and is used in ophthalmology to assess the structures of the eye. M-mode is often used to assess cardiac valve motion.

COMPUTED TOMOGRAPHY

WHAT IS IT?

CT employs a finely collimated **fan-shaped X-ray beam**, where the X-ray tube rotates around

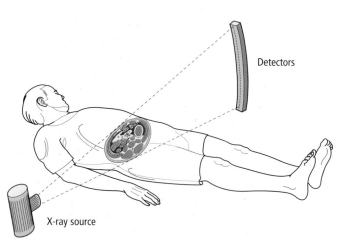

Figure 6.3 *Basis of computed tomography (CT) image production.*

Detectors

X-ray source

the patient and sensitive detectors record the attenuated X-rays that pass through the body (Figure 6.3). Sir Godfrey Hounsfield introduced CT scanning into clinical practice in 1973.

HOW DOES IT WORK?

The CT scanner is comprised of the following parts:

- scanning gantry (housing the X-ray generator and curvilinear detector, opposite each another);
- patient couch;
- computer processor;
- display system.

Each rotation of the gantry produces an axial slice through the patient. Early scanners had to pause after each rotation to move down the body, but modern machines can rotate helically to allow continuous acquisition of data.

Tissues that attenuate the X-ray beam to a higher degree, such as bone, appear denser on a CT image than tissues such as muscle. CT clearly differentiates air, fat, fluid, soft tissue and bone. Each tissue is assigned an **attenuation coefficient** (measured in Hounsfield units, HU)

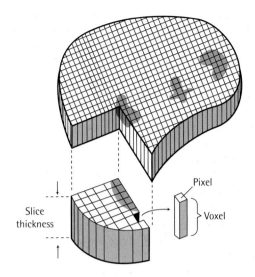

Figure 6.4 *Slice thickness in computed tomography (CT) scanning.*

relative to the value of water (zero HU) (Table 6.1).

Each image is made of a number of **pixels**. However, one should bear in mind that each pixel does not represent only a two-dimensional area: it also represents a volume, the depth of which is determined by a user-definable slice thickness. Thus, if an image has 256×256 pixels, it will have 256×256 **voxels** (Figure 6.4).

The HU of a pixel corresponds to the attenuation coefficient of the tissue that occupies that position in the axial slice through the body. Tissues with high atomic numbers and high X-ray attenuation values, such as bone, appear white; areas of low attenuation, such as air and fat, appear dark. There is a much wider range of attenuation coefficients than the shades of grey that the eye can differentiate between, and so the CT image has to be **manipulated** by **changing window levels** and **window widths** to allow the whole range of CT attenuations to be displayed. For example, different window settings are required to assess the soft tissues and bony structures fully. The majority of currently available CT packages allow multiplanar (MPR) and three-dimensional reconstruction, which can be of great value in musculoskeletal CT. Iodine-based contrast media can be administered intravenously,

Table 6.1 Attenuation coefficients of tissue in computed tomography (CT) scanning

Tissue	CT number (HU)
Bone	1000
Liver	40–60
Brain, white matter	46
Brain, grey matter	43
Blood	40
Muscle	10–40
Kidney	30
Cerebrospinal fluid	15
Water	0
Fat	–50 to –100
Air	–1000

intrathecally (CT myelography), intra-articularly (CT arthrography) and intradiscally (CT discography) in order to improve visualization of soft-tissue components and provide further information.

WHAT IS IT USED FOR?

- **Assessment of fractures**, particularly complex patterns and at sites not easily accessible to X-rays and that are enhanced by the use of three-dimensional reconstruction, e.g. pelvic fractures, tibial plateau fractures, tibial plafond fractures, calcaneal fractures, complex shoulder fractures, vertebral fractures, complex distal radius fractures.
- With **contrast media** to assess **joints** and other **fluid-filled structures**, e.g. CT arthrography, myelography, discography.
- **Bone densitometry** can be performed using quantitative CT.

WHAT ARE ITS ADVANTAGES?

- **Three-dimensional imaging** and **cross-sectional anatomical data** superior to two-dimensional plain radiography.
- **Better than X-rays** for soft-tissue imaging, but not as good as magnetic resonance imaging (MRI).
- **Quantitative data on composition**, e.g. used for bone densitometry.
- Good for **assessing cortical bone**.
- Can be used to **guide interventional procedures**, e.g. biopsy, vertebroplasty.

WHAT ARE ITS DISADVANTAGES?

- Significant dose of **ionizing radiation**.
- **Inferior soft-tissue contrast** resolution to MRI.
- Can be **claustrophobic** for the patient, but this is much rarer than with MRI.

ADDITIONAL TECHNIQUES AND ADVANCES

- **Spiral** (or **helical**) CT allows rapid multi-slicing as the gantry rotates continuously.
- **Multidetector** CT consists of multiple rows of detectors on the opposite side of the X-ray source, such that one rotation allows multiple slices though the body to be imaged at once. Such scanners are now in standard use in radiology.
- Positron-emission tomography (**PET**) CT is a growing field that allows the combination of PET and CT scanning.

MAGNETIC RESONANCE IMAGING

WHAT IS IT?

MRI involves the application of strong **magnetic fields** and **excitation radiofrequency pulses** to the patient, resulting in the emission of radiofrequency signals by the tissues of interest, which are used to build up an image.

HOW DOES IT WORK?

Most MRI sequences are tuned to **detect hydrogen nuclei** (protons) in water. Images therefore reflect the relative concentration of protons in tissues, by measuring the strength of signals from individual voxels in a slice of the patient and reflecting it on a greyscale in the corresponding pixels on the screen. That is, the greater the returned signal from a voxel, the brighter the pixel.

In nature, each proton spins like a top around an axis (known as **nuclear spin**). In the absence of a magnetic field, these axes are **randomly oriented** and produce no net magnetic effect. When a **strong static magnetic field** is applied to the protons in the magnetic resonance (MR) scanner, their axes of rotation **align with the long axis of the magnet** (with a slight excess oriented parallel to the field), resulting in a net magnetic field. Protons also wobble around their long axis with a fixed frequency (known as **precession**) (Figure 6.5).

The scanning process begins with the activation of the **strong magnet**. The protons align with the longitudinal axis of the scanner. Next, a **radiofrequency pulse** is applied for a few milliseconds. This causes the protons to realign at an angle to the longitudinal axis of the scanner, and also causes the precessions of each proton to be pulled into step (or **phase**)

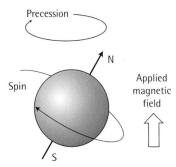

Figure 6.5 *Nuclear spin and precession.*

with each other. The protons act like rotating magnets in a dynamo, inducing currents in the receiving coils of the scanner. The changes in these currents (or signals) are used to characterize the tissue.

When the pulse stops:

- The protons realign with the long axis and the longitudinal magnetization vector increases to its maximum. **T1** is defined as the **time** taken for the **longitudinal magnetization vector** (and corresponding MR signal) to **recover to 63 per cent** of its maximal value.
- The precessions fall out of step with each other (**dephasing**), causing the transverse magnetization vector to decrease from its maximum. **T2** is defined as the **time** taken for the transverse magnetization vector (and corresponding MR signal) to **fall to 37 per cent** of its maximal value.

T1 and T2 values vary for different tissues and therefore are used for forming the image.

The timing of the excitation pulse and the collection of the signal enable different sequence weighting. In simple terms, in **T1-weighted images**, fat, e.g. bone marrow, has a bright signal; on **T2-weighted images**, fluid has a bright signal. Tissues with little fat or water, e.g. cortical bone, ligaments and tendons, are dark on both T1- and T2-weighted images (Table 6.2). Put even more simply, **T1** is good for **anatomy** as it is weighted towards fat, while **T2** is good for **pathology** as it is weighted towards water.

WHAT IS IT USED FOR?

MRI is used increasingly in orthopaedics for a wide variety of indications, including:

- osteonecrosis;
- infection;
- trauma, such as occult fractures (e.g. femoral neck) and soft-tissue injuries (e.g. ligamentous knee injuries);
- tumours, e.g. local staging of primary bone and soft-tissue tumours;
- regional disease, e.g. intervertebral disc disease, rotator cuff pathology.

WHAT ARE ITS ADVANTAGES?

- Ability to image in **any** anatomical plane (**multiplanar imaging**).
- **High-contrast resolution**, therefore good for soft-tissue and bone-marrow imaging.
- **No ionizing radiation**.
- Non-invasive **imaging of blood vessels** without use of contrast media.

Table 6.2 Signal intensities of musculoskeletal tissues

Tissue	Signal on T1-weighted image	Signal on T2-weighted image
Fluid	Low	High
Fat	High	High
Muscle	Intermediate	Intermediate
Cartilage	Intermediate	High
Cortical bone	Low	Low

Note that TR is the time to repetition of a pulse. In general, TR for T1 is <750–1000 and for T2 is about 4000.

WHAT ARE ITS DISADVANTAGES?

The use of MRI is limited by its contraindications. **Absolute contraindications** include the presence of implanted pacemakers and defibrillators, cerebral aneurysm clips, vascular clips (less than 2 weeks old), metal in the orbit of the eye, internal hearing aids and dorsal column stimulators. **Relative contraindications** include the first and second trimesters of pregnancy, claustrophobia, obesity (although open MRI scanners can be used instead), penile prostheses, and children who may not be able to keep still within the scanner.

MRI also has the following disadvantages:

- Not as good as CT for imaging bone.
- **High cost** of equipment.
- **Image artefact problems** from motion and ferromagnetic objects.
- **Claustrophobic** for about 10 per cent of patients.

ADDITIONAL TECHNIQUES AND ADVANCES

- **Paramagnetic agents:** intravenous contrast media containing chelated gadolinium cause an **increased signal on T1-weighted images** due to a paramagnetic effect, thus increasing contrast between areas of high uptake and the surrounding tissues. Gadolinium is a rare earth metal with seven unpaired electrons and therefore has a high net magnetic moment, which affects large numbers of adjacent hydrogen nuclei.
- **Sequences:** detailed knowledge of specific MR sequences is beyond the level expected of the practising orthopaedic surgeon. The following is a brief guide to spotting the common sequences:
  - **Spin echo (SE):** a commonly used pulse sequence for obtaining T1 and T2 images. In T1SE, look for short time to repetition (TR), short time to echo (TE; <10–25 ms), and high signal from fat and low signal from fluid. In T2SE, look for high TR, high TE (about 100 ms) and high signal from fluid. Turbo spin echo

(TSE) and fast spin echo (FSE) are faster than standard spin echo but cannot differentiate between water and fat (use STIR (see below) instead).
  - **Short tau inversion recovery (STIR): inversion recovery pulse sequence with specific timing to suppress the signal from fat.** Look for TI (time of inversion), low signal from bone marrow, and high signal from fluid (e.g. oedema).
  - **Gradient echo (GRE):** a type of pulse sequence with faster T1- and T2-type images. Useful for fibrocartilaginous structures, e.g. triangular fibrocartilaginous complex, menisci.
  - **Proton density (PD):** part of the standard T2SE, but with high TR and short TE. Useful for structures with intermediate signal (e.g. menisci). Gives excellent anatomical detail.
- **Intra-articular contrast media:** MR arthrography is an excellent means of diagnosing articular pathology, such as rotator cuff tears.

RADIONUCLIDE BONE SCANNING

WHAT IS IT?

X-rays generated in X-ray tubes (used in plain radiography, fluoroscopy and CT scanning) are properly called X-rays, while those emitted from radioactive isotopes (radionuclides) are called gamma (γ) rays. Bone scanning involves the **intravenous** injection of **technetium-99m** (^{99m}Tc) phosphonates, which localize at sites of osteoblastic activity.

HOW DOES IT WORK?

Radionuclides are **unstable nuclei** with neutron excess or deficit. The nuclei disintegrate to form other atoms, with the release of alpha, beta or gamma radiation. The Systéme International (SI) unit for radioactivity is the becquerel (Bq), which equals one disintegration per second.

Technetium-99m is a radionuclide with a short half-life (6 h) and is a pure gamma emitter. It is formed from the disintegration of its parent nuclide molybdenum-99 (^{99}Mo). ^{99m}Tc is coupled with phosphate compounds, such as methylene diphosphonate (^{99m}Tc-MDP), and administered intravenously for bone scanning, where it is chemi-absorbed on to hydroxyapatite crystals in bone. Its uptake is a reflection of osteoblastic activity, but vascularity is also important. The phosphorus component interacts with endogenous calcium to produce insoluble technetium calcium phosphate complexes.

Within 24 hours, around 70 per cent of the administered dose (500–600 MBq) is excreted through the kidneys; hence, bladder exposure to radiation must be minimized by patient hydration and frequent micturition.

Photoemission from localized sites (spot images) or the whole skeleton (whole-body images) can be recorded using a **scintillation gamma camera**, which contains crystals of sodium iodide that absorb ^{99m}Tc gamma rays.

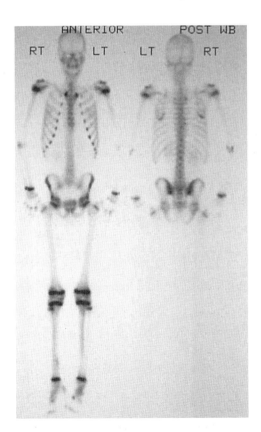

Figure 6.6 *Normal bone scan.*

The signal is **enhanced by photomultiplier tubes** and processed by a computer to produce an image that represents a map of blood flow and osteoblastic activity.

In a **triple-phase bone scan**, the three phases are:

1 **Flow or dynamic images:** images taken immediately (1–2 min), showing arterial flow and hyperperfusion.
2 **Blood pool or equilibrium images:** images taken at 3–5 minutes, showing extracellular fluid volume and thus the extent of bone and soft-tissue hyperaemia.
3 **Static or delayed images:** taken after approximately 4 hours when soft-tissue activity has cleared, highlighting skeletal activity. Separate anterior and posterior scans are obtained.

Normal activity on bone scans is symmetrical, with increased activity seen within the bladder, the kidneys, the ends of the long bones in adults, the sacroiliac joints, the tips of the scapulae, the nasal cavity and the epiphyseal growth areas in children (Figure 6.6).

WHAT IS IT USED FOR?

Radionuclide bone scanning has several indications, including the following:

- Assessment of **occult bone pain**.
- Assessment of **metastatic disease**.
- **Infection:** flow and blood-pool phases are hot in cellulitis; all three phases are hot in osteomyelitis.
- **Trauma:** occult, stress fractures.
- **Tumour,** e.g. osteoid osteoma, osteoblastoma, especially spinal.
- **Arthritis:** activity and extent.
- **Postoperative:** pseudarthrosis, painful prosthesis (bone scan tends to become normal after 1 year in the latter).
- Assessment of **Paget's disease**.

WHAT ARE ITS ADVANTAGES?

- Very **sensitive to increases** in bone turnover.
- Good **general survey** for skeletal pathology.

- Helps to initially **localize bone lesions**, after which further imaging can be performed targeted to the specific anatomical site.

WHAT ARE ITS DISADVANTAGES?

- **Poor spatial resolution**.
- **Non-specific appearance** for elucidating causes of increased activity.
- May be **false negative in myeloma** and **lytic metastases**, due to either decreased blood flow or lack of osteoblastic response.
- Relatively **high radiation dose**, particularly to bone marrow and in children.

ADDITIONAL TECHNIQUES AND ADVANCES

- **Gallium-67** binds to plasma proteins and can be used to **localize areas of inflammation**, e.g. abscesses and neoplasia. It is frequently used in combination with a technetium bone scan (double-tracer technique) and is less dependent on vascular flow than a technetium scan.
- **Indium-111** labels white blood cells and platelets and can be used to **localize areas of infection and inflammation** (but not neoplasia), e.g. abscesses and thromboses.
- **Single photon emission computed tomography** (SPECT) applies tomographic technology to radionuclide scanning, enabling a cross-sectional image to be obtained, which enhances the conspicuity of lesions and helps in their localization. The gamma camera head rotates 360 degrees around the body obtaining multiple planar images, which are then reconstructed in sagittal, coronal and axial planes.

BONE DENSITOMETRY

WHAT IS IT?

Dual-energy X-ray absorptiometry (DEXA) scanning is used to **assess bone mineral density** (BMD) in the central skeleton (femur and lumbar spine). It uses **X-rays of two different energies**, which are absorbed in different proportions by bone and soft tissue.

HOW DOES IT WORK?

The patient lies on the scanning table for 2 minutes, having undressed to light clothing and removed any metal piercings (naval piercings may cover the fourth lumbar vertebra). It is best to scan the femur on the anteroposterior (AP) projection and the lumbar spine on the lateral projection. Note that as the lower ribs cover L2 and the iliac crests cover L4 on the lateral, L3 may often be the only vertebra that can be scanned.

For AP films, the spine is scanned with the patient flat on the back and the knee flexed over a block at right-angles in order to flatten the lumbar lordosis. The femur is scanned with the patient flat on the back with toes together and a heel separation of around 23 cm.

WHAT IS IT USED FOR?

DEXA scanning is used for the following:

- **Assessing bone density in primary and secondary osteoporosis**, both for diagnosis and for monitoring treatment. Also allows assessment of fracture risk.
- **Evaluating the effect of preventive interventions** on other metabolic diseases (e.g. primary hyperparathyroidism) and age-related bone loss.
- **Measuring periprosthetic bone loss**. The literature supports the use of this modality for evaluation of the magnitude and rate of changes in bone mineral content after total hip arthroplasty, particularly in patients with cementless prostheses.

HOW ARE THE RESULTS INTERPRETED?

Values for bone density (g/cm^2) from DEXA are converted into values related to either the peak BMD or the age-matched BMD of the average female or male. When **matched for sex and race** and compared with peak bone mass of young normal adults, this is known as the **T score**:

$$= \frac{\text{(patient's BMD)} - \text{(population peak BMD)}}{\text{standard deviation (SD) of population peak BMD}}$$

When matched for sex, race and age, this is known as the **Z score**:

$$= \frac{\text{(patient's BMD)} - \text{(population age-related BMD)}}{\text{SD of population age-related BMD}}$$

Osteoporosis is diagnosed if the **T score is over −2.5** according to the World Health Organization (WHO) criteria (Kanis *et al.*, 1994). Note that normal is a T score less than −1, osteopenia is a T score greater than −1 but less than −2.5, and severe osteoporosis is a T score less than −2.5 and the presence of one or more fragility fractures.

The **Z score** is used to compare the patient's BMD with the mean value for individuals of the same age. A **low Z score indicates an aetiology other than age-related bone loss**.

WHAT ARE ITS ADVANTAGES?

- Allows **assessment of fracture risk** in osteoporosis and subsequent need for treatment.
- New software allows use of the technique at the forearm and calcaneum and for periprosthetic applications.

WHAT ARE ITS DISADVANTAGES?

- **Does not distinguish between cortical and cancellous** bone density. Fat content is also a confounding factor due to its low density/attenuation coefficient.
- In the spine:
  - In the AP projection, the measured BMD is **falsely increased by intervertebral osteoarthritis**; therefore, lateral scanning is preferred.
  - **False high-density values** may be seen with **fractured vertebrae and calcification**.
  - **False low-density values** may be seen after **posterior element surgical resection**.
- In the femur, the measurement most often used is the total upper femur, which includes the femoral neck, trochanteric region and intertrochanteric region, and is therefore not area-specific.

ADDITIONAL TECHNIQUES AND ADVANCES

Alternative techniques include the following:

Radiogrammetry

This measures predefined bone dimensions (cortex versus total bone width) at **peripheral** tubular bones, e.g. metacarpals. Its clinical value in the axial skeleton is limited. The measurements are crude and do not assess density.

Radiographic absorptiometry

This measures density on a digital radiograph of the hand (**peripheral**) in comparison with an aluminium reference wedge, with the results given in aluminium equivalent values. No distinction is made between cortical and cancellous bone compartments.

Single X-ray absorptiometry

Single X-ray absorptiometry (SXA) is similar to DEXA but uses only a single-energy X-ray. Measured at the radius or calcaneum. No distinction is made between cortical and cancellous bone compartments. SXA is less accurate than DEXA and is now obsolete.

Quantitative computed tomography

Single-energy quantitative computed tomography (QCT) measures an averaged axial ellipse of three to four vertebral bodies (**central**) against a reference standard of different concentrations of hydroxyapatite in plastic, placed under the lumbar spine and scanned simultaneously. Hounsfield units are then converted to bone equivalent values (g/cm^3 of hydroxyapatite). This provides a **true density estimate**, but it may be falsely low as it also measures intravertebral fat (as does DEXA). Dual-energy QCT may also be used, but the radiation dose employed is high. QCT is an expensive technique.

Quantitative ultrasound scanning

Non-invasive **peripheral** measurement (calcaneus, tibia, patella, phalanges) of ultrasound transmission velocities and broadband (multifrequency) ultrasound attenuation. There is no radiation exposure and therefore this technique is increasing in popularity in Europe and Japan.

Quantitative magnetic resonance imaging

This is currently used for research and has major cost and availability implications. High-resolution MRI can be used to assess the density, geometry and architecture of the trabecular network, i.e. distinguishes cortical and cancellous bone.

Viva questions

1 What is an X-ray?

2 What is ultrasound used for in orthopaedics?

3 How does a CT/MRI scanner work?

4 How are bone scan images acquired?

5 How is bone density measured in orthopaedics?

FURTHER READING

Kanis, JA, Melton, LJ, 3rd, Christiansen, C, Johnston, CC, Khaltaev, N. The diagnosis of osteoporosis. *J Bone Miner Res* 1994;**9**:1137–41.
Hain, SF, O'Doherty, MJ, Smith, MA. Functional imaging and the orthopaedic surgeon. *J Bone Joint Surg Br* 2002;**84**:315–21.
Johnson, TR, Steinbach, LS (eds). *Essentials of Musculoskeletal Imaging*. Rosemont, IL: American Academy of Orthopaedic Surgeons, 2003.
Potter, HG, Schweitzer, ME, Altchek, DW. Advanced imaging in orthopaedics: current pitfalls and new applications. *Instr Course Lect* 1997;**46**:521–9.
Watt, I. Magnetic resonance imaging in orthopaedics. *J Bone Joint Surg Br* 1991;**73**:539–50.

7

Orthopaedic oncology

NIMALAN MARUTHAINAR AND STEPHEN CANNON

INTRODUCTION

A **tumour** (neoplasm) is a mass of tissue formed as a result of abnormal, excessive and inappropriate proliferation of cells, the growth of which continues indefinitely regardless of the mechanisms that control normal cellular proliferation.

Tumours may be divided into **benign** and **malignant** lesions. Benign tumours remain as localized single masses. They may cause symptoms by their bulk, or pressure, effect upon adjoining structures. Malignant tumours invade the surrounding tissues and may spread to distant sites via the vascular or lymphatic systems. The distant deposits of malignant tumours are termed **metastases**.

Tumours may present to the orthopaedic surgeon in bone or soft tissue. These neoplasms may be benign or malignant. The lesion may be a primary or a secondary (metastatic) deposit of a malignant tumour.

Primary tumours of bone are relatively uncommon. An estimated 360 new cases were seen in the UK in 2003, and only 8000 new cases were reported to the American Cancer Society in 1995. Timely diagnosis of these neoplasms must depend on the treating physician or surgeon maintaining a high index of suspicion.

DIAGNOSIS

A critical aspect in the management of a tumour in bone and soft tissue is the recognition of its presence by the treating doctor. Once picked up, there is considerable available guidance on appropriate assessment and further management, including possible referral to specialist treatment centres.

The presenting symptoms of **persistent pain**, particularly at night, or **swelling** should lead to a comprehensive clinical assessment and appropriate investigations to exclude neoplasia. The attribution of pain symptoms in children to 'growing pains' is a common pitfall, leading to missed or late diagnoses. Similarly, patients may present with periarticular bone tumours having undergone knee arthroscopy without preoperative X-rays.

A **history of trauma** is often present in patients with bone and soft-tissue tumours. The trauma is likely to be the event that draws the patient's attention to the lesion rather than the precipitant of the lesion. Persisting pain or swelling after trauma should also raise a suspicion of possible neoplasia. Patients may present with **pathological fracture**. Appropriate management of these fractures is often different to that of their traumatic counterparts. On occasion, other symptoms at presentation include **paraesthesia** or **numbness** from neural compression or lesions arising within nerves.

In establishing the likely diagnosis, the patient's age may provide some indication. Lesions of bone in the first three decades are most often primary or haemopoietic in origin. In older patients, metastases are more likely. **Differential diagnosis** at all ages includes **infection**.

A complete history must be taken, establishing the duration of symptoms and any associated weight loss or lethargy. History of **pre-existing malignancy** is crucial, as is a history of **previous radiotherapy treatment**. A history of **smoking** may also point to a possible primary cause. With a few exceptions (e.g. neurofibromatosis, Li–Fraumeni syndrome), family history does not appear to be a significant factor in bone and soft-tissue tumours.

Tumours that most commonly give rise to metastases in bone are carcinomas of the breast, prostate, lung, kidney and thyroid and melanomas. These metastatic lesions are often destructive (osteolytic) in nature, with the exception of prostatic metastases, which are commonly sclerotic. Other tumours, e.g. colorectal carcinoma, may also give rise to metastases in bone, and it has been suggested that improved survivorship through chemotherapy may yield an increase in the incidence of bone metastases.

INVESTIGATIONS

The assessment of a case of suspected neoplasia may include the following:

- **Full blood count** and **inflammatory marker assays**.
- **Serum electrophoresis** in older patients to investigate possible myeloproliferative disorder and, if appropriate, urine analysis for Bence Jones proteins.
- **Urea and electrolytes** and **liver function assays** may establish baseline renal and liver function before potent cytotoxic therapy. In addition, alkaline phosphatase may provide an indication of prognosis in osteosarcoma.

- Prostate specific antigen (**PSA**) assay (and acid phosphatase).
- **Plain radiographs** are invaluable in the diagnosis (see below for interpretation).
- Magnetic resonance imaging (**MRI**) of the lesion, whether bone or soft tissue, further characterizes the pathology and stages the lesion locally, demonstrating the extent of oedematous reaction and presence of skip lesions.
- Computed tomography (**CT**) of the lesion may be of value in tumours of bone. Additionally, CT of the chest is regularly employed in the distant staging of malignant lesions.
- **Tissue biopsy** and **histological analysis** is a critical part of diagnosis. If performed inappropriately, may considerably compromise outcome.
- **Bone scintigraphy** is essential in the assessment of the rest of the skeleton. Approximately 20 per cent of cases of Ewing's sarcoma present with bone metastases. Multifocal osteosarcoma is rare but usually fatal. Scintigraphy is especially useful in the investigation of possible osteoid osteoma.

RADIOGRAPHS

Where a lesion arises in bone, its location may indicate the likely diagnosis. The position within the bone may be considered in relation to the epiphysis, metaphysis and diaphysis and also to the medullary cavity and cortex (Figure 7.1).

Concepts employed in the study of the radiographs are those of the **effect** of the **lesion on the bone** and the effect of the **bone on the lesion**.

Lesions may precipitate a variable reaction of the adjoining bone. Slow-growing lesions tend to allow bone reaction at the margin, leading to a well-demarcated appearance with a **narrow zone of transition** (Figure 7.2). Rapidly enlarging aggressive lesions allow little bone-forming response to develop. These lesions yield a poorly demarcated, **permeative** appearance with a **wide zone of transition** (Figure 7.3).

Rapidly growing subperiosteal lesions, such as some osteosarcomas, may elevate the

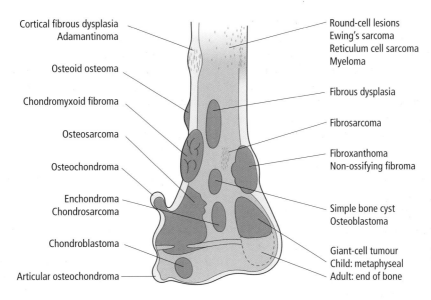

Cortical fibrous dysplasia
Adamantinoma

Osteoid osteoma

Chondromyxoid fibroma

Osteosarcoma

Osteochondroma

Enchondroma
Chondrosarcoma

Chondroblastoma

Articular osteochondroma

Round-cell lesions
Ewing's sarcoma
Reticulum cell sarcoma
Myeloma

Fibrous dysplasia

Fibrosarcoma

Fibroxanthoma
Non-ossifying fibroma

Simple bone cyst
Osteoblastoma

Giant-cell tumour
Child: metaphyseal
Adult: end of bone

Figure 7.1 *Common anatomical location of bone tumours.*

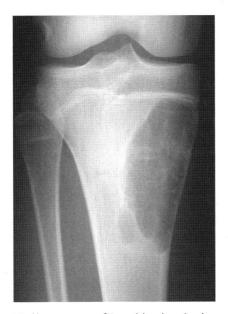

Figure 7.2 *Narrow zone of transition in a benign tumour (non-ossifying fibroma).*

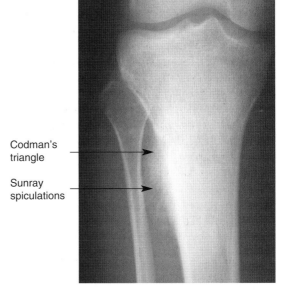

Codman's triangle

Sunray spiculations

Figure 7.3 *Wide zone of transition in osteosarcoma, with Codman's triangle and sunray speculation.*

periosteum so quickly that bone deposition is allowed only at the margin with normal bone, creating the **Codman's triangle** appearance (Figure 7.3). Some attempt at bone formation by the periosteum overlying the lesion may result in streaks of calcification, termed **sunray spiculation** (Figure 7.3).

Relatively slow-growing lesions within bone may result in bony expansion. More aggressive lesions from within the medulla may result in cortical resorption (**endosteal scalloping**).

Characteristic radiographic features of some tumours are given in the tumour descriptions below. Note that for a lesion to become apparent as lytic on plain radiographs, there must be loss of at least 50 per cent of the bone mass in comparison with the surrounding bone.

BIOPSY

Tissue may be obtained for histological analysis by **excisional**, **incisional** or **percutaneous** biopsy techniques. The potential complications of incomplete attempted excisional biopsy have led to this technique being reserved for lesions where there is a very low probability of malignancy.

Percutaneous sampling may be by **core-needle biopsy** or **fine-needle aspiration cytology**. Instruments such as Jamshedi or Trucut needles may be used to obtain core specimens. Tumours may have a necrotic core with viable tissue of histological use confined to the periphery. It is therefore vital that tissue from the appropriate zone of the lesion is obtained. Later excision of any tumorous lesion will need to include the biopsy tract. The potential for seeding of tumour tissue into joint cavities during biopsy needs to be recognized.

The selection of biopsy path and positioning of the biopsy needle within a lesion is a process best undertaken following consultation with the surgeon likely to undertake any later definitive resection and with specialist pathologists.

The analysis of bone and soft-tissue tumour tissue requires knowledge and techniques not always available to the general pathologist. Initial processing of tissue in the laboratory differs from that of the specimens handled routinely in a general hospital environment. For example, bone tumour tissue may be required fresh and without preservative in order to allow imprint and immunohistochemical analysis. The establishing of the precise origin and nature of bone and soft tissue tumours often requires special expertise; bone tumour centres may request that any biopsy material and histological slides be forwarded for review. It is not unusual for tissue to be studied collectively by pathologists from more than one tumour centre.

Even in large tumours, the area from which the biopsy is obtained can greatly influence the ease of tissue diagnosis and accuracy of initial grading. The centre of large lesions may comprise necrotic non-specific tissue. It is becoming common practice to obtain core-needle biopsies under ultrasound, CT or MRI guidance, allowing accurate targeting of the volume of tissue to be sampled. Expertly performed needle biopsy, with appropriate image guidance, can yield a 97–98 per cent diagnostic accuracy.

STAGING

To be useful, the surgical staging system for sarcomas should:

- incorporate the most significant prognostic factors into a system that describes the patient's progressive degree of risk;
- delineate progressive stages of disease that have specific implications for surgical management;
- provide guidelines for the use of adjuvant therapies.

Based on these principles, Enneking (1986) proposed a staging system that has become recognized by the Musculoskeletal Tumour Society for the management of bone and soft-tissue tumours. The factors considered in the staging are **histological grade (G)**, **local extent (T)** and the **presence or absence of distant metastases (M)**. Although strictly this system is based on the findings following surgical resection of the lesion, a representative preoperative biopsy and appropriate imaging may yield an accurate approximation of the surgical stage.

The surgical staging system of Enneking stratifies bone and soft-tissue tumours by grade, site and presence/absence of metastases (Table 7.1).

TREATMENT

REFERRAL TO A SPECIALIST CENTRE

The complexity of the management of bone tumours, diagnosis, staging and treatment dictates referral to specialist centres. These

Enneking staging system

Grade

G₁:

- low-grade;
- lower risk for metastases;
- well differentiated;
- few mitotic figures;
- moderate cytological atypia.

G₂:

- high-grade;
- higher incidence of metastases;
- poorly differentiated;
- high mitotic rate;
- high cell/matrix ratio;
- necrosis;
- microvascular invasion.

Site (local extent)

Is lesion contained within a well-delineated anatomical compartment?

T_1: intracompartmental
T_2: extracompartmental

The definitions of compartments are debatable, but in principle the anatomical compartments are those natural barriers to tumour extension, such as cortical bone and the major fascial septae.

Metastases

Presence of regional or distant metastases:
M_0: no metastases
M_1: metastases present

units often have **specialist radiologists, pathologists, oncologists, support professionals** and **surgeons** experienced in the management of these rare lesions. Optimum management of a potential tumour must entail an **appropriate selection of biopsy tract**, such that prognosis and any future reconstructive surgery are not compromised. This factor is proposed as a further reason for referral of these cases to specialist centres. Yet another benefit of

Table 7.1 Surgical staging system of Enneking

Stage	Grade	Site	Metastases?
IA	Low (G_1)	Intracompartmental (T_1)	No (M_0)
IB	Low (G_1)	Extracompartmental (T_2)	No (M_0)
IIA	High (G_2)	Intracompartmental (T_1)	No (M_0)
IIB	High (G_2)	Extracompartmental (T_2)	No (M_0)
III	Any	Any	Yes (M_1)

specialist referral is that the **chemotherapeutic regimens** employed in bone and soft-tissue tumours can be undertaken by dedicated oncologists following **international treatment programmes** and trials. Chemotherapy in osteosarcoma, for example, has been the subject of a pan-European study, currently extended to include the USA.

TUMOUR EXCISION

The options for tumour excision and their results may best be evaluated by consideration of the surgical plane of the dissection.

Intralesional

The **path of excision** passes through the **pseudo-capsule** (reactive zone) and **directly into the lesion**. The entire operative field is to be considered as potentially contaminated. All incisional biopsies are intralesional procedures. An intralesional definitive procedure may be appropriate where the tumour is of a **benign nature** or as **palliation** to overcome a mass effect.

Marginal

The entire lesion is **excised in one piece**, with the plane of dissection in the pseudo-capsule around the lesion.

Wide (intracompartmental)

The **lesion is removed** together with its **pseudo-capsule** and a **cuff of normal tissue**. The entire structure of origin of the tumour is not removed. This is also termed **en bloc resection**.

Radical (extracompartmental)

The **entire lesion** and its structure of origin are **removed**. The plane of dissection is outside the limiting fascia or bone.

AMPUTATION VERSUS LIMB SALVAGE

The treatment of a tumour should **not compromise its prognosis**. Treatment should also **preserve function** as best as possible. It should be noted that amputation does not equate to an equal or better prognosis than limb-salvage surgery. An amputation where the level is planned inadequately or where its execution is suboptimal will yield a guarded prognosis. Planning of an amputation must consider the possibility of skip lesions proximally in a bone, and the proximal anatomy of any affected compartment.

The indications for amputation are decreasing due to improved survivorship of patients treated by appropriate resection, limb salvage and adjuvant techniques. In general, amputation is now **reserved for a few select indications**, including:

- patients in whom **perivascular or neurological invasion renders resection of the tumour impossible** without sacrificing distal function or viability;
- patients in whom tumour excision, including biopsy tracts, **cannot be achieved without extensive excision of muscle**;
- **pathological fractures** where there has been significant contamination by the tumour.

RECONSTRUCTION IN LIMB-SALVAGE SURGERY

The reconstruction options for bony resection with limb-salvage surgery include massive **endoprostheses**, **autograft** and **allograft**. Local recurrence of malignant tumours after limb-

salvage surgery may be addressed by amputation without compromise of the overall prognosis.

Massive endoprosthetic replacement

The most commonly used method of reconstruction for bony resection is that of massive endoprosthetic replacement. This may be by **custom-made implants** (often with computer-aided design and manufacture) or by **modular systems**. These implants serve to replace the significant bulk of bone resected and often also an adjacent joint (Figure 7.4).

Early complications include **vascular injury**, **unpredicted neurological injury**, **thromboembolism**, **infection** and, if the implant has a subcutaneous location, **necrosis of overlying tissues**. Late complications include **implant loosening** and **failure**, **infection**, **pathological fracture** and **local recurrence**.

As the bony resection for tumour usually requires excision of juxtarticular bone, the endoprosthetic replacement includes a joint reconstruction. As an extensive amount of bone and ligaments is sacrificed, these endoprosthetic joints are often fully constrained. Wear of the joint surfaces may require procedures to 're-bush' or renew their components.

Endoprosthetic replacements to the lower limbs in the immature skeleton require extending mechanisms to minimize final limb-length discrepancies. Extending prostheses have

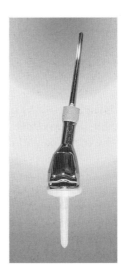

Figure 7.4 *Custom-made distal femoral endoprosthetic replacement. Image courtesy of Stanmore Implants, Royal National Orthopaedic Hospital Trust, Stanmore, UK. www.stanmoreimplants.com.*

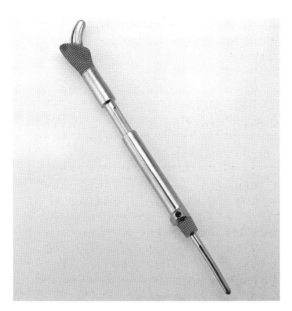

Figure 7.5 *Growing endoprosthetic midshaft femoral replacement. Image courtesy of Stanmore Implants, Royal National Orthopaedic Hospital Trust, Stanmore, UK. www.stanmoreimplants.com.*

evolved from requiring repeated major surgery in order to insert lengthening sleeves, to needing smaller incisions in order to allow manual turning of in-built extending rack-and-pinion mechanisms (Figure 7.5). More recent systems employ pulsed magnetic fields in order to turn in-built motors.

Autograft

Reconstruction using the patient's own bone may be considered, particularly where **only resection of diaphyseal bone** is required. Here, a **strut graft**, typically from the **fibula**, may be interposed. This technique has been of use in **tibial tumours**, where the grafted fibulae have been shown to subsequently enlarge in response to loading. The fibula has also been employed in osteo-articular reconstruction for excision of **tumours of the distal radius**.

Autograft reconstruction may also be achieved by **resection of the pathological bone, irradiation** and **re-implantation**. This bone is **non-viable** when implanted and therefore has **reduced mechanical properties**. There are, however, limited indications for this technique,

e.g. where a **resection of a large segment of the pelvic ring** is required.

Allograft

As in autograft reconstruction, a large bulk of the bone may be **non-viable**. In addition, there are risks of **disease transmission** from the donor and problems of the availability of **cadaveric** bone of the appropriate size. Bulk allograft reconstruction is uncommon in the UK.

Chemotherapy (adjuvant and neo-adjuvant)

The improved survivorship of patients with osteosarcoma in the past few decades has been through the development of multi-agent adjuvant chemotherapy treatment protocols. Further significant increase in survival has resulted from the use of neo-adjuvant chemotherapy. In this, the patient has a number of cycles of chemotherapy before surgery. After neo-adjuvant therapy, restaging investigations are undertaken. These may even demonstrate shrinkage of the tumour and its reactive zone where the response has been good.

Radiotherapy

Radiotherapy may be considered as adjuvant treatment for primary bone and soft-tissue tumour resection where a **histological marginal resection** is demonstrated or where **patient factors** limit the surgical resection that can be achieved. Radiotherapy is also indicated in the management of **bone metastases** or **pathological fracture** after surgical stabilization. The effectiveness of radiotherapy is limited in osteosarcoma and chondrosarcoma.

TREATMENT OF BENIGN BONE TUMOURS

Where a lesion can be confidently diagnosed as benign, more conservative treatments may be considered. The lesion may be **observed for further growth** or **spontaneous re-ossification**. Surgical intervention should be considered if there is **thinning of the cortex** by at least 50 per cent (associated with significantly increased risk of pathological fracture) or if there is a mass effect on adjacent structures due to the size and location of the lesion. The surgical armamentarium for benign bone tumours includes **intralesional resection** and **curettage**. This may be augmented by **local cytotoxic therapies**, such as **phenolization**, **cryotherapy** and **cement in-filling**. Cementomas work via a local chemical and thermal effect and provision of mechanical support to the remaining bone. Occasionally, recurrence of benign tumours may be addressed by **endoprosthetic replacement** or **amputation**.

KEY FEATURES OF SELECTED BENIGN BONE TUMOURS

BENIGN EPIPHYSEAL TUMOURS

Chondroblastoma

- Usually arise in the immature skeleton.
- Aggressive benign condition with high local recurrence rate.
- Local recurrence may be reduced by curettage with cryosurgery, avoiding the need for joint resection and reconstruction.

Giant-cell tumour (GCT)

- Occur after skeletal maturity (80 per cent).
- Arise on the metaphyseal side of the physis but cross it, appearing as eccentric lytic lesions in the epiphysis.
- Present as an expanding mass in the region of the epiphysis or with pathological fracture.
- Aggressive, locally recurrent tumour.
- Rarely malignant from outset (giant-cell sarcoma). Malignant transformation may occur and is seen particularly after local recurrence and treatment with radiotherapy.
- **Radiological grading system:** latent, active and aggressive.
- **Grading system:** GI and GII (benign), and GIII (malignant).
- **Treatment:** usually curettage and augmentation by bone graft/cement or

cryosurgery. Consider resection or amputation for recurrence or lesions demonstrating malignant features histologically.

BENIGN METAPHYSEAL AND DIAPHYSEAL TUMOURS

Simple (unicameral) bone cysts

- Arise in growing skeleton.
- Most common in the proximal humerus (67 per cent) and proximal femur (15 per cent).
- Usually asymptomatic until they fracture.
- Well-demarcated lytic lesions, expanding bone.
- Diagnosis usually made reliably on radiological features and site of lesion. If uncertain, consider bone scintigraphy, which should demonstrate a cold spot corresponding to the radiographic lesion.
- If diagnosis can be made confidently and lesion is detected on incidental X-ray, lesion may be monitored for spontaneous ossification. May consider invasive techniques if lesion fails to resolve or pathological fracture is impending. In case of pathological fracture, initiate supportive measures for fracture and observe healing. If ossification is not triggered, consider invasive techniques.
- Invasive treatment options include aspiration with instillation of steroid/bone marrow.
- Intramedullary nails may also be used.

Osteochondroma (exostosis)

- Most common benign bone tumour.
- Usually solitary, except in patients with hereditary multiple exostoses.
- Pedunculated lesions arising from juxtaphyseal location and growing away from the joint.
- May cause local irritation and pain. Growth of lesion or new pain in adulthood may signify malignant change.
- Malignant change occurs in approximately 1 per cent of lesions.
- Radiological appearance of lesion may appear smaller than clinically palpable mass due to the presence of a cartilaginous cap.

- Malignant transformation occurs in the cartilaginous cap. If this exceeds 1 cm in thickness on MRI, consider resection.

Enchondroma

- May be solitary or multiple (Ollier's disease).
- Often incidental findings.
- Those occurring in hands or feet are benign, irrespective of radiological appearance (only case reports of malignancy here).
- Lesions in pelvis or shoulders should prompt high suspicion of malignancy (chondrosarcoma).

Osteoid osteoma

- Characteristic symptoms of localized pain, worse at night and relieved by salicylates.
- Can affect any bone, although femur, tibia and spine are most often involved.
- May affect any part of bone, although usually intracortical.
- Lesion itself is radiolucent but gives rise to surrounding sclerotic reaction.
- CT may be necessary to demonstrate lesion.
- Bone scintigraphy demonstrates markedly increased uptake.
- Treatment is surgical excision of the lytic lesion or percutaneous thermal ablation under image guidance.

KEY FEATURES OF SELECTED MALIGNANT BONE TUMOURS

Osteosarcoma

- Bimodal age distribution of incidence. First peak in childhood and adolescence, and further peak in later years. Second peak may be associated with Paget's disease, irradiation or polyostotic fibrous dysplasia.
- Most often affects bones about the knee (50 per cent) or humerus (25 per cent). Rarely affects the axial skeleton.
- Radiological features of increased intramedullary sclerosis with permeative destruction. Elevation of periosteum gives rise to appearance of Codman's triangle (see Figure 7.3). Extra-osseous component gives

rise to ossification in the soft tissues.
- Histologically a high-grade spindle-cell tumour.
- Variants of classical osteosarcoma described may occur. There may be a predominantly lytic appearance to the lesion. Lesion may also arise in cortex giving rise to parosteal or periosteal osteosarcomas.
- Neo-adjuvant chemotherapy has been demonstrated to improve survivorship following surgical resection.

Chondrosarcoma

- Malignancy of cartilaginous tissues.
- Peak incidence in middle life.
- Radiologically may demonstrate patchy calcification, giving rise to 'popcorn' appearance. Where central (intramedullary) in site, may give rise to endosteal scalloping. Narrow zone of transition may lead to misdiagnosis as benign.
- Variable histological grade.
- Treatment is by surgical resection, with little effective adjuvant chemotherapy or radiotherapy. In long-standing lesions, dedifferentiation may occur.

Ewing's sarcoma/primitive neuroectodermal tumour (PNET)

These are small round-cell tumours believed to be of the same aetiology. The tissue type of origin is uncertain, although the condition is associated with the gene translocation (11:22).

- Occur in children and adolescents (80 per cent of cases in first two decades), with median age 13 years.
- Most frequently affects the femoral diaphysis.
- Male-to-female ratio 3 : 2.
- Radiological studies may demonstrate pathognomonic onion skin appearance due to episodes of periosteal reaction and new bone formation. Often have a large soft-tissue element.
- Neo-adjuvant chemotherapy is highly effective in reducing tumour mass.

Haemopoietic tumours

These tumours (multiple myeloma, plasmacytoma) may present to the orthopaedic surgeon as incidental findings, with pain or after pathological fracture. Diagnosis should follow the principles outlined above, with appropriate referral for further management, such as surgical stabilization of pathological fractures.

Secondary tumours of bone

- Metastatic disease affecting bone is common and may be increasing in incidence with improved overall tumour survivorship.
- Long-established tumours with a predilection for spread to bone are those of the lung, breast, prostate, kidney and thyroid.
- Initial management of tumours presenting as bony metastases should follow the principles outlined above.
- Guidance on the role of the orthopaedic surgeon in these cases has been published by the British Orthopaedic Association (see Further reading).
- In treating the osseous element, the key is avoidance of pathological fracture. Assessment of risk of fracture may be performed (Mirels, 1989) and prophylactic stabilization undertaken if appropriate.
- Where fracture through the lesion is already present, surgical fixation by a load-bearing prosthesis may be required, as union of the fracture may not occur. Mechanical and fatigue properties of the implant selected should preferably exceed the patient's predicted survival.

CONCLUSION

Orthopaedic surgeons are likely to encounter bone malignancy (primary or secondary) infrequently in their practice. A detailed knowledge of individual tumours is not expected of the general orthopaedic surgeon, and only a brief summary of the more common

neoplasms is given in this chapter. The management, including diagnosis, should follow the simple principles outlined, avoiding compromise of the prognosis. If a primary bone tumour is suspected or there is any uncertainty regarding diagnosis, early referral to a specialist centre should be considered.

Viva questions

1 Describe this tumour. [Prop-based question using plain radiographs or other imaging modalities.]

2 How would you investigate a patient who presents with a possible malignant bone tumour?

3 How are bone tumours staged?

4 What are the principles of treatment of bone tumours?

5 What surgical options are available in the treatment of bone tumours?

FURTHER READING

British Orthopaedic Association. *Metastatic Bone Disease: A Guide to Good Practice*. London: British Orthopaedic Association. www.boa.ac.uk/PDF%20files/Metastatic%20bone%20disease.pdf.

Enneking, WF. A system of staging musculoskeletal neoplasms. *Clin Orthop Relat Res* 1986;**204**:9–24.

Mirels, H. Metastatic disease in long bones: a proposed scoring system for diagnosing impending pathologic fracture. *Clin Orthop Rel Res* 1989:**249**;256–64.

Saifuddin, A, Mitchell, R, Burnett, SJ, Sandison, A, Pringle, JA. Ultrasound-guided needle biopsy of primary bone tumours. *J Bone Joint Surg Br* 2000;**82**:50–4.

Tillman, RM. The role of the orthopaedic surgeon in metastatic disease of the appendicular skeleton. *J Bone Joint Surg Br* 1999:**81**:1–2.

8

Ligaments and tendons

CHEH CHIN TAI AND ANDREW WILLIAMS

INTRODUCTION

Tendons and ligaments play essential roles in joint motion. **Ligaments connect bone with bone** and function:

- to augment the static mechanical stability of joints;
- to prevent excessive or abnormal motion;
- as a sensory source for protective reflexes and to provide proprioceptive feedback about movement and posture, thereby contributing to the neuromuscular dynamic control of stability.

Tendons attach muscle to bone and function:

- to transmit tensile loads from muscle to bone;
- to enable the muscle belly to be at an optimal distance from the joint without an extended length of muscle between origin and insertion;
- as a store of energy (analogous to a spring).

STRUCTURE

Ligaments and tendons are composed of **cells** and **extracellular matrix** (largely collagen). In general, the cells (fibroblasts) occupy only 20 per cent of the total tissue volume, while the extracellular matrix accounts for the remaining 80 per cent. Approximately 30 per cent of the matrix is solid, comprising primarily collagen but also ground substance (including proteoglycans, which are critical to function) and a small amount of elastin. There is **more elastin in ligaments** than in tendons.

The **collagen content is high** (over 70 per cent) and is greater in tendons than in ligaments. In extremity tendons, the solid material may consist almost entirely of collagen (up to 99 per cent of dry weight). There are two notable exceptions: the ligamentum nuchae and the ligamentum flava along the spinal column, which contain large amounts of elastic fibres (almost 75 per cent of dry weight).

COLLAGEN

Collagen is synthesized as a precursor, pro-collagen, by fibroblasts. Pro-collagen is secreted and cleaved extracellularly to form collagen fibres (Figure 8.1).

More than **90 per cent of collagen in tendons and ligaments is type I**, and less than 10 per cent is type III. Type IV is present in small quantities. Type I collagen consists of **three polypeptide chains**; two (alpha 1) are identical and one differs slightly (alpha 2). The three alpha chains are combined to form a **right-handed triple helix**, which gives the collagen molecule a rod-like shape. The intra- and interchain bonding, or **cross-linking**, which

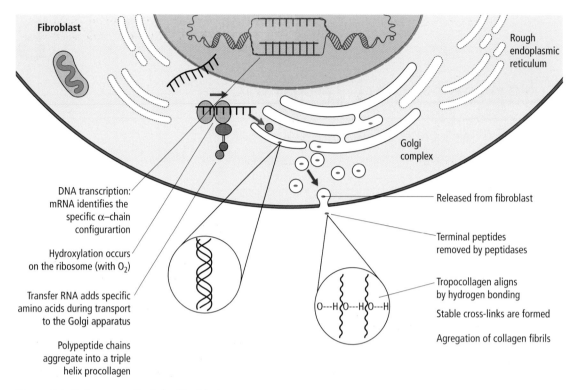

Figure 8.1 *Collagen synthesis in fibroblasts.*

are due mainly to hydrogen bonds, provide stability to the molecule.

Several collagen molecules aggregate in a **quarter-staggered array** to form microfibrils (each 0.02–0.2 μm in diameter) (Figure 8.2).

Further aggregation of the microfibrils results in the formation of collagen **fibres** (each 1–20 μm in diameter) and **bundles**. Fibroblasts are aligned between these bundles in the direction of ligament or tendon function. The arrangement of the collagen fibres is nearly **parallel in tendons**, allowing them to handle high unidirectional (uni-axial) tensile loads (Figure 8.3).

The **less parallel arrangement of the collagen fibres in ligaments** and the **layered arrangement** allows these structures to sustain predominantly tensile stresses in one direction but also smaller stresses in other directions for any applied external force. In any single layer the fibres lie parallel to each other, but in subsequent layers they lie in different directions. As a result of

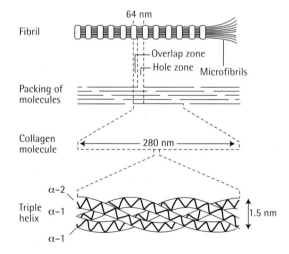

Figure 8.2 *Quarter-staggered array of collagen-forming microfibrils.*

this arrangement, a ligament can resist applied forces from many directions. In addition, the fibres in ligaments are arranged in a **wavy**

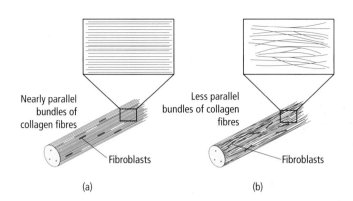

Nearly parallel bundles of collagen fibres

Less parallel bundles of collagen fibres

Fibroblasts

Fibroblasts

(a)

(b)

Figure 8.3 *Arrangement of collagen fibres in (a) tendon and (b) ligament.*

pattern (**crimp**), increasing their capacity to absorb tension.

GROUND SUBSTANCE

Ground substance consists of **proteoglycans (PG)**, **glycoproteins**, **plasma proteins** and a variety of **small molecules**. PGs are composed of sulphated polysaccharide chains (glycosaminoglycans) bound to a core protein, which in turn is bound via a link protein to a hyaluronic acid chain to form an extremely high-molecular-weight PG aggregate. These PG aggregates bind most of the extracellular water of the ligaments and tendons, making the matrix a highly structured gel-like material. By acting as a cement-like substance between the collagen microfibrils, they help to **stabilize the collagenous skeleton** of tendons and ligaments and contribute to the **overall strength** of these composite structures. However, only a small number of these molecules exist in tendons.

ELASTIN

Elastin consists of **hydrophobic non-glycosylated proteins** secreted by fibroblasts into the extracellular matrix. These proteins form an **extensive network** with highly **cross-linked filaments** and **sheets**, which allows the network to **stretch** and **coil** (up to 200 per cent of their unloaded length at relatively low loads). Elastic fibres are of great importance to the recovery of tissues after loading. Their function, however, diminishes towards maximal loading levels because their maximum strength is about five times lower than that of collagen.

SURROUNDING CONNECTIVE TISSUE

Tendons and ligaments are surrounded by **loose areolar connective tissues**, known as the **paratenon** in tendon (no specific name in ligaments). These form a sheath, which can either run the entire length of the tendons or exist only at the point where the tendon bends in concert with a joint. The paratenon protects the tendon and facilitates gliding. It is also the major source for remodelling and healing responses, as it contains abundant cells and blood vessels (**vascular tendons**). In some tendons, a true synovial sheath replaces the paratenon (**avascular tendons**).

A synovium-like membrane, called the **epitenon**, is found just beneath the paratenon in tendons that are subjected to particularly high friction forces (e.g. in the palm and wrist). The epitenon enhances gliding of the tendon by producing synovial fluid from its synovial cells. The epitenon surrounds the endotenon, which in turn binds together the fascicles (groups of collagen bundles).

INSERTION SITE

Tendons and ligaments are **highly resistant to lengthening**. Tendons in particular are also relatively flexible and can therefore be angulated around bone surfaces or deflected beneath retinacula to alter the direction of muscular pull. In ligaments, due to the organization of the fibres in layers, not all fibres are stretched when loaded along the main fibre axis. Consequently, **ligaments are less strong** than tendons.

The structure of the insertion into bone is similar in ligaments and tendons and consists of four **zones of indirect insertion**:

- **Zone 1:** parallel collagen fibres at the end of the tendon or ligament.
- **Zone 2:** collagen fibres intermesh with unmineralized fibrocartilage.
- **Zone 3:** fibrocartilage gradually becomes mineralized.
- **Zone 4:** mineralized fibrocartilage merges into cortical bone.

The **perforating fibres of Sharpey** cross all four zones. The gradual change in structural properties results in increased stiffness and decreased stress concentration, minimizing injuries at insertion sites. In addition, the collagen fibres of ligaments can also insert directly into bone by blending with the periosteum at an oblique or orthogonal angle.

In tendons, the musculotendinous junction is of equal importance, since high local stresses can occur here, predisposing to injury. Frequently, tendons have an internal portion within the muscle fascia known as the **aponeurosis**. The aponeurosis provides a large surface area for load transfer from muscle to tendon; the orientation of this junction enhances its strength.

BLOOD SUPPLY

Compared with other connective tissues such as bone and skin, ligaments and tendons are poorly vascularized and have a lower metabolic rate. The blood supply of ligaments **originates mainly at the insertion sites**, runs longitudinally through the ligament and is **uniform**. The blood supply of paratenon-covered tendons is provided by a relatively **sparse array of small arterioles**, which run longitudinally from the adjacent muscular tissues and surrounding areolar connective tissue. In sheathed avascular tendons, a **vincula (mesotenon)** carries a vessel to supply one tendon segment; adjacent avascular areas receive nutrition via diffusion.

As a result of these differences, **paratenon-covered tendons heal better** than other tendons.

NERVE SUPPLY

The nerve supply is mainly **afferent**, with specialized afferent receptors. When these receptors are activated (during rapid increase in tension), myotactic reflexes are initiated, which inhibit the development of excessive tension during muscular contraction. Hence, tendons and ligaments play an important proprioceptive role in overall neuromuscular control of the limb.

FUNCTION

LOAD–ELONGATION CURVES

The biomechanical properties can be measured in tensile loading experiments using isolated cadaveric tendon or ligament–bone complexes of human or animal origin. The tissue is elongated until it ruptures and the load–elongation curve plotted (Figure 8.4).

The first region of the load–elongation curve is concave and is usually called the **non-linear toe region**. The reasons for this behaviour are multifactorial. During the stretching of ligament or tendon, an increasing number of fibres are recruited under tension and **crimped fibres begin to straighten**. Initially, there is little resistance to tension as the fibres lengthen, but as elongation progresses an increasing number

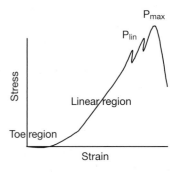

Figure 8.4 *Stress–strain curve for ligaments and tendons. P_{lin}, linear yield point; P_{max}, maximum power (or ultimate tensile strength).*

of fibrils become taut and carry load. Some studies suggest that sliding and shear of the interfibrillar ground substance may cause this elongation.

As elongation continues at higher loads, the stiffness of the tissue increases, and progressively greater force is required to produce equivalent amounts of elongation. This is known as the **linear region**, as the deformation of the tissue has a more or less linear relationship with load. At the end of this region, the load value is designated as P_{lin}, the yield point for the tissue. The energy to P_{lin} is represented by the area under the curve up to the end of the linear region.

Small force reduction (**dips**) can sometimes be observed at the end of the linear region in the loading curves for tendons and ligaments. These dips are caused by the **early sequential failure** of a few greatly stretched fibre bundles. Ultimately, as elongation exceeds the capacity of the fibres, yield and failure of the tissues result from **progressive fibril failure**. This is when the curve begins to bend toward the strain axis and reaches a point of ultimate stress. With attainment of the maximum load, P_{max}, which reflects the ultimate tensile strength of the specimen, complete failure occurs rapidly. The strain to failure is usually only a few percentage points of total length. However, in real life, ligaments and tendons are rarely stretched significantly, as muscular reflexes initiated by proprioceptive feedback provide protection.

The modulus of elasticity for tendons and ligaments is based on a linear relationship between load and deformation (structural property), or stress and strain (mechanical property). The stress (force or load divided by the cross-sectional area) is proportional to the strain (change in length or deformation divided by the original length):

$$E = \delta/\varepsilon$$

where E is the modulus of elasticity (slope of the stress–strain curve), δ is stress and ε is strain.

In the toe region of the graph, the modulus is not constant but increases gradually. The modulus stabilizes in the fairly linear region of the curve.

Not all ligaments and tendons are identical. The curve for ligamentum flavum, with its high proportion of elastic fibres, is different. When tensile testing human ligamentum flavum, elongation of the specimen reaches 50 per cent before the stiffness increases appreciably. At 70 per cent elongation, the stiffness increases greatly with additional loading, and the ligament fails abruptly with little further deformation. This is very uncommon, as most tendons and ligaments fail after a length increase of only a few percentage points of the original.

VISCO-ELASTICITY

Visco-elastic materials exhibit stress–strain behaviour that is time- and rate-dependent, i.e. the material deformation depends on the load and its rate and duration of application of load. In a tissue that is viscous (fluid-like), constant loading results in a progressive deformation over an extended period of time, known as **creep**. In contrast, a more elastic (solid-like) tissue returns to its original shape or length after load is removed and its stress–stain behaviour remains unchanged with cycled loads. Tendons and ligaments maintain the capacity for both viscous and elastic responses: at **low loads**, **viscous** behaviour dominates; at **higher loads**, **elastic** behaviour dominates. This balance allows normal ligaments and tendons to function within a fairly wide range of loads without damaging their fibres.

When ligaments and tendons are repetitively loaded, the stress–strain curve shifts to the right, indicating that the tissues have become less stiff and more compliant. However, when subjected to increased strain rates, the linear portion of the stress–strain curve becomes steeper, indicating greater stiffness of the tissue and more energy storage, thus requiring more force to rupture.

The three main features of visco-elastic behaviour are:

- **Hysteresis:** the load–elongation curve differs during loading and unloading, resulting in net internal energy loss, usually as heat.
- **Stress relaxation:** this is a decrease in stress

in the tendon or ligament subjected to constant strain over an extended period. However, when the stress–relaxation test is repeated cyclically, the decrease in stress gradually becomes less pronounced. This is used as an argument for cyclic loading of hamstring grafts before fixation in cruciate ligament reconstruction.

- **Creep:** this is an increase in deformation or strain that occurs when a constant load is applied over an extended period. When this test is repeated cyclically, the increase in strain gradually becomes less pronounced. Clinically, this behaviour is applied in the application of plaster casts for deformity correction, e.g. the Ponseti method for treatment of congenital talipes equinovarus.

Under normal physiological conditions in vivo, ligaments and tendons are subjected to a stress magnitude that is only about one-quarter to one-third of the ultimate tensile load. The upper limit for physiological strain in tendons and ligaments (e.g. during running and jumping) is 2–5 per cent.

Factors affecting the biomechanical properties of ligaments and tendons include the following:

- **Ageing effect:** during maturation (up to age 20 years), the number and quality of cross-links increases, resulting in increased tensile strength of tendons and ligaments. After maturation, as ageing occurs, the mean collagen diameter and content decrease, resulting in the gradual decline of mechanical properties. Before puberty the weakest link in the ligament bone complex is the developing bone, but once skeletal maturity is reached mid-substance failure of the ligament usually occurs. Similarly, in the growing skeleton tendon avulsion may occur, but in adolescent and older age groups failure tends to occur at the musculotendinous junction due to stress concentration and the relatively weak muscular tissue.
- **Endocrine effect:** increased laxity and decreased stiffness of the tendon and ligaments are noted in the pelvic region during the latter stages of pregnancy and in the postpartum period. It is also thought that the incidence of anterior cruciate ligament ruptures in females varies according to the phase of the menstrual cycle.
- **Pharmacological effect:** some studies have shown that short-term treatment with indomethacin increases the tensile strength of tendons, probably due to an increased cross-linkage of collagen molecules. Other studies have shown that the rate and strength of tissue healing decreases as a result of such treatment. Corticosteroid injections have been shown to weaken the biomechanical qualities of both normal and healing tissues. The association of Achilles and patellar tendon ruptures with local steroid injections is well known. There are also many case reports of tendon ruptures associated with the abuse of anabolic steroids.
- **Mobilization and immobilization effect:** see Healing below.

INJURY

The degree of injury is related to the rate of loading and the amount of load. There are two main mechanisms of injury:

- **Repetitive micro-trauma:** fatigue failure occurs due to repetitive loading well below the normal ultimate tensile strength. These injuries result in **micro-tears** followed by an **inflammatory reaction** (in an attempt to heal) and sometimes **calcification**, which alters the biomechanical properties of the tissues. This type of injury is common and is more likely to occur in tendons, since these structures tend to carry higher loads in vivo than ligaments.
- **Macro-trauma:** acute failure due to forces (excluding laceration) above the ultimate tensile strength results in partial or complete rupture. These injuries tend to have well-documented mechanisms of injury and are associated with forces resisted by specific tendons or ligaments, e.g. injury to the lateral collateral knee ligament by a varus force. In ligaments, ruptures of sequential series of collagen fibre bundles tend to be

distributed throughout the ligament rather than being localized to one specific area.

Failure of a ligament or tendon – either an acute rupture or micro-tears – can occur at insertion sites (avulsion), with or without a bony fragment, within the substance itself, or a combination of both. At a **low loading rate** the bony insertion is the weakest component of the **tendon/ligament–bone complex**, but at a **high loading rate** the **tendon or ligament** is the weakest link. This suggests that with increasing strain rate, the increase in tissue strength is higher at the tendon/ligament–bone complex junction than in the tendon or ligament itself. However, some studies have shown that failure modes are independent of strain rate and merely depend on the maturation of the loaded tendon/ligament–bone complex and so may be age-specific. Note that ligament avulsions typically occur between the mineralized and unmineralized fibrocartilage layers.

In tendons, two additional factors contribute to the nature of injury:

- **Cross-sectional area of the tendon in relation to its muscle:** the strength of both the muscle and the tendon depends on their physiological cross-sectional areas. The larger the cross-sectional area of the muscle, the stronger the force produced by the contraction, and therefore the greater the tensile loads transmitted through the tendon. Similarly, the larger the cross-sectional area of the tendon, the greater the load it can bear. If the tensile strength of a tendon is greater than that of its muscle, then muscle ruptures are more likely to occur.
- **Amount of force produced by the contraction of the muscle to which the tendon is attached:** when the muscle is maximally contracted, the tensile stress on the tendon is at its highest. This stress can be increased if eccentric contraction of the muscle rather than concentric contraction takes place. As a result, the load imposed on the tendon may exceed the yield point, causing tendon rupture.

Clinically, injuries to tendons and ligaments can be categorized according to their degree of severity:

- **Grade I (mild):** some pain is felt, but no joint laxity can be detected clinically, even though micro-failure of collagen fibres may have occurred.
- **Grade II (moderate):** severe pain and some joint laxity can be detected clinically. Progressive failure of the collagen has taken place, resulting in partial rupture. The joint laxity is often masked by muscle activity, and hence the clinical test for joint laxity is often positive only if performed with the patient under anaesthesia.
- **Grade III (severe):** severe pain occurs at the time of trauma, with less pain after injury. Clinically, the joint is found to be completely unstable. Most collagen fibres have ruptured, but a few may still be intact. However, the tissue can still be in continuity, even though it has undergone extensive macro- and micro-failure and elongation.

HEALING

The response to injury of different tendons and ligaments differs significantly. This could be due to differences in intrinsic fibroblastic response to injury, the mechanical environment, intra-articular versus extra-articular environment (inhibitory effect of synovial fluid), blood supply and the degree of inflammatory response.

Unlike skin and bone, ligaments and tendons are believed to have a slower and more limited healing response (ligaments and tendons are not as well vascularized or innervated as skin and bone). Healing can be divided into three phases (analogous to healing in other connective tissues):

- **Phase one – haemorrhagic/inflammatory phase:** this phase is characterized by the formation of a **haematoma** within the damaged region and the initiation of a rapid **inflammatory response**. This results in invasion by polymorphonuclear cells and monocytes/macrophages, with the release of a complex cascade of cytokines and growth factors. The monocytes remove debris and fibroblastic cells begin to appear. This phase of ligament healing lasts for **hours to a few days**.

- **Phase two – proliferative phase:** in this phase, **new blood vessels** are formed and fibroblasts are recruited from the local environment or circulation to produce **new matrix material**, mainly collagen (type III is predominant initially). The new matrix then increases in mass and become less viscous and more elastic as the inflammation decreases over the next few weeks of healing.
- **Phase three – remodelling phase:** this phase starts within **weeks** after the injury and can last up to several years. It is characterized by **progressive maturation** and **conversion of collagen fibres** (to type I), alignment in a more physiological orientation (in response to loads) and reorganization of the matrix. Surgical tendon repairs are at their weakest in the first week, regaining most of their original strength by 3–4 weeks and achieving **maximum strength at 6 months**.

Ideally, healing should lead to complete restoration of the original tissue with identical morphological and functional characteristics. Unfortunately, even after years of remodelling, healed matrix remains different from normal tissue biochemically, mechanically and histologically (collagen is more disorganized and less oriented, more defects exist between collagen fibres, and the number of collagen fibres of larger diameter is reduced).

Factors affecting healing include the following:

- **Mobilization:** ligaments and tendons appear to remodel in response to the mechanical demands placed upon them. Controlled movement of a joint appears to have a beneficial effect on healing, increasing the tensile strength of tendons and of the ligament–bone interface by stimulating synthesis of collagen and proteoglycan, and by promoting proper collagen fibre orientation. In animal studies of healing of ligament injury, immobilization results in decreased strength and stiffness of tendons and ligaments; the tissue metabolism also increases, leading to proportionally more immature collagen, with a decrease in the amount and quality of the cross-links between collagen molecules. This decline in structural properties is reversible, but the process is slow.

- **Surgery:** the calibre of suture, the number of suture strands, the suture technique and the use of peripheral epitendinous or sheath repair can all affect the strength of the healing process. Suturing of mop-end tears with extensive overlapping of tissue ends and minimal gapping confers little benefit.

- **Biological and biochemical manipulation:** the use of growth factors, e.g. epidermal growth factor (EGF) and platelet-derived growth factor (PDGF), increases fibroblast proliferation in vitro. Other agents such as steroids and hyaluronate have been shown to decrease adhesion formation in the healing process. However, the latter also decrease the rate and strength of tendon healing and increase the rate of infection.

- **Joint instability:** in an unstable joint, the healing of ligament is inferior, especially if instability is due to multiple ligament injury.

Viva questions

1 What is the structure of collagen?

2 Describe the blood supply of tendons and ligaments.

3 How do tendons and ligaments heal after injury?

4 Draw the stress–strain curve of a ligament/tendon and explain its various parts.

5 Discuss injuries to tendons and mechanisms of fatigue failure.

FURTHER READING

Buckwalter, JA, Hunziker, EB. Orthopaedics: healing of bones, cartilages, tendons, and ligaments – a new era. *Lancet* 1996;**348**: sII18.

Butler, DL, Grood, ES, Noyes, FR, Zernicke, RF: Biomechanics of ligaments and tendons. *Exerc Sport Sci Rev* 1978;**6**:125–81.

Fleming, BC, Beynnon, BD. In vivo measurement of ligament/tendon strains and forces: a review. *Ann Biomed Eng* 2004;**32**:318–28.

Noyes, FR, DeLucas, JL, Torvik, PJ: Biomechanics of anterior cruciate ligament failure: an analysis of strain-rate sensitivity and mechanisms of failure in primates. *J Bone Joint Surg Am* 1974;**56**:236–53.

Sharma, P, Maffulli, N. Tendon injury and tendinopathy: healing and repair. *J Bone Joint Surg Am* 2005;**87**:187–202.

9

Meniscus

VIJAI RANAWAT AND JOHN SKINNER

INTRODUCTION

The menisci are two **crescentic fibro-cartilaginous structures** interposed between the condyles of the femur and tibia in the knee. Note that menisci or labra are also found deepening the articular surfaces of other synovial joints, such as the acromioclavicular, sternoclavicular, glenohumeral and hip joints, although this chapter concentrates on the knee.

ANATOMY

Each meniscus covers approximately the peripheral two-thirds of the corresponding

articular surface of the tibia (Figure 9.1). The **peripheral border** is **thick, convex and attached to the capsule** of the joint. The **inner border** tapers to a **thin free edge**. The proximal surfaces are concave and in contact with the femoral condyles. The distal surfaces are flat and rest on the tibial plateau.

The **medial meniscus** (MM) is nearly **semicircular** in shape and about 3.5 cm in length. It has a **triangular cross-section** and is **asymmetrical**, having a considerably wider posterior than anterior horn. It is attached firmly to the **posterior intercondylar fossa** of the tibia directly anterior to the posterior cruciate ligament (PCL) attachment. The anterior attachment is more variable but is usually attached 7 mm anterior to the anterior

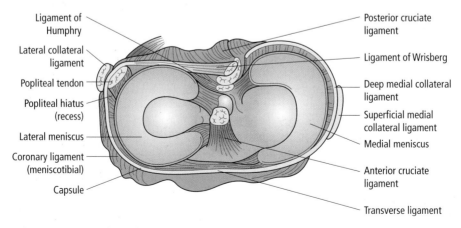

Figure 9.1 *Superior aspect of the tibial plateau.*

cruciate ligament (ACL) insertion in line with the medial tibial tubercle. Peripherally, the MM is continuously attached to the capsule of the joint, being associated most firmly at a condensation in the capsule known as the deep medial collateral ligament.

The **lateral meniscus** (LM) is almost **circular** and covers a larger area than the MM. The anterior horn attaches to the intercondylar fossa adjacent to the ACL. The posterior horn is attached to the intercondylar fossa adjacent and anterior to the posterior horn of the MM. Unlike that of the MM, the attachment of the LM to the capsule is interrupted by the popliteus tendon. In addition, the LM does not have a direct attachment to the lateral collateral ligament and has only a loose peripheral attachment to the joint capsule. Additional ligaments run from the posterior horn of the lateral meniscus to the medial femoral condyle, either in front of (the **anterior meniscofemoral ligament of Humphry**) or behind (the **posterior meniscofemoral ligament of Wrisberg**) the PCL.

EMBRYOLOGY

The menisci appear by **day 45**, when they differentiate directly from **blastemal cells** connected to the capsule and immediately assume their semilunar shape. At birth, the menisci are **completely vascularized**, but this regresses so that by age 10 years an avascular central third of the meniscus is present. The transition from vascular (red zone) to avascular (white zone) regions progresses, and by adulthood only the peripheral 10–30 per cent of the meniscus remains vascular.

ULTRA-STRUCTURE

Histologically, the meniscus is a fibrocartilaginous structure whose **extracellular matrix** is composed primarily of **water** (approximately 70 per cent) and an interlacing network of **collagen fibres** (mainly type I, 55–65 per cent of dry weight) surrounded by **elastin**, **proteoglycans** and **glycoproteins**. The cellular component consists of **fibrochondrocytes**, anaerobic cells with few

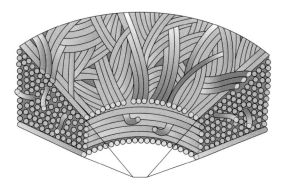

Figure 9.2 *Collagen fibre arrangement in a meniscus, with most fibres oriented circumferentially but some oriented radially and acting as ties.*

mitochondria, which synthesize and maintain the extracellular matrix. Microscopically, these cells are of two types – **fusiform** cells (found in the superficial zone of the meniscus in lacunae) and **ovoid** cells (found elsewhere in the meniscus). Both contain abundant endoplasmic reticulum and Golgi apparatus.

Ultra-structural studies demonstrate three layers of collagen fibres: **superficial**, **surface** and **middle**. The **majority of collagen fibres** (particularly in the middle layer) have a **circumferential orientation** following the C-shaped curve of the meniscus. However, there are a **few small radially arranged fibres** (mainly in the superficial layer) that may act as ties, providing structural rigidity against compressive forces and preventing longitudinal splitting (Figure 9.2).

FUNCTION

The menisci perform several functions:

- load transmission across the knee;
- enhancement of articular conformity;
- distribution of synovial fluid across the articular surface;
- prevention of soft-tissue impingement during joint motion;
- role in anteroposterior (AP) stabilization of the knee.

Meniscal function was first clinically inferred by the severe degenerative changes that

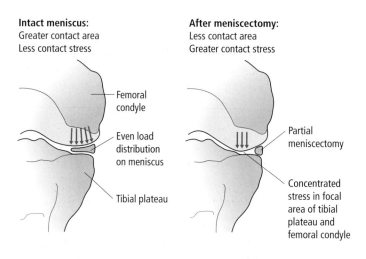

Intact meniscus:
Greater contact area
Less contact stress

After meniscectomy:
Less contact area
Greater contact stress

Femoral condyle

Even load distribution on meniscus

Tibial plateau

Partial meniscectomy

Concentrated stress in focal area of tibial plateau and femoral condyle

Figure 9.3 *Load transmission in the normal and post-meniscectomized knee.*

followed meniscectomy; it is this role of load transmission that is the most important.

LOAD TRANSMISSION

The meniscus has been shown to play a vital role in load transmission across the knee joint. Biomechanical studies have shown that at least 50 per cent of the compressive load of the knee joint is transmitted in extension and approximately 85 per cent of the load in 90-degree flexion. In the meniscectomized knee, the contact area is reduced to approximately 50 per cent and so load per unit area increases drastically, resulting in articular cartilage degeneration (Figure 9.3).

Partial meniscectomy also significantly **increases contact pressures**. Studies have shown that resection of as little as 15–34 per cent increases contact pressures by more than 350 per cent.

ARTICULAR CONFORMITY

As the knee passes through its range of motion, the menisci move with respect to the tibial articular surface. During **flexion**, both menisci (but LM more then MM) **displace in an AP direction** along the tibial plateau in the mid-condylar parasagittal plane. In addition to the AP translation, the menisci **deform** to remain in constant congruity to the tibial and femoral articular surfaces. This deformable property of the meniscal tissue not only aids load transmission but also is thought to play a role in

shock absorption. This is due to the frictional drag exerted by the interstitial fluid as it is forced through the porous permeable solid matrix.

JOINT LUBRICATION

The menisci serve to increase the congruity between the femoral and tibial condyles, and so they contribute to joint conformity. It has been proposed that this conformity promotes a viscous hydrodynamic action required for full fluid-film lubrication and assists in overall lubrication and circulation of synovial fluid around the joint (see Chapter 25).

JOINT STABILITY

The MM plays a role in **AP stability**. This is demonstrated by the significantly greater anterior laxity in ACL-deficient knees with medial meniscectomy compared with ACL-deficient knees with the MM present. Medial meniscectomy alone has no effect on AP laxity.

PROPRIOCEPTION

The menisci may serve a proprioceptive role as demonstrated by the presence of **type I and II nerve endings** concentrated in the **anterior** and **posterior horns**. These neural elements, in addition to similar structures seen on and within the adjacent cruciate ligaments, may be part of a complex proprioceptive reflex arc that contributes to the functional stability of the knee. As they are concentrated anteriorly and posteriorly, they may contribute to afferent feedback at the extremes of flexion and extension.

ANATOMICAL AND DEVELOPMENTAL ABNORMALITIES

ANOMALOUS ATTACHMENTS

A variety of abnormal attachments of the MM have been described, including insertion of the anterior horn into the ACL, intercondylar notch and infrapatellar fold and of the posterior horn into the ACL.

HYPOPLASIA AND CONGENITAL ABSENCE

The incidences of hypoplasia and congenital absence are unknown but invariably occur in association with ipsilateral knee abnormalities. This is probably due to the common mesenchymal origin of these structures.

DISCOID MENISCI

Lateral

Discoid lateral meniscus is the most common, with a reported incidence of 4–15.5 per cent. It usually presents in childhood with a classical complaint of 'snapping' and pain. Magnetic resonance imaging (MRI) scans are diagnostic. Arthroscopic partial meniscectomy gives good short-term results.

Medial

Discoid medial meniscus is very rare, with a reported incidence of 0.06–0.3 per cent.

MENISCAL AND GANGLION CYSTS

Ganglion cysts associated with the menisci are common and are related to cystic degeneration of that tissue. Meniscal cysts are a subgroup that occurs in association with trauma.

MENISCAL TEARS

CLASSIFICATION

Two methods of classification exist:

- based on location with reference to blood supply;
- based on tear pattern.

Location

The menisci of the knee are relatively avascular structures whose **peripheral blood supply**

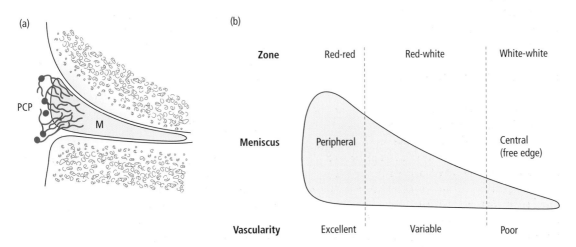

Figure 9.4 *Diagrams of (a) the blood supply of the meniscus and (b) the zones of vasculature. M, meniscus; PCP, premeniscal capillary plexus.*

originates primarily from the **lateral** and **medial genicular arteries**. Branches of these vessels give rise to a **perimeniscal capillary plexus** (PCP) within the synovial and capsular tissues of the knee joint.

These perimeniscal vessels are oriented in a predominantly circumferential pattern, with radial branches directed towards the centre of the joint. Studies have shown that the degree of **vascular penetration** is 10–30 per cent of meniscal width (the **red zone**) (Figure 9.4a). This gives rise to different **zones of meniscal vasculature** (Figure 9.4b).

The clinical importance of the blood supply is that peripheral tears are suitable for repair whereas central tears are unsuitable due to lack of healing potential. The cell responsible for mensical healing is the fibrochondrocyte. When injury occurs in the peripheral vascular zone, a **fibrin clot** rich in inflammatory cells forms, through which vessel and undifferentiated mesenchymal cell proliferation occurs, with the creation of a fibrovascular cellular scar tissue. This process does not occur in the inner zones.

Tear pattern

Tears can be subdivided into the following:

- **Vertical:**
  - Longitudinal: commonly peripheral; 'bucket-handle' tears are extensive longitudinal tears with subluxation of the free edge between the articular surfaces.
  - Radial: occur in the vertical plane, commonly at lateral aspect of LM; asymptomatic when small.
- **Horizontal:**
  - Pure cleavage.
  - Partial cleavage (flap tears): most commonly observed pattern.
- **Complex:** combination of above patterns; normally associated with degenerate meniscal tissue.

WHEN TO REPAIR?

Suggested criteria for repair are:

- **Location:** the red zone (0–3 mm from periphery) and some tears in the red-white zone (3–5 mm from periphery).
- **Tear pattern:** vertical longitudinal tears longer than 1 cm and radial tears extending into red zone.
- **Tissue quality:** not indicated in macerated and degenerate tissue.

Following the above criteria, 85 per cent healing rates have been reported.

Viva questions

1 Describe the anatomy of a meniscus.

2 Describe the vascular zones of the menisci.

3 What are the functions of the meniscus?

4 What is the usual mechanism of injury for a meniscal tear?

5 What are the indications for operative intervention for a meniscal tear?

FURTHER READING

Arnoczky, SP, Warren, RF. Microvasculature of the human meniscus. *Am J Sports Med* 1982;**10**:90–5.

Bullough, PG, Vosburgh, F, Arnoczky, SP, Levy, IM. The menisci of the knee. In JN Insall and WN Scott (eds), *Surgery of the Knee*. New York: Churchill Livingstone, 2001, pp. 135–46.

Kocher, MS, Klingele, K, Rassman, SO. Meniscal disorders: normal, discoid, and cysts. *Orthop Clin North Am* 2003;**34**:329–40.

Mow, VC, Arnoczky, SP, Jackson, DW (eds). *Knee Meniscus: Basic and Clinical Foundations*. New York: Raven Press, 1992.

Wojtys, EM, Chan, DB. Meniscus structure and function. *Instr Course Lect* 2005;**54**:323–30.

10

Articular cartilage

TIM WATERS AND GEORGE BENTLEY

INTRODUCTION

Hyaline (literally, 'glass-like') cartilage coats the articular surfaces of synovial joints. It is composed of individual chondrocytes bound together by an extracellular matrix. The function of hyaline cartilage is to distribute weight-bearing forces and reduce friction. It is **avascular**, **aneural**, **alymphatic** and almost **non-immunogenic**. It is nourished entirely via diffusion from the synovial fluid.

The major constituent of the extracellular matrix is **water** (75 per cent wet weight of articular cartilage), which is held in place by the negative charge of the proteoglycans (10–15 per cent wet weight). **Collagen** fibres (almost exclusively type II) constitute around 10–20 per cent wet weight (40–70 per cent dry weight), forming a meshwork with high tensile strength. **Chondrocytes** (5 per cent wet weight) manufacture and maintain the extracellular matrix.

Constituents of articular cartilage

- **Cells (chondrocytes)**
- **Extracellular matrix**
  - Fibres
    - Collagen
      - Type II, IX, XI
      - Type VI, X
    - Elastin
  - Ground substance
    - Water
    - Proteoglycans and glycosaminoglycans
      - Aggrecan
      - Hyaluronan
      - Decorin, byglycan, fibromodulin, syndecan, lumican, superficial zone protein
  - Glycoproteins
    - Cartilage oligomeric protein (COMP), laminin, lubricin, chondro-adherin
    - Cartilage matrix protein (CMP), cartilage matrix glycoprotein (CMGP), chondronectin, fibronectin, anchorin CII
  - Degradative enzymes (matrix metalloproteinases)
  - Extracellular ions

Approximately 90 per cent of the dry mass of the tissue is made of the proteoglycan aggrecan, type II collagen and hyaluronan.

STRUCTURE

LAYERS

The structure of articular cartilage can be divided into layers as seen on histological examination (Figure 10.1). The uppermost superficial layer is almost entirely collagen, with a few elongated cells. The **collagen concentration decreases** through the deeper

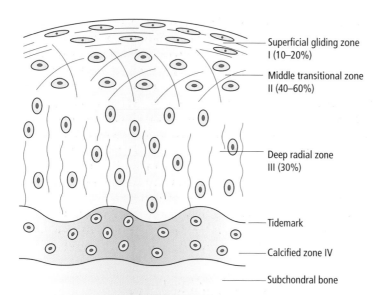

Superficial gliding zone
I (10–20%)

Middle transitional zone
II (40–60%)

Deep radial zone
III (30%)

Tidemark

Calcified zone IV

Subchondral bone

Figure 10.1 Layers of articular cartilage seen on histological section.

layers, as does the water concentration, from 80 per cent in the superficial layer to 65 per cent in the deep zone. Conversely, the proteoglycan concentration increases with depth.

The **superficial zone** (zone I, gliding zone) separates the cartilage from the surrounding tissue and fluid. This zone consists of a **lamina splendens**, a clear film of small collagen fibrils and a cellular layer of flattened chondrocytes one to three cells thick. The chondrocytes produce their own specific proteins and exhibit macrophage-like features, including phagocytosis and inflammatory characteristics. The superficial zone is the **thinnest layer**. It has the highest water and collagen content and the lowest level of proteoglycan synthesis. The superficial zone may also function as a barrier to the passage of large molecules from the synovial fluid. The **collagen fibres** lie parallel to the articular surface, and this tangential orientation allows the articular surface to resist shear stresses. In osteoarthritis, this zone is the first to show degenerative changes.

In the **transitional zone** (zone II, middle zone), the fibres are arranged obliquely and the proteoglycan concentration is higher. This zone forms the transition between the shearing forces of surface layer to compression forces in the deeper layers.

The **radial zone** (zone III, deep zone) is the largest part of the articular cartilage. The perpendicularly arranged collagen fibres distribute loads and resist compression.

The chondrocytes in zones II and III produce all the components of the extracellular matrix. The chondrocytes are spherical in shape. Although there are no intercellular junctions between chondrocytes, communities of two or more cells form **chondrons**. These share the same pericellular matrix, which differs in its composition and has a higher rate of turnover compared with the inter-territorial extracellular matrix between the chondrons.

The **tidemark** is the boundary between the calcified and uncalcified cartilage made visible by histological staining. It is cell-free and represents a **calcification front** that tends to migrate towards the surface with age.

In the **calcified zone** (zone IV), hydroxyapatite crystals anchor the cartilage to the subchondral bone. It forms a barrier to diffusion from blood vessels supplying the subchondral bone. **Type X collagen** is present mainly in the calcified cartilage layer.

COLLAGEN

Collagen synthesis takes place in stages both within and outside the chondrocyte. Polypeptide chains are formed and modified following messenger ribonucleic acid (mRNA) translation within the rough endoplasmic reticulum. The signal peptide is cleaved, lysine and proline residues are hydroxylated, and hydroxylysine residues are glycosylated. N-linked sugars are added to the terminal portion, and the modified polypeptide chains form **triple-helical molecules**. Disulphide bonds between and within the chains define the shape of the molecule. In the Golgi apparatus, the resultant **pro-collagen** is packed into secretory granules and released into the extracellular matrix via microtubules. Outside the cell, the terminal ends of pro-collagen uncoil and are cleaved to form **tropo-collagen fibrils**. These molecules combine via the cross-linkage of lysine and hydroxylysine residues. The resulting fibrils aggregate to form **collagen fibres**.

Approximately 90 per cent of the collagen in articular cartilage is type II. The collagen fibres are comprised of a core of types XI and II collagen surrounded by multiple layers of type II collagen. **Type XI collagen** is thought to regulate the diameter of the fibres, which is greater in the deeper zones.

Type IX collagen is found on the surface of the fibre. It has a chondroitin sulphate side chain and may act as a link to form collagen–proteoglycan complexes and regulate type II fibril formation.

Type VI collagen does not form fibres but is found in the pericellular region in a three-dimensional meshwork. It may help to carry some of the shear stresses and is probably involved in cell–matrix interactions. Its levels increase significantly in early osteoarthritis.

Type X collagen similarly forms a meshwork and is present in the calcified cartilage layer. It is associated with **cartilage calcification** and is produced by hypertrophied chondrocytes during endochondral ossification. It is therefore found in the physis, fracture callus, heterotopic ossification, calcifying cartilaginous tumours and osteoarthritis (see below).

Type I collagen is not found in normal articular cartilage but is present following injury in the subsequently formed fibrocartilage.

PROTEOGLYCANS AND GLYCOSAMINOGLYCANS

Proteoglycans are responsible for most of the water content of cartilage and also provide compressive strength to cartilage. They are large **hydrophilic** molecules containing chains of **glycosaminoglycans** (GAG) (chondroitin sulphate, keratan sulphate) bound by sugar bonds to a linear core of protein (Figure 10.2). GAGs have high negative charges from attached carboxyl and sulphate groups, which attract cations and water, thus increasing the osmotic pressure in the tissue. **Aggrecan** is the predominant proteoglycan in articular cartilage. Lesser proteoglycans present include decorin,

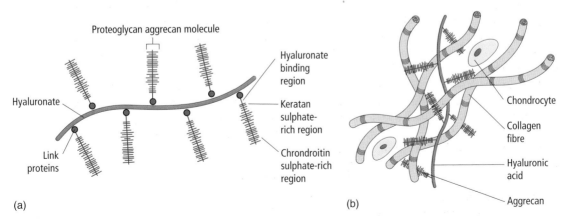

Figure 10.2 *(a) Structure of a proteoglycan aggregate and (b) relationship between cells and matrix components in articular cartilage.*

byglycan, fibromodulin, syndecan, lumican and superficial zone protein.

Aggrecan is heavily glycosylated with GAG components such as chondroitin sulphate and keratan sulphate. Aggrecan interacts with hyaluronic acid, stabilized via a link protein, to form a large (up to 50×10^6 MW) proteoglycan aggregate (Figure 10.2). Influx of water is limited to approximately 40 per cent of maximum hydration by the collagen meshwork, which physically prevents further expansion. These properties provide the compressive strength of the tissue to mechanical loading.

DEGRADATIVE ENZYMES

The matrix metalloproteinases are classified into **collagenases, stromelysins, gelatinases and membrane-associated metalloproteinases**. These degrade collagen and proteoglycan aggregates as part of the normal turnover of the matrix constituents. Balancing this action are the proteinase inhibitors. **Tissue-induced metalloproteinase inhibitors** (TIMPs) are acidic polypeptides that prevent degradation by the metalloproteinases by binding to the matrix proteins. The avascular nature of articular cartilage is maintained by TIMPs that inhibit the proteases produced by migrating vascular endothelium. TIMPs may form the basis of future drugs that inhibit the excessive expression of matrix metalloproteinases, which may be responsible for the progression and severity of osteoarthritis.

IONS

Cartilage typically has a high **sodium** and **potassium** ion content. The sulphate residues on proteoglycans attract these cations. Extracellular calcium tends to be highly concentrated in the calcified zone. In the deep and superficial zones, calcium ions are in lower concentrations than in the plasma and are buffered by the sulphate residues.

GLYCOPROTEINS

Sparsely distributed through the extracellular matrix, these macromolecules act as 'tissue glue',

binding to various constituents of the matrix and the chondrocyte surface. Glycoproteins include COMP, which binds to various matrix proteins, chondrocalcin, a calcium-binding glycoprotein, and laminin, which is found in the pericellular matrix of chondrocytes. Lubricin, found in synovial fluid, is thought to act as a joint lubricant. Other glycoproteins involved with the anchorage of chondrocytes include chondro-adherin, CMP, CMGP and chondronectin.

CHONDROCYTES

The articular chondrocyte is derived from uncommitted mesenchymal stem cells. Chondroblasts proliferate during fetal development, and the majority of cartilage transforms into bone through endochondral ossification, with the growth plate and cartilaginous epiphyses persisting after birth. At skeletal maturity, the articular surface is the only remaining cartilaginous part. Articular chondrocytes and growth plate chondrocytes represent different pathways of terminal differentiation. The matrix and synovial fluid environment play extremely important roles in the maintenance of the phenotype of articular chondrocytes. Once committed to one of these pathways, the cell phenotype is not usually reversible, although if growth plate chondrocytes are positioned in an articular defect the surface layers take on the appearance of articular cartilage.

Being avascular, cell nutrition takes place via diffusion from the synovial fluid. Although the exact mechanism is poorly understood, a simple explanation is that when the joint is not under load, the cartilage (being highly hydrophilic) absorbs synovial fluid. Under load, fluid is squeezed out, and with it metabolic waste. Absence of joint loading fails to maintain adequate nutrition and therefore predisposes to degeneration.

In **osteoarthritis**, chondrocytes mimic the events of endochondral bone formation, with **chondrocyte proliferation**, and hypertrophy, with expression of **type X collagen, alkaline phosphatase, matrix vesicles** and **matrix calcification**. This may explain the subchondral sclerosis seen on radiographs, as endochondral ossification occurs in the deep layer of the articular cartilage.

The metabolic rate of chondrocytes is generally very low. Deeper cartilage zones contain chondrocytes with decreased rough endoplasmic reticulum and increased degenerative products (increased intraplasmic filaments). The half-life of proteoglycans is weeks to months; that of collagen is several years or possibly even longer. The extracellular matrix in the immediate vicinity of the chondrocytes or chondron may, however, have a relatively high turnover. A large proportion of chondrocyte energy utilization is via the lactic-acid pathway, even in the presence of high oxygen and glucose concentrations.

Various hormones, growth factors and cytokines influence chondrocytes. Fibroblast growth factor (FGF) stimulates adult chondrocyte deoxyribonucleic acid (DNA) synthesis. Insulin-like growth factor I (IGF-I) stimulates adult chondrocyte DNA and matrix synthesis. Parathyroid hormone (PTH) and thyroxine stimulate matrix synthesis. Abnormal production of some of these factors has been implicated in the pathogenesis of rheumatoid arthritis and osteoarthritis.

FUNCTION

The main functions of articular cartilage are **joint lubrication** (allowing movement between opposing surfaces with the minimum of friction and wear) and **shock absorption** (distributing joint loads and therefore reducing the stresses experienced). Articular cartilage has a very low coefficient of friction (0.002), 30 times smoother than most modern joint replacements. This coefficient of friction can be lowered further by fluid-film formation, elastic deformation of articular cartilage, synovial fluid and efflux of fluid from cartilage. The coefficient of friction can be increased by fibrillation of articular cartilage.

BIOMECHANICAL PROPERTIES

Cartilage is ten times more effective a shock absorber than bone. Cartilage protects bone by diffusing the load. Cartilage is a **biphasic** material that is **visco-elastic** (like a water-soaked sponge). With respect to its visco-elasticity, cartilage undergoes **creep** (under constant load, it initially deforms rapidly, increasing the surface area through which to dissipate the force, followed by slow deformation until a steady state is reached) and **stress relaxation** (under constant deformation, high initial stress is followed by progressively decreasing stress to the level required to maintain the deformation). These properties occur through **macromolecular** and **water movement**. Seventy per cent of the water present is intermolecular and can move when a load or pressure gradient is applied.

Cartilage is freely permeable to water, but under high compressive loads water movement is hindered by the frictional drag of the macromolecules. This decreases the flow and stiffens cartilage, allowing greater resistance to higher loads. Cartilage is also **anisotropic**, having different mechanical properties depending on the direction in which it is loaded. This is due to the collagen fibre arrangements, cross-links and collagen–proteoglycan interactions.

In tension, the molecular structure of articular cartilage, the organization of collagen fibres, and the collagen fibre cross-links are altered. Cartilage is pulled apart, which increases water permeability. This in turn decreases compressive stiffness.

LUBRICATION

In classical engineering terms, there are two types of lubrication: **boundary** and **fluid-film**. The ideas behind joint lubrication have been extrapolated from these, although the exact mechanisms have not been elucidated fully in humans. Each type of lubrication probably comes into play at a different point in the movement of the joint.

Boundary lubrication involves a monolayer of lubricant molecule (probably the glycoprotein lubricin) adsorbed on each surface (boundary) of the joint. This prevents direct articular contact and is most important at rest or under load. In **fluid-film lubrication**, a thin layer of fluid increases the separation of the two surfaces. The following methods are described:

- **Hydrodynamic lubrication:** the two surfaces are at an angle to each other. The viscosity in the resulting wedge of fluid separates the two surfaces.
- **Squeeze-film lubrication:** the two surfaces are parallel and move perpendicularly to each other. The viscosity of the incompressible fluid maintains the lubrication. High loads can be carried for short lengths of time. As the layer of fluid lubricant is forced out, it becomes thinner and the joint surfaces come into contact, but they are still protected by the lubricin.
- **Elastohydrodynamic lubrication:** this occurs as speed increases and is similar to squeeze film, but the yielding articular surface creates a larger surface area when compressed by the fluid. There is less dissipation of the fluid-film, and therefore the load is sustained for a longer period. This is the predominant lubrication mechanism in synovial joints during dynamic joint function.

Synovial joints, being non-rigid structures, exhibit modified forms of boundary and fluid-film lubrication. When movement begins, boundary lubrication is exhibited at points of close contact of the two surfaces and fluid-film elsewhere.

Two other forms of lubrication are also thought to occur between the static state with boundary lubrication and the elastohydro-dynamic lubrication seen at speed:

- **Weeping or self-lubrication:** articular cartilage is variably permeable to fluid, depending on whether it is loaded. As the articular cartilage of the joint slides under compression, fluid is exuded under and in front of the leading edge of the load, enhancing lubrication. As the load decreases after maximum compression, water is once again imbibed and the articular cartilage reforms its shape.
- **Boosted lubrication:** the solvent part of the lubricant enters the articular cartilage, which leaves behind the concentrated hyaluronic

acid complexes as a lubricant in 'trapped pools' of concentrated synovial fluid.

INJURY AND HEALING

SUPERFICIAL INJURIES

Superficial lacerations (above the tidemark) do not heal. This region is completely avascular. Although peripheral chondrocytes may increase matrix synthesis and proliferate, they do not migrate actively enough into the defect to effect repair.

DEEP INJURIES

Lacerations that extend below the tidemark to subchondral bone result in haematoma, fibrin clot and activation of the inflammatory response. This acts as a scaffold for the formation of fibrocartilage, produced by the undifferentiated mesenchymal cells that have migrated into the defect. This differs from hyaline cartilage in that it consists of disorganized bundles of type I collagen and is therefore not really suitable for repetitive load-bearing.

INFECTION AND INFLAMMATION

Infection can be devastating to the articular surface. This can be as a direct result of the organism itself, such as the chondrocyte proteases of *Staphylococcus aureus*, or due to the host's inflammatory response. Polymorphs stimulate production of cytokines and other inflammatory products, which cause hydrolysis of collagen and proteoglycans. Destruction of cells and the release of lysosomal enzymes (e.g. collagenases, proteases, galactosidases) further injures the joint.

CHANGES IN OSTEOARTHRITIC CARTILAGE

Collagen is disrupted either by direct trauma or by an increase in degrading enzyme concentration. Interference with the collagen meshwork allows the proteoglycans to attract more water. This 'softens' the articular cartilage and decreases its Young's modulus of elasticity, reducing its ability to bear load. The increased permeability also allows the **loss of lubricant**, which in turn leads to increased interfacial wear.

In addition, cartilage bearing surface deformation occurs under load with repetitive stressing, leading to fatigue wear and accumulation of microscopic damage. Fatigue wear occurs due to either high stress and low cycle loading or low stress and high cycle loading. This causes damage by three mechanisms:

- disruption of the collagen–proteoglycan matrix (occurs with increasing age);
- leaching out of proteoglycan by repeated large interstitial fluid movements in the superficial layer, leading to increased permeability and decreased stiffness;
- rapid repeat high loading, where there is no

time for stress relaxation, leading to collagen–proteoglycan matrix damage.

Chondrocytes attempt to compensate by increasing their rate of synthesis of DNA, collagen and proteoglycans. Chondrocytes proliferate and hypertrophy with expression of type X collagen, alkaline phosphatase and matrix vesicles and increased matrix calcification. However, the levels of proteoglycans eventually decrease, and the chains become shorter. The **chondroitin/keratan sulphate ratio** is **increased**. Levels of metalloproteinases and interleukin 1 (IL-1) increase, which has a further catabolic effect on the matrix.

Table 10.1 shows the biochemical changes seen with ageing and osteoarthritis in cartilage.

Table 10.1 Biochemical changes seen with ageing and osteoarthritis in cartilage

	Ageing	Osteoarthritis
Water content	Decreases	Increases (90% compared with normally 65–80%)
Synthetic activity	Decreases	Increases
Collagen	Unchanged	Breakdown of matrix framework leads to decrease in collagen, but relative concentration increases due to loss of PGs
PG content	Decreases (length of protein core and GAG chains decreases)	Decreases
PG synthesis	Decreases	Increases
PG degradation	Decreases	Increases very significantly
Chondroitin sulphate (both 4- and 6-)	Decreases	Increases
Keratan sulphate	Increases	Decreases
Chondrocyte size	Increases	
Chondrocyte number	Decreases	
Modulus of elasticity	Increases	Decreases due to increased water content; increased water content also causes increased permeability and decreased strength
Enzymes		Increased activity of MMPs
Matrix subunit molecules		Increased levels, e.g. COMP, aggrecan (in synovial fluid and serum)

COMP, cartilage oligomeric protein; GAG, glycosaminoglycans; MMP, matrix metalloproteinase; PG, proteoglycan.

The collagen–proteoglycan matrix may be disrupted by mechanical damage (as shown above, but also accelerated by factors such as ligament rupture and joint incongruity) and biochemical damage (such as proteolytic enzyme degradation, disordered collagen metabolism and abnormal collagen production). The water content decreases due to the loss of the hydrophilic components. Macroscopically, the surface exhibits fibrillation (vertical splits) followed by the development of deep fissures and erosions.

TREATMENT

NON-OPERATIVE TREATMENT

Physical therapy

The maintenance of motion is vital to nutrition and healing of the damaged joint. As detailed above, loading of the joint is essential in order to allow diffusion of synovial fluid and thus metabolic turnover of the cartilage. Hence, immobilization leads to cartilage atrophy, whereas physical therapy is therapeutic. Salter (1989) has shown that continuous passive movement may be beneficial in the healing of full-thickness articular defects in rabbits, although this has yet to be demonstrated in humans.

Oral visco-supplementation

Nutritional supplements, especially those advertised as being beneficial to joints, constitute a multi-million-pound industry. **Glucosamine** is an amino-monosaccharide sugar and is a naturally occurring component of the glycosaminoglycans keratan sulphate and hyaluronate. **Chondroitin** is another glycosaminoglycan. Of these, glucosamine is the only substance to have been evaluated in clinical trials and to have shown some benefit. Produced either synthetically or from shells, glucosamine is sold as glucosamine sulphate and glucosamine hydrochloride. In vitro studies have demonstrated the **effect of glucosamine in reversing the inhibition of proteoglycan synthesis by IL-1 and suppressing the inflammatory response of neutrophils.** Several randomized studies have shown the efficacy of glucosamine in knee osteoarthritis, but the methodology and outcome measures used have been criticized widely in the literature. Nonetheless, it is likely that some benefit is obtained from glucosamine, and in view of the very low risk of side effects (shellfish allergy, occasional gastrointestinal symptoms) and the low cost of glucosamine, it is worth trying. Most trials used a dose of 1500 mg/day, but there is variety in the consistency of available formulations.

Intra-articular visco-supplementation

This aims to replace lost hyaluronan and improve the visco-elastic properties of the articular cartilage. Several products have been produced. Preparations are of relatively low molecular weight (e.g. Hyalgan™), intermediate molecular weight but lower than that of normal healthy synovial fluid (e.g. Orthovisc™), or cross-linked hyaluronan of high molecular weight (e.g. Synvisc™). As with oral supplements, many of the studies showing efficacy have an element of publication bias, with poor numbers and outcome measures. An independent randomized study by Leopold et al. (2003) concluded no significant difference between hylan G-F 20 (Synvisc™) and corticosteroid injection and it was therefore not cost-effective. This study excluded osteoarthritis with bone-on-bone contact, and the authors agree that visco-supplementation may have a role to play in patients with this condition.

OPERATIVE TREATMENT

Abrasion arthroplasty

This is essentially **cartilage repair** from subchondral bone. By turning the cartilage defect into a 'deep injury', undifferentiated mesenchymal stem cells (MSCs) proliferate in the defect when the subchondral bone plate is penetrated. They subsequently differentiate into fibrocartilage. This repair tissue initially has a moderately high proportion of proteoglycan and some type II collagen, but, as mentioned above, the proteoglycan content decreases and the disorganized collagen reverts to predominantly type I collagen. Moreover, there is usually incomplete integration of the fibrocartilaginous tissue with the adjacent normal articular cartilage, and the resultant tissue therefore is not very resistant to shear stress. However, this crude repair may still alleviate symptoms for several years.

Autograft/mosaicplasty

Full-thickness osteochondral grafts from the least weight-bearing periphery of the articular surface (superomedial margin of the femoral notch) are transplanted into the cartilage defect. This method was found to be of most benefit in the medial compartment of the knee and of less value for patellar lesions. However, modern tissue engineering therapies appear to be superseding this form of treatment. The use of other autografts, such as a portion of the patella in the recreation of the tibial articular surface, has generally had poor results.

Allograft

Cadaveric osteochondral allografts have been used most extensively for reconstruction after resection of malignant tumours. The cartilage is usually frozen with a cryoprotectant such as glycerol, which prevents rupture of the cell membranes during the freezing process. Some of the chondrocytes will therefore remain viable when the tissue is thawed. The bony part of the graft acts as a scaffold for the allograft cartilage surface, which can integrate into the adjacent host bone. It is this integration that is crucial for the graft's survival, and therefore it is important to size it correctly. Any mismatch increases degradation due to excessive contact forces. Since the collagen and proteoglycan matrix makes the cells inaccessible to antibodies and T-cells, cartilage is considered an immunogenically privileged tissue. However, several reports of infection with spore-forming organisms following transplant have been published, and there is concern regarding the possibility of viral or prion transmission.

PERIOSTEAL/PERICHONDRIAL MESENCHYMAL STEM CELLS

Periosteum and perichondrium both contain significant numbers of stem cells, which can be used to differentiate into hyaline cartilage. Rib perichondrium or periosteum can be used. The cambium layer (the layer next to the bone or cartilage from which it is harvested) contains the greatest number of MSCs and is positioned towards the synovial side of the defect. In the case of deep defects, the periosteum is sutured into place on top of the bone graft. The periosteum or perichondrium may differentiate into hyaline cartilage under these circumstances. Unlike abrasion arthroplasty, type II collagen and high levels of proteoglycan are seen in the repair tissue. There are no convincing reports of the efficacy of this method in clinical practice.

CHONDROCYTES FROM MESENCHYMAL STEM CELLS

MSCs are isolated from bone marrow using tissue culture plates. The stromal cells, including the MSCs, adhere and can then be cultured. Using periosteum, the MSCs are released from the cambium layer using an enzymatic treatment. By placing the MSCs in a three-dimensional matrix (e.g. collagen or alginate), the MSCs will differentiate into chondrocytes. These continue to proliferate when introduced into a collagen gel, which is inserted into the defect and forms hyaline cartilage. The deep part undergoes endochondral ossification, leading to a normal bone–cartilage interface.

AUTOLOGOUS CHONDROCYTE IMPLANTATION

Brittberg et al. (1994) first reported the autologous chondrocyte implantation (ACI) technique. A small amount of cartilage from a non-weight-bearing articular surface can be harvested and the cells isolated. Although the rate of chondrocyte proliferation is extremely low in vivo, chondrocytes can undergo many cell divisions in tissue culture, expanding the population considerably. After 4–5 weeks, the cells are suspended in a collagen gel carrier and re-implanted at a subsequent operation. A periosteal or collagen flap is sutured over the articular cartilage defect, and the cultured chondrocytes are injected beneath it. Needle biopsies have demonstrated histologically normal hyaline cartilage grown in the defect after 1–2 years. More recent techniques involve growing the cells on a collagen membrane before implantation – matrix-induced autologous chondrocyte implantation (MACI) – and suspending the cells in a three-dimensional polymer fleece or hyaluron-based scaffold, which is implanted into the defect without the need for a covering flap.

ROLE OF GROWTH FACTORS

A variety of growth factors are produced by chondrocytes, including FGF, IGF-1, transforming growth factor (TGF), platelet-derived growth factor (PGDF) and bone morphogenic proteins (BMPs). There have been limited studies into the effect of these factors on articular cartilage repair. Although promising, none of these studies has shown any overall efficacy in human trials.

TGF, IGF-1 and FGF stimulate chondrocyte proliferation. IGF-1 appears to stimulate collagen and proteoglycan production; TGF stimulates proteoglycan synthesis while suppressing type II collagen synthesis. TGF, when injected subperiosteally, leads to chondrocyte differentiation from the periosteum; unfortunately, when administered intra-articularly, TFG causes a synovitis that masks any therapeutic effect on the articular cartilage.

Intra-articular FGF has been shown to increase the amount of articular cartilage, but it enhances proteoglycan degradation and essentially weakens the overall cartilage. However, FGF injected into partial-thickness defects has been shown to stimulate filling of the defect with fibroblasts from MSCs recruited from the synovium. No differentiation to hyaline cartilage occurred.

Some success in reconstituting relatively normal-appearing hyaline cartilage has been shown with defects implanted with BMPs and also filled with a collagen gel containing liposomes of encapsulated TGF.

Viva questions

1 What is the composition of articular cartilage?

2 Draw the structure of articular cartilage.

3 What are the functions of articular cartilage? How is structure related to function?

4 What pathological processes are involved in the development of osteoarthritis?

5 What are the different options available for treating cartilage defects?

FURTHER READING

Bentley, G, Biant, LC, Carrington, RW, *et al.* A prospective, randomised comparison of autologous chondrocyte implantation versus mosaicplasty for osteochondral defects in the knee. *J Bone Joint Surg Br* 2003;**85**:223–30.

Brittberg, M, Lindahl, A, Nilsson, A, *et al.* Treatment of deep cartilage defects in the knee with autologous chondrocyte transplantation. *N Engl J Med* 1994;**331**:889–95.

Leopold, SS, Redd, BB, Warme, WJ, *et al.* Corticosteroid compared with hyaluronic acid injections for the treatment of osteoarthritis of the knee: a prospective, randomized trial. *J Bone Joint Surg Am* 2003;**85**:1197–203.

Salter, RB. The biologic concept of continuous passive motion of synovial joints: the first 18 years of basic research and its clinical application. *Clin Orthop* 1989;**242**:12–25.

Ulrich-Vinther, M, Maloney, MD, Schwarz, EM, Rosier, R, O'Keefe, RJ. Articular cartilage biology. *J Am Acad Orthop Surg* 2003;**11**:421–30.

Nerve

CAROLINE HING AND ROLFE BIRCH

INTRODUCTION

An understanding of the structure and function of nerves is important in appreciating how the body reacts to changes in its environment. The microstructure of a nerve relates to its function and also determines how well the nerve recovers from injury.

STRUCTURE OF A NERVE

Components of the nervous system

- **Central nervous system:** brain and spinal cord.

- **Peripheral nervous system:** cranial, spinal and peripheral nerves.

- **Autonomic nervous system:** sympathetic and parasympathetic systems.

The **central nervous system** controls somatic and visceral function. The **peripheral nervous system** relays information from the periphery to the brain, and vice versa. **Afferent** (sensory) nerve fibres transmit somatic and visceral information from the periphery to the brain. **Efferent** (motor) nerve fibres transmit somatic and autonomic information from the brain to the periphery (Figure 11.1). Nerves can be classified according to their degree of myelination, diameter and speed of conduction (Table 11.1).

The macroscopic structure of a nerve is related to its function. The basic functional unit of a nerve is a **neuron** comprising of a **cell body** (perikaryon) and an **axon**. The **axolemma** (cell membrane) encloses the **axoplasm** (cytoplasm). The contents of the nerve cell include microtubules, vesicles, axoplasmic reticulum, and lamellar and multivesicular bodies that comprise the cytoskeleton and are involved in axonal transport and nutrition. **Dendrites** branch out from the cell body and conduct impulses to other cell bodies.

A nerve is composed of **fascicles** or **bundles** (groups of sheathed axons) of nerve fibres (axon embedded in a Schwann cell). The **endoneurium** is the connective tissue covering the nerve fibre; it consists of longitudinally arranged collagen fibres, fibroblasts and blood vessels. The **perineurium** envelops the nerve fibre bundles, forming a fascicle; it consists of alternating layers of collagen and cell processes acting as a diffusion barrier. Finally, the **epineurium**, consisting of collagen and fibroblasts, acts as a supporting structure for the nerve fascicles grouped into a nerve trunk (Figure 11.2).

The blood supply of nerves consists of **intrinsic** and **extrinsic plexuses**. The extrinsic vessels are segmental and found in the **paraneurium**, a layer external to the perineurium. The intrinsic vessels are

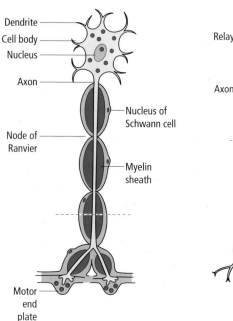

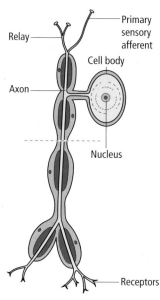

Figure 11.1 *Motor and sensory units.*

Table 11.1 Classification of nerves

Axon type	Myelination	Diameter(μm)	Speed(m/s)	Function
Aα	Myelinated	20	100	Efferent to skeletal muscle; afferent from muscle spindles and tendon stretch organelles
Aβ	Myelinated	10	50	Organized sensory receptors, e.g. Merkel, Meissner, Pacinian, Ruffini, hair follicles
Aγ	Myelinated	5	20	Efferent to muscle spindles
Aδ	Myelinated	5	20	Fast pain (e.g. knife), cold sensation, touch
B	Myelinated	3	10	Preganglionic autonomic
C	Unmyelinated	1	2	Postganglionic autonomic slow pain (e.g. nettles), thermoreceptors

distributed in a longitudinal fashion in the epineurium, perineurium and endoneurium.

The neuron is supported in the extracellular space by **glial cells**. In the central nervous system, glial cells comprise **oligodendrocytes** (responsible for **myelination**), **astrocytes** and **microglia**. The myelin sheath is formed by cytoplasmic extensions from the oligodendrocytes; unlike the myelin sheaths of the peripheral nervous system, the central

nervous system myelin sheath does not possess a neurilemma. Astrocytes regulate extracellular potassium concentration and neurotransmitters as well as storing and transfer metabolites from blood vessels to the neurons. Microglia are thought to play a phagocytic role, defending the central nervous system from noxious stimuli.

Schwann cells are the glial cells that arise from the **neuroectoderm** and are responsible for myelination of peripheral nerves. The size of

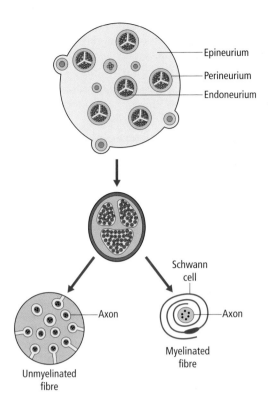

Figure 11.2 *Cross-section of nerve.*

the axon determines whether it will be myelinated. Larger axons are invaginated into a series of Schwann cells that lay down the myelin sheath in spiral layers and form a **neurilemma** on the outside, with each Schwann cell contributing myelin to one segment (**internode**) of the axon. The myelin sheath has a multilaminar structure that is high in lipids and proteins and is traversed by cytoplasmic channels that facilitates conduction. The smaller axons are arranged in bundles enveloped by Schwann cell cytoplasm with no myelin sheath.

At the end of the internode, the axon has an increased diameter and forms the **paranode**. In this region, the axon and its myelin sheath are crenated with the myelin lamellae, ending in terminal loops of Schwann cell cytoplasm.

The **nodes of Ranvier** are gaps between adjacent Schwann cell internodes along myelinated axons. The nodes are important in **saltatory conduction** (see Figure 11.1). In this region, the axon diameter is reduced slightly, the diameter of the axon being inversely proportional

to the length of the node of Ranvier. The concentration of sodium channels is increased in this region to facilitate saltatory conduction.

Axonal transport occurs in both an antegrade and a retrograde fashion along the axon. Axonal transport is important in maintaining the structure of nerves and the supply of neurotransmitters. Transport can occur in a fast or slow fashion and is adenosine triphosphate (ATP) energy-dependent, making it vulnerable to injury, anoxia and ischaemia. Microtubule and microfilament components are transported slowly in an antegrade direction. Neurotransmitters are also transported in an antegrade direction, but by a faster mechanism. Once the neurotransmitters have been released at the synapse, the neurotransmitter vesicles are transported in a retrograde direction for recycling by the cell body.

ACTION POTENTIALS AND THEIR PROPAGATION

Neurons are bound by a lipoprotein cell membrane and possess a **membrane potential** of $-70\,mV$ due to the voltage difference between the intracellular and extracellular space. This voltage difference is due to the high concentration of potassium ions $[K^+]$ and low concentration of sodium ions $[Na^+]$ and chloride ion $[Cl^-]$ within the cell. In the extracellular space, there is a low concentration of $[K^+]$ and a high concentration of $[Na^+]$ and $[Cl^-]$. The different ionic concentrations in the intracellular and extracellular spaces are maintained by:

- a **lipid membrane**, which prevents the passage of water-soluble ions;
- **selectively permeable** ion channels;
- a metabolically active Na^+/K^+ **exchange pump**;
- **Donnan equilibrium** (irregular distribution of permeant ions across an impermeant membrane when a large impermeable organic ion is present on one side).

Cl^- ions diffuse out of the cell through the lipid membrane. The Na^+/K^+ exchange pump maintains a high concentration of $[K^+]$ in the

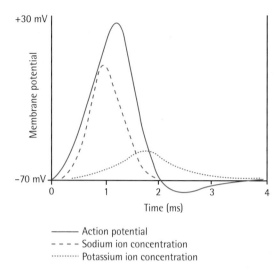

Figure 11.3 *Relationship of membrane potential to Na⁺ and K⁺ concentrations.*

cell and a high concentration of [Na⁺] in the extracellular space. Voltage-dependent ion channels exist for both K⁺ and Na⁺ ions. The voltage-gated Na⁺ channel can be in a resting closed state, or an active open state following membrane depolarization, or an inactivated closed state. The voltage-gated K⁺ channels can be open when the membrane is depolarized or closed during the resting potential (Figure 11.3).

The **threshold stimulus** is the minimum stimulus intensity needed to produce an action potential. A smaller stimulus (**subthreshold**) will not produce a stimulus. However, **summation** of a number of subthreshold stimuli may be sufficient to incite a response.

An **action potential** occurs when a neuron is stimulated, resulting in the opening of the Na channels and an in-rush of Na⁺ ions into the cell. The channels are dependent on oxygen and ATP. This results in **depolarization** of the membrane from its initial resting state of –70 mV due to **ionic conductance**, and the polarity across the cell membrane becomes **positive**. This also triggers the opening of more Na⁺ channels. The Na⁺ channels remain open for 1 ms before closing. For a few milliseconds after closing, they cannot reopen (the **refractory period**), thus limiting the number of stimuli to which a nerve can respond.

Repolarization of the membrane results from the passage of K⁺ ions out of the cell through K⁺ channels. The **electrical potential** falls to below the original –70-mV resting potential due to the delay in closure of the K⁺ channels and the time taken for the Na⁺ channels to convert from an inactive to a resting state. The Na⁺/K⁺ exchange pump then restores the cell to its original resting potential.

The local change in potential of an area of the nerve fibre membrane compared with an adjacent area at resting potential generates a current, resulting in the **propagation** of the action potential. The speed of propagation will depend on the axon fibre diameter and the degree of myelination. In myelinated fibres, the action potential cannot propagate across the myelin and instead 'jumps' (**saltatory conduction**) across the nodes of Ranvier. This increases the efficiency of the cell, resulting in fast conduction with minimum metabolic activity. Saltatory conduction is analogous to the electrical conduction of a capacitor, in contrast to the wave of chemical depolarization present in non-myelinated fibres.

Neurons communicate with each other via a **synapse**, which can be chemical or electrical. In humans, chemical synapses predominate. Synapses occur between the terminal branch of one axon and the cell body dendrites of another axon. An action potential causes the release of **neurotransmitters** from synaptic vesicles. The neurotransmitter diffuses across the synaptic cleft to the postsynaptic membrane, which it either excites (**excitatory postsynaptic potentials**) or inhibits (**inhibitory postsynaptic potentials**). Examples of neurotransmitters include acetylcholine (preganglionic synapses, parasympathetic postganglionic synapses, sympathetic efferent to sweat glands, somatic efferent synapses), adrenaline (sympathetic postganglionic synapses), noradrenaline (sympathetic postganglionic synapses), serotonin and histamine.

FUNCTION OF NERVES

As described previously, the nervous system consists of the central, peripheral and

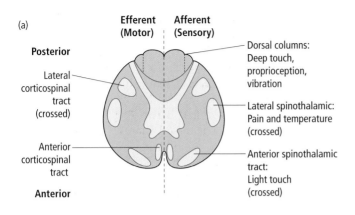

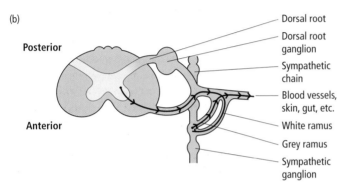

Figure 11.4 *(a) Cross-section of spinal cord and (b) autonomic pathways.*

autonomic nervous systems. The central nervous system consists of the brain and spinal cord, which terminates at the level of the first lumbar vertebra. The peripheral nervous system consists of 12 pairs of **cranial nerves** and 31 pairs of **spinal nerves**.

PERIPHERAL NERVOUS SYSTEM

The spinal nerves divide close to the spinal cord, forming a **sensory dorsal root** and a **motor ventral root**. The cell body of the sensory nerve is situated in the dorsal root ganglion. The motor nerve's cell body is situated in the spinal cord (Figure 11.4).

The sensory (afferent) nervous system relays impulses from superficial and deep sensory receptors. There is a functional specificity of nerve fibres and their organelles. Superficial sensory receptors can be divided further into **mechanoreceptors**, **thermoreceptors** and **nociceptors**.

Examples of mechanoreceptors in and below human skin are given in Table 11.2.

Table 11.2 Examples of mechanoreceptors in and below human skin

	Receptor status	Sensitive to	Innervated by
Merkel cell	*Slowly adapting*	*Sustained pressure*	*Fast, myelinated Aβ*
Meissner's corpuscle	*Rapidly adapting*	*Changing stimuli*	*Fast, myelinated Aβ*
Ruffini's corpuscle	*Slowly adapting*		*Fast, myelinated Aβ*
Pacinian corpuscle	*Rapidly adapting*		*Fast, myelinated Aβ*
Hair follicle receptor			*Fast, myelinated Aβ and Aδ*

Thermoreceptors are of two types – **cooling receptors** and **warming receptors**. These receptors detect changes in the environmental temperature and are innervated by myelinated fast Aδ and unmyelinated slow C fibres.

Nociceptors respond to noxious stimuli and consist of **mechanical**, **thermal**, **mechanothermal** and **polymodal** receptors. Myelinated fast Aδ and unmyelinated slow C fibres innervate these receptors.

Deep sensation from muscles, ligaments, tendons and joints occurs via free nerve endings and receptors, such as the following:

- **Muscle spindles:** consist of intrafusal nuclear bag fibres and nuclear chain fibres within the muscle itself. Innervated by myelinated afferent sensory Aα fibres and efferent motor Aγ fibres (Figure 11.5).
- **Golgi tendon organs:** found near neuromuscular junctions. Consist of small bundles of tendon fibres enclosed in a capsule of concentric cytoplasmic sheets. The capsule is pierced by myelinated Aα nerve fibres that divide and wrap around the tendon fasciculi. Activated by passive stretch and important in proprioception. Slowly adapting.

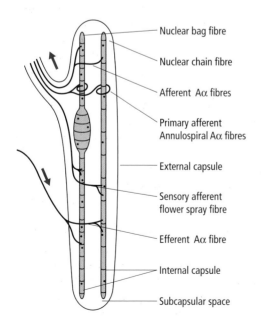

Figure 11.5 *Muscle spindle.*

- **Paciniform receptors:** lamellated receptors. Smaller than Pacinian corpuscles. Rapidly adapting low-threshold mechanoreceptors found in joint capsules. Supplied by myelinated Aα afferent fibres.

In the motor system, transmission of impulses to the muscle is via the **motor end plate**. The motor end plate consists of a **neural ending** and a **muscle sole plate**. There are two types of neural ending – the extrafusal Aα (**en plaque**) ending and the intrafusal Aγ (**plate**) ending. The muscle action potential is initiated by acetylcholine release at these endings.

AUTONOMIC NERVOUS SYSTEM

The autonomic nervous system can be divided into the **sympathetic** and **parasympathetic** systems. The autonomic nervous system comprises both central and peripheral components and forms the visceral part of the nervous system. The visceral and somatic afferent pathways are similar, with neurons from the periphery passing without interruption through autonomic ganglia or plexuses before accompanying somatic afferents in the dorsal spinal roots to the central nervous system. Unlike the somatic counterpart, the visceral efferent pathways are comprised of multiple preganglionic and postganglionic neurons with corresponding synapses. This facilitates the relay of many autonomic effects.

The sympathetic system controls sweating, vasoconstriction, contraction of erector pilae, sphincteric contraction, bronchial dilation, papillary dilation, reduction of gut motility and cardiac stimulation. The **sympathetic nervous system** consists of **preganglionic myelinated efferent axons** from the grey matter of the first thoracic to second lumbar levels of the spinal cord. The axons emerge from the spinal cord through the ventral spinal roots, before passing via the **white rami communicantes** to synapse in the paravertebral or axial ganglia. The ganglia function as relay stations, where axons traverse or synapse with other axons, allowing amplification and dissemination of signals. The ganglia consist of a connective tissue capsule surrounding groups of neurons, fibroblasts, satellite cells and capillaries. Postganglionic

Labels for Figure 11.5:
- Nuclear bag fibre
- Nuclear chain fibre
- Afferent Aα fibres
- Primary afferent Annulospiral Aα fibres
- External capsule
- Sensory afferent flower spray fibre
- Efferent Aα fibre
- Internal capsule
- Subcapsular space

neurons leave the ganglia and reach their target in one of several ways:

- Pass direct to the viscera.
- Pass direct to adjacent blood vessels.
- Pass via the grey rami communicantes, the axons return to their originating spinal nerve and on to blood vessels, erector pilae and sweat glands.
- Pass along the sympathetic trunk to another level.

The functional difference between white and grey rami communicantes is illustrated by **Horner's syndrome**. Interruption of the white rami communicans of the cervicothoracic ganglion interrupts the preganglionic fibre pathways to the superior cervical ganglion, which supplies postganglionic fibres to muscles of the eyelid, dilator pupillae and secretory glands. Hence, injury to the white ramus causes ptosis, meiosis, enophthalmos and loss of sweating – Horner's syndrome. Interruption of the grey rami communicans at this level sympathectomizes the limb alone and does not cause Horner's syndrome, as the axons have already synapsed in the cervicothoracic ganglion.

The parasympathetic nervous system consists of efferent myelinated preganglionic fibres from nuclei in the brain (via the **oculomotor**, **facial**, **glossopharyngeal**, **vagus** and **accessory** nerves) and second to fourth sacral spinal nerves. The peripheral ganglia of the parasympathetic system include the cranial ganglia (**ciliary**, **pterygopalatine**, **submandibular** and **otic**), which are efferent. Afferent and postganglionic parasympathetic fibres also pass through these ganglia but do not synapse within them. The postganglionic parasympathetic non-myelinated axons synapse close to their target organs. The parasympathetic nervous system has an inhibitory effect on the heart (as well as causing dilation of blood vessels), bladder and bowel.

NERVE INJURY AND REPAIR

Aetiology of nerve injury

- physical: traction, trauma, injection, thermal;
- inflammation;

- infection;
- ischaemia;
- pharmacological;
- tumour;
- systemic disease;
- iatropathic.

The mechanism of nerve injury includes:

- open/closed injuries;
- acute/chronic injuries;
- single/continuing/repeated injuries;
- whole/part of a nerve;
- depth of the lesion;
- nerve state (healthy/diseased).

Nerve injury has been classified by **Seddon** (1943), **Sunderland** (1951) and **Thomas and Ochoa** (1964) (Table 11.3). Sunderland's classification is based on an anatomical description of the lesion, rendering it a retrospective diagnosis with less clinical relevance than Seddon's or Thomas and Ochoa's classification systems. Thomas and Ochoa's classification system divides injuries into those resulting in neuronal degeneration and those that do not. This has been expanded further by **Birch and Bonney** (1998) into injuries with no block to conduction and those leading to a conduction block. Birch and Bonney's classification has direct relevance to clinical practice and prognosis, making it the most useful of the classification systems.

The degree of nerve injury affects the outcome. A **neurapraxia** comprises a transient concussion or crushing of the nerve. There is no **Wallerian degeneration**, but instead there is a block to flow of nerve impulses, with consequent interruption of physical function. A neurapraxia has a favourable outcome, provided the source of the injury is removed. **Axonotmesis** and **neuronotmesis** have less favourable outcomes, as they are degenerative lesions.

Distinguishing between degenerative and non-degenerative lesions on clinical grounds is therefore possible. A **degenerative lesion** manifests as a **progressive loss** of all peripheral function. This includes peripheral autonomic function (sudomotor and vasomotor) due to interruption of postganglionic sympathetic

Table 11.3 Classification of nerve injury

Classification system Thomas and Ochoa, Birch and Bonney	Seddon	Sunderland	Pathology
Transient conduction block (non-degenerative)	Neurapraxia	I	Anoxia with recoverable disturbance of membrane potentials at molecular level
Prolonged conduction block (non-degenerative)	Neurapraxia	I	Distortion of myelin sheath
Degenerative (favourable prognosis)	Axonotmesis	II	Axonal disruption; basal lamina, endoneurium and perineurium intact
Degenerative (intermediate)	Axonotmesis	III	Axonal disruption; basal lamina and endoneurium damaged
Degenerative (unfavourable prognosis)	Axonotmesis	IV	Axonal disruption; endoneurium and perineurium damaged; epineurium intact
Degenerative (unfavourable prognosis)	Neuronotmesis	V	Loss of continuity of all elements of nerve

fibres. A **non-degenerative lesion** comprising a block of nerve transmission preserves some elements of peripheral function, such as the sympathetic fibres and deep-pressure sensation.

The duration of injury also affects the type of nerve lesion sustained and its outcome. With the example of the radial nerve trapped within a fracture of the humeral shaft, if the nerve is not freed, the lesion to the radial nerve progresses rapidly from one of simple conduction block to prolonged conduction block and ultimately to what is effectively neuronotmesis.

Nerve fibres react differently to injury. A clinical example is the effect of a tourniquet left on a limb, with the severity of symptoms and potential recovery related to the duration of the tourniquet. A transient ischaemia (causing neurapraxia) results in a loss of superficial sensibility, followed by pain and finally a loss of motor power. This is due to the initial effect on large myelinated fibres followed by C fibres, with little effect on autonomic fibres, reflected in the preservation of pilomotor and vasomotor function.

Neurapraxia in essence involves a local conduction block. The nerve and axon are in continuity, and **segmental demyelination** is the only histological finding. Full recovery is likely with this degree of nerve injury, which is a non-degenerative non-progressive lesion resulting in a conduction block only. **Pure neurapraxia** is rare in clinical practice and should not be diagnosed in the presence of complete palsy, Tinel sign, neuropathic pain, sympathetic paralysis or progressive symptoms when an open wound lies over the course of a nerve. In such cases, a working diagnosis of neuronotmesis or axonotmesis (degenerative lesions) should be made. However, distinguishing between a degenerative lesion capable of recovery with a favourable prognosis (axonotmesis) from a degenerative lesion of unfavourable prognosis (neuronotmesis) is not possible on clinical grounds alone.

More severe injuries with axonal damage or interruption cause a degenerative type of lesion, first described by Waller (1850) as **Wallerian degeneration**. Waller's work on the hypoglossal nerve of the frog after transection showed that distal degeneration of the nerve axon occurred, with later regeneration of neural tissue from the proximal stump. This was later confirmed by Ramon y Cajal.

Degenerative lesions correspond to axonotmesis or neuronotmesis (Sunderland second-, third-, fourth- and fifth-degree injury). With a **second-degree Sunderland injury** (axonotmesis), the axon is disrupted, but the endoneurium and perineurium remain intact. Wallerian degeneration occurs distal to the site of injury, but the Schwann cells around the distal segment of injured axon remain intact and the regenerating axon follows its normal course to its normal target. Regeneration occurs at a rate of 1 mm/day and complete recovery is possible.

In **neuronotmesis**, the connective tissue envelopes of the nerve are interrupted and above all the basal lamina is transected or ruptured. Recovery, if any, is poor. Only repair of the nerve offers any chance of useful recovery. The **Sunderland third**, **fourth** and **fifth degrees** indicate deepening injury to the connective tissue envelope. Third- and fourth-degree lesions are seen in long traction injuries without complete rupture. Fifth degree represents complete loss of continuity in all elements of the nerve and is the most severe lesion.

On **sectioning** a nerve, the axon atrophies proximally, the cell body dendrites retract and the axon distal to the site of injury degenerates. The cell body's role changes from that of neurotransmission to the production of components for nerve regeneration. The cell nucleus migrates to the periphery of the cell body and **chromatolysis** occurs. The cell volume increases and production of ribonucleic acid (RNA) and regenerative enzymes also increases.

Distal to the site of injury, the myelin sheath degenerates, a haematoma forms and macrophages are stimulated to remove the axonal debris. Although the endoneurium and basement membrane may be intact, the neural tube will collapse once the myelin and axonal debris have been phagocytosed. Schwann cells and macrophages eventually replace the neural tube. Next, Schwann cells start to proliferate and migrate, forming columns (**bands of Bungner**). The mitotic activity of the Schwann cell increases, and the cell starts to produce growth factors as its phenotype changes and it becomes non-myelinating. Myelination occurs at

a later stage in the regeneration process.

The axon proximal to the site of injury forms multiple axon sprouts with a **growth cone** situated at the tip of each sprout. **Filopodia** in the growth cone use **contact guidance** for **fibronectin** and **laminin** in the Schwann cell basement lamina to facilitate regeneration at a rate of 1 mm/day. Regeneration of axons can be followed by the presence of an advancing **Tinel sign**.

If the axon does not regenerate, permanent changes occur to the target organs. This is a time-dependent phenomenon, with the motor end plates the first to disappear after 3 months, followed by the muscle spindles and cutaneous sensory organs.

Factors determining prognosis following nerve injury include the following:

- **Violence of injury:** high-energy injuries have worse prognosis. A cleanly divided nerve repaired accurately has a better prognosis than a repaired nerve following a violent traction injury because of the extensive damage to nerve, connective tissue and bone.
- **Delay between injury and repair:** there is a worse prognosis with delay of repair due to a time-dependent degeneration of the target organs and because of the severe effects upon neurons within the central nervous system following axonotomy.
- **Age:** there is generally a better prognosis in younger patients due to the plasticity of the developing nervous system, although the immature nervous system is also more vulnerable to injury.
- **Gap between nerve ends:** the larger the gap, the worse the prognosis.
- **Level of injury:** repairs of nerve injuries at a distal level (e.g. posterior interosseous nerve) have a better prognosis than those at a more proximal level (e.g. radial nerve in the axilla).
- **Condition of nerve ends:** a tidy knife wound has a better prognosis than an untidy crush injury.
- **Association with arterial/bony injury:** nerve injuries associated with injury to bone or major vessels at the same level have a worse prognosis.

- **Type of nerve:** nerves that innervate one or two muscles (e.g. accessory and musculocutaneous nerves) have a better prognosis than those with mixed cutaneous and muscle innervation (e.g. median nerve). Some nerves (e.g. superficial radial nerve) have a poor prognosis following injury because of poor sensory recovery, often complicated by pain.

The type of neuropathic pain following nerve injury can aid in the diagnosis of nerve injury and can be divided into the following:

- **Post-traumatic neuralgia:** pain after nerve injury with no sympathetic involvement. Pain is spontaneous but may be worsened by physical stimulus. Pain is expressed within the territory of the nerve. Treatment is to repair the nerve but outcome may be poor, e.g. following repair of the superficial radial nerve.
- **Neurostenalgia:** pain caused by persistent nerve compression/distortion/ischaemia of a nerve that is anatomically intact. Pain is severe and usually confined to the territory of the nerve. It indicates that the nerve is still subject to a damaging lesion. Examples include compression of the sciatic nerve from expanding haematoma and entrapment of the radial nerve within a humeral shaft fracture. Treatment of the cause carries a good prognosis, with early relief from pain and full recovery of the nerve.
- **Causalgia/chronic regional pain syndrome (type 2):** burning pain with allodynia, hyperpathia, disturbance of skin colour, altered temperature and sweating. This is a rare but severe injury, often seen with partial division of a nerve. The pain is intense and extends beyond the territory of the damaged nerve. Sympathetic involvement is characteristic. Examples include penetrating missile injury to the root of the upper or lower limb. Repair of the nerve carries a good prognosis, as does repair of the commonly associated vascular injury such as false aneurysm or arteriovenous fistula.
- **Central pain:** caused by root avulsions. Two types of pain are described: a constant crushing or burning pain felt within the anaesthetic part, and a sharp shooting pain within the dermatome of the affected nerve.

Terms used to describe patient symptoms with nerve injuries

- **Paraesthesia:** spontaneous abnormal sensation.
- **Dysaesthesia:** unpleasant spontaneous normal sensation.
- **Allodynia:** pain from stimulation that does not normally cause pain.
- **Hyperalgesia:** increased response to a stimulus that is normally painful.
- **Hypersensitivity:** overreaction sensitivity of regeneration.
- **Hyperpathia:** deep-seated, poorly localized, fiery pain radiating throughout the limb that is induced by palpation of the muscles.

NERVE-CONDUCTION STUDIES

Diagnosis of nerve injury relies primarily on clinical examination but can be supplemented by **nerve-conduction** studies (NCS) and **electromyography** (EMG). Surface or needle electrodes are used to record the action potential travelling along a nerve or the electrical activity in muscle. NCS utilizes an electrode to stimulate large, fast, myelinated conducting fibres and a recording electrode to measure the motor or sensory action potentials (Figure 11.6). Measurements of **latency**, **amplitude** and **conduction** velocity can then be made:

- **Latency:** measures the time between onset of the stimulus and the response in milliseconds (ms).
- **Amplitude:** measures the size of the response in microvolts (μV) or millivolts (mV).
- **Velocity:** distance between the stimulating and recording electrodes divided by the time, measured in metres per second (m/s).

The amplitude of the response indicates the **quantity** of axons contributing to the action

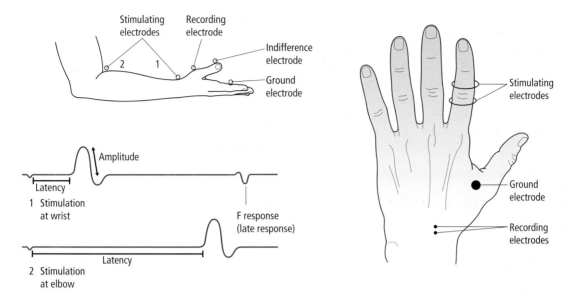

Figure 11.6 *(a) Motor and (b) sensory nerve conduction study for carpal tunnel syndrome.*

potential. The latency and velocity indicate the **quality** of conduction along the axons.

Supramaximal stimulation of a motor nerve is recorded as the motor unit action potential (MUAP) from the muscle (see also Chapter 12). Hence, the **amplitude** (mV) of the MUAP indicates the number of functioning motor units. The **latency** (ms) of the MUAP records the time taken from motor nerve stimulation to muscle response and includes synaptic transmission and muscle depolarization. The **conduction velocity** (m/s) is calculated by stimulating the motor nerve at two different sites. The distance between the distal stimulation site and the recording electrode is subtracted from the distance between the proximal stimulation site and the recording electrode. This distance is then divided by the distal latency subtracted from the proximal latency to give velocity for the motor nerve.

Sensory nerve action potentials (SNAP) are measured by stimulating and recording at separate sites along the same sensory nerve. The recording electrode is the more proximal of the two, with the SNAP recorded for antidromic (distal to proximal) conduction. Amplitude (µV) and latency (ms) can be measured directly, and velocity (m/s) is calculated by dividing the distance between the electrodes by the latency.

Compound nerve action potentials (CNAP) are usually measured antidromically (distal to proximal) from mixed sensory and motor nerves, with the recording electrode situated proximal to the stimulating electrode. The CNAP has a larger amplitude than the SNAP and thus may be easier to record.

The amplitude and conduction velocity vary according to several factors:

- Upper limb nerves conduct faster than lower limb nerves (50–70 m/s upper limb, 40–50 m/s lower limb).
- Conduction is faster proximally along a nerve.
- Certain nerves conduct faster than others.
- There is a reduction in velocity at lower temperatures.
- Conduction velocity is related to myelination, with slower velocities in very old and very young people.

One of the most common examples of the application of NCS is for suspected carpal tunnel syndrome (CTS). Motor studies consist of a **stimulating electrode** placed over the median nerve proximal to the carpal tunnel, a **recording electrode** placed over a muscle in the hand supplied by the median nerve (abductor pollicis brevis, APB), an **indifference electrode**

Table 11.4 Normative data for common nerve-conduction studies in the upper limb

Nerve	F wave (ms)	Distal latency (ms)	Amplitude	Velocity (m/s)
Median (motor conduction)	<32	<4	>5 mV	>50
Median (sensory action potential)			>5 μV	>50
Ulnar (motor conduction)	<32	<3	>5 mV	>50
Ulnar (sensory action potential)			>5 μV	>50

placed a few centimetres away, and a **ground electrode** placed over an inactive muscle. The stimulus is turned on until a threshold CMAP is recorded, and the current is then increased to supramaximal to ensure that all the motor units are activated.

In CTS, sensory latency studies are more sensitive than motor studies and are also included for completeness. Routine testing for CTS also includes stimulation of the ulnar or radial nerve for comparison. In severe cases of CTS, the sensory potentials may be absent, and motor studies are then essential to demonstrate delayed conduction. In general, NCS are abnormal in 60 per cent of patients with CTS. Indications for surgery based on NCS include prolonged distal motor latency, denervation of the APB and absence of a median digital SNAP. Normative data for NCS of the median and ulnar nerves are shown in Table 11.4.

In contrast to distal NCS, nerve conduction in the most proximal segments of the nerve is difficult to measure due to anatomical constraints; therefore, in this situation, late responses such as the **F response** (or wave) and the **H reflex** are measured. These are low-amplitude responses with long latencies, including conduction in the proximal and distal sections of a nerve.

The **F response** measures the antidromic conduction of an impulse from a peripheral nerve to the anterior horn cells along with reflex orthodromic conduction down the motor nerves to the muscle. The F response does not cross any synapses and can be thought of as an **echo**. It is useful in detecting early proximal nerve lesions. A prolonged F response latency with normal peripheral motor nerve conduction would imply slowing over proximal motor

fibres at the plexus or root level. The F response may be abnormal immediately after nerve root injury, even when the EMG is normal. However, muscles are innervated by multiple roots, and so an abnormal F response is present only with multiple severe motor root compromise, e.g. Guillain–Barré syndrome, and extensive proximal neuropathies such as plexopathies.

The **H reflex** is the electrophysiological equivalent of a deep tendon reflex. It is elicited by a submaximal stimulation of Aα afferent fibres from muscle stretch receptors that enter the dorsal horn and synapse with alpha motor neurons, resulting in a motor response on completion of the monosynaptic reflex arc (apart from in the soleus muscle). The H reflex can be difficult to record, which limits its applicability. It is absent or delayed in polyneuropathies and radiculopathies, but it may also be absent in patients over 60 years of age.

Somatosensory evoked potentials (SSEP) can also be used to investigate proximal lesions and for spinal cord monitoring. Surface electrodes are used to stimulate a mixed nerve. The resultant evoked potential from the central nervous system can be recorded at a specific site such as Erb's point in the supraclavicular fossa or more proximally, from the skin overlying the cervical vertebrae and from the scalp overlying the sensory cortex. The pattern of abnormality may be used to diagnose the level of injury.

The timing of NCS and EMG affects the results obtained, reflecting the degree of injury and the extent of recovery. With respect to nerve injury, the patterns shown in Table 11.5 are found.

Table 11.5 Nerve conduction and electromyographic (EMG) changes seen with varying degrees of nerve injury

Injury	SNAP/CNAP	Conduction velocity	EMG
Conduction block (neurapraxia)	Reduced amplitude proximally, normal distally	Conduction block at injury site, preserved below level of injury	No/sparse fibrillations, MUAP firing at rapid rates, reduced interference pattern
Degenerative lesion, favourable prognosis (axonotmesis)	Absent or reduced	Absent or normal if present	Fibrillations, reduced interference pattern, increased firing rate of MUAP
Degenerative lesion, unfavourable prognosis (neuronotmesis)	Absent	Absent	Fibrillations, no voluntary MUAP

CNAP, compound nerve action potential; MUAP, motor unit action potential; SNAP, sensory nerve action potential.

SUMMARY

An understanding of the anatomy and physiology of nerves is important in the diagnosis of nerve injury, prediction of resultant recovery and performing a repair if necessary.

Viva questions

1 Draw a cross-section of a nerve. Describe its structure and how this may vary along its course.

2 Classify nerve injuries. What does 'axonotmesis' mean? What is the mode of degeneration? What affects speed of recovery? What is the value of the Tinel sign?

3 What is the pathology of carpal tunnel syndrome?

4 Interpret a nerve conduction study.

5 What are the F wave and the H reflex? What is their clinical significance?

FURTHER READING

Birch, R, Bonney, G, Wynn Parry, CB. *Surgical Disorders of the Peripheral Nerves*. Edinburgh: Churchill Livingstone, 1998.

Flores, AJ, Lavernia, CJ, Owens, PW. Anatomy and physiology of peripheral nerve injury and repair. *Am J Orthop* 2000;**29**:167–73.

Maggi, SP, Lowe, JB, Mackinnon, SE. Pathophysiology of nerve injury. *Clin Plastic Surg* 2003;**30**:109–26.

Robinson, LR. Traumatic injury to peripheral nerves. *Muscle Nerve* 2000;**23**:863–73.

Woodruff, MI, Lavalette, DP. Neurophysiology for the orthopaedic surgeon. *Curr Orthop* 2000;**14**:347–55.

12
Skeletal muscle

MICHAEL FOX AND SIMON LAMBERT

STRUCTURE

Skeletal muscle cells are of **mesodermal** origin. Mature cells in adult skeletal muscle are **myotubes** or muscle fibres. They are differentiated multinucleated cells formed by cytoplasmic fusion of immature mononucleated myoblasts. In muscle growth, these mononucleated precursor cells also fuse to the myotubes, adding to both the ends and the side of the cell. Muscle fibres vary in size and length between the sexes and between differing muscle groups. Fibres in muscles that have a precision requirement, such as the small muscles of the hand, tend to be smaller than in power muscles, such as the quadriceps. The fibre size is likely to be related intimately to the innervation of the muscle. Muscle fibres are bounded by a plasma membrane, the **sarcolemma**, and have a cytoplasm termed the **sarcoplasm**.

All cells have genes coding for contractile proteins. In non-muscle cells, these proteins have a role in cell motility and cytoskeletal adaptation. In muscle cells, contractile proteins are present in great numbers, forming around 80 per cent of the cell volume and lying in a highly ordered form, with the cell nuclei marginalized. By convention, muscle fibres are termed mature when nuclear marginalization is seen. Cell nuclei are congregated particularly densely at the neuromuscular junction.

Many muscle fibres grouped together are termed **fascicles** (Figure 12.1). In turn, groupings of fascicles give structure to the muscle itself. The fascicle is the smallest unit of structure visible to the naked eye. It is the ability of the fascicle to contract that determines the character of the muscle.

In muscle, support cells and connective tissue run between fibres. **Endomysium** surrounds individual fibres, **perimysium** encloses the functional fascicular unit, and **epimysium** surrounds the muscle in its entirety.

MUSCLE CELL MEMBRANES

Sarcoplasmic reticulum

Surrounding each myofibril is a membranous sac called the **sarcoplasmic reticulum**. This membrane serves as a repository for calcium, which is released to stimulate contraction.

T-tubules

The outer membrane of each muscle fibre gives off multiple invaginations. These form tubes that run in a network that connect every sarcomere. The **T-tubules** connect at a membranous junction with the sarcoplasmic reticulum of each myofibril. The function of the T-tubules is to carry the depolarization of the surface membrane deep inside the muscle fibre.

VASCULAR SUPPLY OF MUSCLE

In mammalian muscles, vascular architecture follows a relatively constant pattern. A main,

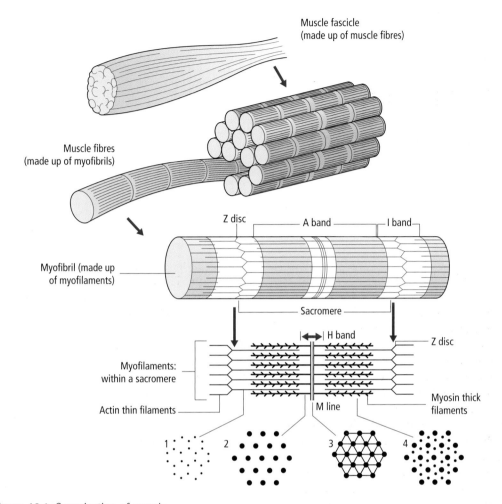

Figure 12.1 *Organization of muscle.*

rapidly branching artery enters the muscle and creates a series of arcades. As in peripheral nerve, from these arcades, arterioles penetrate the sheath surrounding the fascicle. In muscle, this is the perimysium. The arterioles enter obliquely or at right-angles to the muscle fibres and then run parallel. The terminal capillaries are associated with muscle fibre nuclei.

ULTRA-STRUCTURE

The major contractile proteins in skeletal muscle are **actin** and **myosin**. The grouped functional unit of these filaments is termed the **myofibril**. Myofibrils are segmented into functional contractile units called **sarcomeres**. Sarcomeres are visible under electron

microscopy. Sarcomeres are 2–2.5 microns in length and 1 micron in diameter when not contracted. The length of the sarcomere varies with muscle activity but also shows variance along the length of the myofibril. Sarcomeres in the myotendinous junction tend to be shorter. This may have a pre-tensioning or protective role. It is also responsible for variation in the force/velocity curve.

The bands visible on either light or electron microscopy correspond to the contractile protein components:

- **A bands** represent the myosin filaments (**anisotropic** on light microscopy).
- **I bands** represent actin filaments in adjacent sarcomeres where there is no overlap with

myosin filaments (**isotropic** on light microscopy).

- **H bands** correspond to the myosin filament segment where there are no interdigitating actin filaments.
- **M lines** represent the connections between adjacent **myosin** filaments in their central region. These are termed the **M-band proteins**.
- **Z discs** represent the attachment of adjacent sarcomeres. The disc lies between sarcomeres (from *Zwischen* = between [German]).

The arrangement of actin and myosin filaments is that of a hexagonal lattice in the centre of the sarcomere, i.e. each myosin filament is bounded by six actin filaments. This hexagonal arrangement becomes more square towards the end of each sarcomere, i.e. at the Z bands.

Other important proteins have a role in maintaining the structure of the sarcolemma, such as dystrophin (absent in Duchenne's muscular dystrophy). As a group, these proteins are termed **structural proteins**, as they maintain the overall architecture of the sarcomere during contraction.

CONTRACTILE PROTEINS

Actin

This is a globular protein (molecular weight 42 000) that is a chief constituent of the thin filaments of the sarcomere (Figure 12.2). Other proteins that constitute the thin filament are **tropomyosin** and **troponin** subunits (troponin C, troponin T, troponin I).

Tropomyosin extends across seven actin subunits and blocks the binding sites of the myosin head unit until unblocked by calcium binding to the troponin C subunit. The activated troponin C subunit counteracts the inhibitory effect of the troponin I subunit. Troponin T assists troponin C binding to tropomyosin.

Myosin

Myosin molecules have six distinct subunits (two heavy chains, four light chains). The light

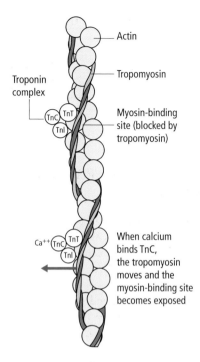

Figure 12.2 *Diagram of actin filament. TnC, troponin C; TnI, troponin I; TnT, troponin T.*

chains are of uncertain function in humans. The heavy chains have distinctive parts, including one part that articulates with actin filaments, the S1 segment or **cross-bridge**. Another part, the **S2 segment**, forms the flexible neck, which moves to allow articulation of the S1 head segment.

FUNCTION

SLIDING FILAMENT CONTRACTION MECHANISM AND FORCE GENERATION

The cross-bridge theory was propounded by Huxley in 1957. In this theory, the filaments of myosin and actin move relative to each other because of an oscillating binding site on the myosin molecule, which binds to the actin molecule at differing rates. At the molecular level, the following sequence occurs:

1 In-rush of Ca^{2+}.
2 Ca^{2+} binds troponin C.
3 Activated troponin C displaces inhibitory

troponin I from site on tropomyosin/actin complex.

4 Troponin T assists.
5 Tropomyosin undergoes conformational change to allow myosin head engagement.
6 Myosin head engages.
7 Force generation occurs due to S1 head segment rotation.

FORCE, SPEED AND POWER OF CONTRACTION

The **force** of a muscle at any given length is proportional to the cross-sectional area of the muscle. The more sarcomeres there are acting in parallel to each other, the higher the force generated.

Conversely, the **speed** of muscular contraction is related to the length of the muscle. Upon stimulation of a muscle, all sarcomeres contract at the same time. For a long muscle, there will be a greater change in length per unit time, i.e. the greater the muscle velocity. The sarcomeres act in series.

The **power** of a muscle is the product of its force and velocity. Short fat muscles produce high force but low maximum velocity. Long thin muscles produce low force but high maximum velocity. These represent opposite ends of the spectrum. Note that it is possible that both types of muscle could generate the same amount of power.

INNERVATION OF SKELETAL MUSCLE

Muscle develops with its motor nerve supply. Initially, each developing muscle fibre or myotube is multiply innervated by several axons. As the muscle develops, all but one of the axons lose their synaptic connection with the fibre. Each motor neuron therefore innervates a muscle fibre with every one of its axons. Because of the seemingly random establishment of the dominant axon to the fibre in development, muscle fibres lying next to each other are not usually innervated by the same parent motor neuron. All muscle fibres innervated by the same motor neuron are termed a **motor unit**.

The size of an action potential recorded from the surface of a muscle is proportional to the number of muscle fibres innervated by the motor neuron being stimulated.

THE NEUROMUSCULAR JUNCTION

In the motor neuron, action potentials propagate an influx of Ca^{2+} through voltage-sensitive channels. Increased concentrations of intracellular Ca^{2+} cause preformed vesicles of acetylcholine to fuse with the presynaptic nerve membrane. Acetylcholine in the synaptic cleft binds to postsynaptic receptors on the sarcolemma (Figure 12.3). The binding of acetylcholine depolarizes the muscle fibre membrane.

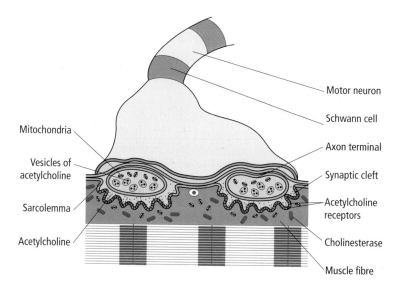

Figure 12.3 *Neuromuscular junction.*

Mitochondria

Vesicles of acetylcholine

Sarcolemma

Acetylcholine

Motor neuron

Schwann cell

Axon terminal

Synaptic cleft

Acetylcholine receptors

Cholinesterase

Muscle fibre

Depolarization is dependent on the amount of acetylcholine released into the synaptic cleft. Depolarization is also dependent on the rate of release of acetylcholine into the cleft, as it is broken down rapidly by cholinesterases from the postsynaptic membrane.

THE MYOTENDINOUS JUNCTION

The myotendinous junction is the area where insertion of every skeletal muscle fibre into its tendon occurs. This area has a specific morphology, which is adapted to its function. Specific features include shorter sarcomere lengths, greater number of organelles per cell, greater synthetic ability, interdigitation of cell membrane and extracellular connective tissue, and a high degree of membrane folding. The latter increases resistance to stress by increasing surface area and reducing the angle of the force vector applied. The net result is that the junction is very strong.

MUSCLE FIBRE TYPES

Muscle fibres in humans are of three main types. The types differ from each other in their size, speed and resistance to fatigue. These characteristics are a function of their relatively aerobic or anaerobic metabolism:

- Type 1 (mnemonic 'slow red ox'):
  - slow fibres;
  - large concentration of myoglobin (red in colour);
  - oxidative;
  - very fatigue resistant.
- Type 2a:
  - fast fibres;
  - oxidative and glycolytic (relatively white in colour);
  - fatigue-resistant.
- Type 2b:
  - fast fibres;
  - glycolytic (relatively white in colour);
  - fatiguable.

The pattern of activity imposed on the muscle is the single most important factor in fibre type expression. Athletes who train extensively for endurance can reach proportions of up to 80 per cent of type 1 fibres in their muscles.

Other muscle fibre types have also been described in smaller quantities. These probably represent interim fibre types that have not had sufficient stimulus to differentiate fully.

INJURY

MECHANISM OF INJURY

Muscle cells damaged by, for example, physical trauma have raised intracellular calcium concentrations. Once the cell is damaged, the process continues via calcium-activated enzymes, such as **protease** and **phospholipase**, which in turn further damage the cell structure. In addition, damage also occurs via free radicals and oxidation of liberated free fatty acids.

MODES OF MUSCLE INJURY

- Muscle belly tear.
- Muscle laceration.
- Musculotendinous junction injury.
- Ischaemic damage and compartment syndrome.
- Denervation.
- Crush injury and rhabdomyolysis.
- Malignant hyperpyrexia: skeletal muscle reaction to halothane, with prolonged contraction of muscle, leading to metabolic disintegration of muscle. Potassium is released first, and therefore there is a risk of myocardial infarction, followed by massive myoglobin load, leading to renal failure if the patient survives the initial insult.
- Delayed muscle soreness: defined as soreness that develops 24–72 h following intense exercise and associated with measurable muscle weakness. The pain occurs mainly at the myotendinous junction. It has been shown to be associated with intramuscular damage but is readily reversible. Connective tissue breakdown products such as hydroxyproline can be identified in the urine.

REPAIR

Muscle needs a blood supply and stimulation in the form of a nerve supply. Repair thus relies on rapid re-establishment of a vascular supply and innervation. In a complete muscle belly transaction, the distal portion of muscle wastes rapidly. Muscle regeneration can occur without a nerve supply, but permanent muscle atrophy will develop if re-innervation fails. Note the following:

- The more proximal the belly tear, the worse the prognosis, as more bulk is denervated.
- Muscle laceration results in dense fibrous scar tissue formation. Myotubes regenerate across scar tissue in small numbers. Partial lacerations predictably have better functional outcomes than complete belly lacerations. A complete laceration in the mid-substance can recover to only around 50 per cent of the previous force that was generated by the muscle.

COMPLETE MUSCLE TEARS

These have been poorly studied to date. Animal studies suggest that tears tend to occur near the myotendinous junction, with a segment of adjacent muscle avulsed when stretched to failure.

INCOMPLETE MUSCLE TEARS

Tears occur near the myotendinous junction in the area of relatively stiffer sarcomeres.

ELECTRODIAGNOSIS IN MUSCLE INJURY

Electromyography (EMG) is the recording of electrical activity in skeletal muscle. Needle electrodes are inserted into the muscle to be studied. The electrode records any spontaneous activity within the muscle at rest and the signal given by the firing of motor units when the muscle is activated. There is generally no spontaneous activity at rest in a healthy muscle after the needle has been inserted. The patterns of motor unit activity (seen as the **motor unit action potential**, MUAP) are related to the nerve supply to the muscle in question (Figure 12.4).

Summary of findings in motor nerve injury

Denervation:
- Spontaneous activity:
  - acute denervation: sharp waves;
  - chronic denervation: fasciculations.

Re-innervation:
- Early:

continued

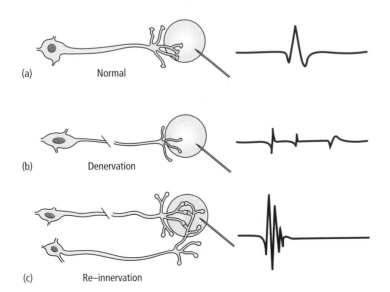

(a) Normal

(b) Denervation

(c) Re–innervation

Figure 12.4 *(a) Normal motor unit action potential (MUAP) recorded by a needle electrode from muscle fibres within its recording area. (b) After denervation, single muscle fibres discharge spontaneously, producing fibrillations and positive sharp waves. (c) When re-innervation by axon sprouting has occurred, the newly formed sprouts conduct slowly, producing temporal dispersion (i.e. prolonged MUAP duration) and MUAP polyphasicity. The higher density of muscle fibres within the recording area of the needle belonging to the enlarging second motor unit results in an increased-amplitude MUAP.*

- reduced amplitude motor action potentials, longer duration;
- poor recruitment.
- Late:
  - large amplitude, stable, consistent firing motor action potentials;
  - good recruitment of units gives polyphasic signal.

Viva questions

1 Describe the basic structure of skeletal muscle.

2 What is the mechanism of contraction of skeletal muscle?

3 What are the events that occur at the neuromuscular junction?

4 What different types of skeletal muscle fibre do you know of?

5 How does injured muscle heal?

FURTHER READING

Beiner, JM, Jokl, P. Muscle contusion injuries: current treatment options. *Am Acad Orthop Surg* 2001;**9**:227–37.

Jarvinen, TA, Jarvinen, TL, Kaariainen, M, Kalimo, H, Jarvinen, M. Muscle injuries: biology and treatment. *Am J Sports Med* 2005;**33**:745–64.

Kirkendall, DT, Garrett, WE, Jr. Clinical perspectives regarding eccentric muscle injury. *Clin Orthop Relat Res* 2002;**403**:S81–9.

Lieber, RL, Friden, J. Clinical significance of skeletal muscle architecture. *Clin Orthop Relat Res* 2001;**383**:140–51.

Peterson, GW, Will, AD. Newer electro-diagnostic techniques in peripheral nerve injuries. *Orthop Clin North Am* 1988;**19**:13–25.

13

Basics of bone

PETER BATES AND MANOJ RAMACHANDRAN

FUNCTION

Bone performs three main functions:

- Bone is the **primary reservoir of calcium** in the body, continuously exchanging calcium with the extracellular environment. The concentration of calcium in the body fluids is regulated tightly, and the supply of calcium in bone is critical to this control.
- The **haematopoietic marrow** located in cancellous bone supplies the body's cells, tissues and organs with erythrocytes, leukocytes and platelets.
- Bone has a **mechanical role** in supporting the body's tissues, protecting the soft internal viscera and providing sites of attachment for the muscles that effect body movement and locomotion.

STRUCTURE

WOVEN (IMMATURE) BONE

In woven bone, **collagen fibres** are aligned randomly and have no lamellae, making the bone weaker and more flexible than lamellar bone. This irregular arrangement affords it **isotropic** characteristics, i.e. it has uniform properties in all directions, independent of the direction of load application. Woven bone exhibits a rapid rate of deposition and turnover, with more cells per unit volume than lamellar

bone. It is found in the **embryonic** and **neonatal skeleton**, the **metaphyseal region of growing bones** up to age 4 years, and in the **fracture callus of children**. It is absent in the normal adult but appears in the **early hard callus** following fracture. It is also found in **pathological bone**, e.g. in tumours, Pagetic bone and osteogenesis imperfecta.

LAMELLAR (MATURE) BONE

This forms the structural component of **cortical** and **cancellous** bone with **stress-oriented collagen fibres** contributing to its **anisotropic** characteristics. **Osteoblasts** lay down collagen matrix in microscopic thin-layered sheets called **lamellae**. Within each lamella, collagen fibres run parallel to each other. Fibres in adjacent lamellae run at oblique angles to each other (**herring-bone structure**), with cement lines separating the lamellae. Lamellar bone is composed predominantly of matrix with a small cell population of **osteocytes** (trapped osteoblasts) encased within bony **lacunae** and resting **bone-lining cells** (with osteoblastic potential) covering the bony surfaces.

Cortical (compact) bone

This comprises 80 per cent of the adult skeleton forming the envelope of cuboid bones and the diaphyses of long bones. Lamellae are laid down as concentric rings forming tubular lamellar systems called **osteons** or **Haversian systems**, which are approximately 50 μm in

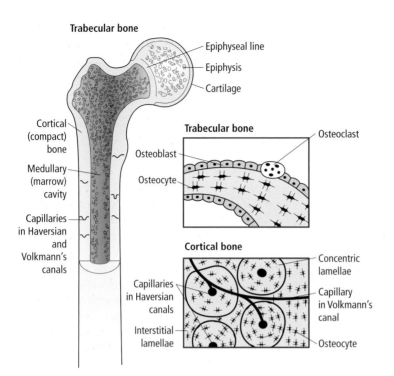

Figure 13.1 *Cortical and cancellous bone lamellar structure. In cortical bone, the lamellae are arranged in concentric rings around Haversian canals. In cancellous bone, the lamellae are arranged as layers within the trabeculae, which are themselves aligned along lines of force.*

diameter (Figure 13.1). Individual osteons are aligned along lines of force (usually parallel with the long axis of the bone). Each osteon has a central neurovascular channel (**Haversian canal**) surrounded by five to seven concentric layers (lamellae) of bone matrix. Rings of trapped osteocytes intercommunicate via gap junctions within channels called **canaliculi**, which spread out radially from the central canal like spokes of a wheel. **Cement lines** separate osteons, with neither canaliculi nor collagen fibres crossing them, forming areas of relative weakness along which cracks may propagate.

A second system of canals called **Volkmann's canals** penetrates and runs perpendicular to the long bone axis, connecting the inner and outer surfaces of the bone. These canals carry blood vessels to and from the Haversian systems. At the periosteal and endosteal surfaces, lamellae run parallel to the surface, forming **circumferential** and **endosteal lamellae**.

Cortical bone is denser and has a higher Young's modulus of elasticity (around 20 GPa) than cancellous bone (around 1 GPa). Cortical bone is also more resistant to bending and torsion.

Cancellous (trabecular) bone

This is found mainly in the metaphyses and epiphyses of long bones and centrally in cuboid bones. It has a three-dimensional lattice of interconnecting trabeculae, which are aligned along axes of mechanical stress, enclosing elements of the bone marrow. Each of the trabeculae is made up of parallel sheets of **lamellae**. Osteocytes, lacunae and canaliculi in cancellous bone resemble those in cortical bone. However, Haversian systems are not present in cancellous bone. Cancellous bone has eight times the metabolic turnover rate of cortical bone due to its large surface area. It is less dense, less elastic (less brittle) and less strong than cortical bone.

Periosteum

This circumferential connective tissue covering bone is responsible for growth in bone diameter and therefore is more prominent in children. It has two layers – an **inner cambial layer,** which is loose, vascular and osteogenic, and an **outer fibrous layer**, which is more structural, less cellular and continuous with joint capsules. With age, periosteum thins and has less osteogenic capability.

CELLS AND MATRIX

Bone is a composite material consisting of cells (10 per cent) within a matrix (90 per cent) that has inorganic and organic components.

Cells

Osteoblasts

These are bone-forming cells derived from **undifferentiated mesenchymal stem cells** in marrow, which produce osteoid (or bone matrix) containing Type I collagen, depositing it on pre-existing mineralized surfaces (known as the **mineralization front**). Osteoblasts line the surfaces of bone, have great **synthetic capacity** (abundant rough endoplasmic reticulum, Golgi apparatus and mitochondria) and show high **alkaline phosphatase activity**. Cell differentiation is mediated by a large number of bone morphogenic proteins (BMPs), growth factors and cytokines. Osteoblasts have **three fates**: they may become **inactive bone-lining cells**, surround themselves with matrix and become **osteocytes**, or disappear from the site of bone formation as a result of **apoptosis**.

Osteocytes

Osteoblasts that become entrapped by calcified bone matrix are known as osteocytes. They comprise 90 per cent of the bone cell population and interconnect with other bone cells via long cytoplasmic processes in the canaliculi. They are important in **controlling calcium** and **phosphorus metabolism**, responding to chemical stimuli such as parathyroid hormone (PTH) and calcitonin and also to **mechanical** and **electrical potential stimuli** (which is likely to be the basis of Wolff's law and of the electromechanical effects on fracture healing).

Bone-lining cells

These flat cells lying on the surface of bone possess cytoplasmic extensions that penetrate bone matrix and **communicate with osteocytes**.

They are considered **inactive osteoblasts** that may be reactivated to become osteoblasts during periods of new bone formation. They are also thought to have a **gatekeeper function**: when stimulated by PTH, they undergo cyclic adenosine monophosphate (cAMP)-mediated morphological changes that expose the bone surface and allow osteoclasts to start resorption.

Osteoclasts

These are mononuclear osteoclast precursor cells (**preosteoclasts**) arising from the **haematopoietic macrophage** and **monocyte stem-cell line**. They may be found in the marrow and circulating blood. When stimulated, these cells proliferate and fuse to form **large multinucleated osteoclasts**, typically having 3–20 nuclei and large numbers of mitochondria and lysosomes and producing acid phosphatase. Osteoclasts resorb bone within pits or depressions known as **Howship's lacunae** on endosteal and periosteal surfaces of bone. In dense cortical bone, they lead osteonal **cutting cones** that tunnel through the bone, creating resorption cavities. On completing their resorptive activities, they may divide into mononuclear cells that can be reactivated to form new osteoclasts.

When lying on the bone surface, their contact area has a **ruffled (brush) border** that increases surface area from membrane in-foldings, which binds to the bone surface via integrins, sealing the area. A low pH is produced beneath this layer (via the carbonic anhydrase system, adenosine triphosphate (ATP)-dependent proton pumps and the Na^+/H^+ exchange system), which dissolves the inorganic apatite crystals. Acidic proteolytic lysosomal enzymes, such as the tartrate-resistant isoenzyme of acid phosphatase (TRAP), and cysteine proteinases, such as the cathepsins, then hydrolyse the organic matrix components. Control of osteoclast function is related closely to that of osteoblasts.

Lack of osteoclast activity is implicated in osteopetrosis, while overactivity is found in Paget's disease (see Appendix).

Bone remodelling unit

A bone remodelling unit (BRU) is an area of bone remodelled by a set of osteoblasts, osteoclasts and stromal supporting tissue. In normal bone, formation matches resorption with continual turnover of bone. Osteoclast precursors are activated to form osteoclasts, which resorb bone. This is followed by reversal, whereby osteoblast precursors are activated to form osteoblasts, which lay down osteoid (collagen and non-collagenous proteins). The osteoid subsequently undergoes mineralization to form bone.

Bone matrix

The inorganic matrix (60 per cent) resists compressive forces, while the organic matrix (40 per cent) resists tensile forces.

Inorganic matrix

This is composed mainly of calcium phosphate crystals, analogous to calcium hydroxyapatite $[Ca_{10}(PO_4)_6(OH)_2]$, and is responsible for the **compressive strength** of bone. The formation of solid calcium phosphate crystals (known as **mineralization**) occurs as a result of phase transformation of soluble calcium and phosphate within specific hole and pore zone regions of the collagen fibrils in the organic matrix of bone, with progressive mineral deposits eventually occupying all of the available space within the fibrils. **Osteocalcium phosphate (brushite)** is also found in bone.

In addition, the inorganic matrix serves as a reservoir for approximately 99 per cent of the body's calcium, 85 per cent of the body's phosphorus and 40–60 per cent of the total body sodium and potassium. Bone also contains numerous impurities, such as strontium, lead and fluoride.

Organic matrix

Collagen (type I), constituting 90 per cent of the organic matrix, consists of a triple helix of two alpha$_1$ chains and one alpha$_2$ chain (with a repetitive GlyXY sequence, where glycine is in the first position and X and Y are often proline and hydroxyproline) arranged in a quarter-staggered structural array producing single fibrils. After synthesis in osteoblasts and fibroblasts, the alpha chains are modified by hydroxylation of lysine and proline residues;

hydroxyproline is a good indicator of **bone turnover**. The modified alpha chains are exported from the cell; **pro-collagen** extensions are removed from the chains (pro-collagen is a good indicator of **bone formation**, along with collagen telopeptides, e.g. carboxy-terminal (CTX). Finally, cross-linkages form between adjacent triple helices; **cross-linked collagen-derived peptides**, e.g. pyridinoline and deoxypyridinoline, are a good indicator of **bone breakdown**. Collagen is primarily responsible for the **tensile strength** of bone. Small amounts of collagen types V and XI are also found in bone.

Note that in addition to the **bone resorption markers** mentioned above, bone formation can be assessed with pro-collagen type I pro-peptides, e.g. CTX extension peptide (P1CP) and amino-terminal extension peptide (P1NP) along with **bone-specific alkaline phosphatase** and **osteocalcin** (see below).

Mineralization in **immature bone** (e.g. during preliminary ossification of cartilage and fetal bone) occurs as a result of alkaline phosphatase activity in mineralizing vesicles, derived from osteoblasts or chondroblasts, which breaks down pyrophosphate (an inhibitor of mineralization) and initiates mineralization. In **mature bone**, the more important mechanism is the deposition and propagation of apatite crystals in the **hole zones** that exist between the ends of fibrils and the **pore zones** that lie between the sides of fibrils of collagen.

Other organic constituents of bone include:

- **Bone-specific proteoglycans:** involved in mineralization, organization of collagen fibres and binding of growth factors.
- **Non-collagenous matrix proteins:**
  - **Osteocalcin:** produced by osteoblasts and involved in the control of osteoclasts (gene on chromosome 1).
  - **Osteonectin:** secreted by osteoblasts and platelets for regulation of mineralization (gene on chromosome 5).
  - **Osteopontin (bone sialoprotein I):** a non-bone-specific cell-binding protein anchoring osteoclasts to the mineralized matrix (gene on chromosome 4).

- **Bone sialoprotein II:** bone-specific (gene on chromosome 4).
- **Others:** e.g. thrombospondin (important in cell attachment) and serum proteins (in same concentration as serum but with increased albumin).
- **Growth factors and cytokines:**
  - **BMP 1–17:** members of the transforming growth factor beta (TGF-β) family of multifunctional molecules.
  - **Insulin-like growth factor** (IGF) I and II.
  - **Interleukins** 1 (IL-1) and 6 (IL-6).

BLOOD SUPPLY

The skeletal system receives 5–10 per cent of cardiac output. Individual long bones have three **interactive circulatory systems** (Figure 13.2), all of which communicate in the adult. In the child, the metaphyseal–epiphyseal system separates when the ossific nucleus is formed.

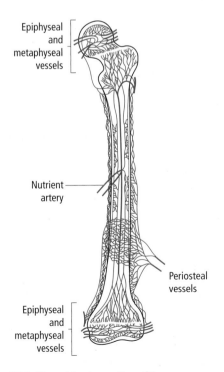

Epiphyseal and metaphyseal vessels

Nutrient artery

Periosteal vessels

Epiphyseal and metaphyseal vessels

Figure 13.2 *Three blood supplies of bone.*

Nutrient artery system (high-pressure system)

A major artery of the systemic circulation enters the **mid-diaphysis** through a nutrient foramen. Once in the medullary canal, it divides into **ascending** and **descending** arteries or arterioles, which anastomose with metaphyseal vessels and directly penetrate the **endosteal surface**, supplying the inner two-thirds of the cortex. In the child, these vessels end on the metaphyseal side of the physis, contributing to the process of endochondral ossification. At the microscopic level, arterioles run in Volkmann's canals with branches to the Haversian systems, draining into venules, and then into central venous sinus and out via the nutrient vein.

Metaphyseal–epiphyseal system

The periarticular vascular complex penetrates the thin cortex and supplies the **metaphysis**, **physis** and **epiphysis**. The metaphyseal vessels anastomose with the medullary and epiphyseal arteries after growth plate fusion. In epiphyses with large articular surfaces, such as the radial and femoral heads, vessels enter the bone between the articular cartilage and the physis, making the supply relatively tenuous.

Periosteal system (low-pressure system)

Capillaries enter at the sites of **major muscle attachments**, normally supplying the outer third of the cortex. This is the dominant system in the child and is responsible for circumferential growth.

These three systems are interconnected, and each is able to become the dominant supply if another is damaged. The normal direction of flow is **centrifugal** (inside to out), but if the endosteal system is damaged, e.g. after intramedullary reaming, the periosteal system becomes dominant and the flow becomes **centripetal** (outside to in). Note that the venous system is normally centripetal in nature.

BONE METABOLISM

Serum calcium levels and bone mineral homeostasis are related intimately and controlled by the synchronized actions of vitamin D3 metabolites, PTH, calcitonin and other hormones. Feedback mechanisms play an important role in regulating plasma calcium and phosphate levels.

CALCIUM

Ninety-nine per cent of total body calcium is **sequestered** in bone, leaving 1 per cent circulating in the extracellular fluid. Intracellular calcium levels are negligible in comparison. Calcium is also important for **nerve**, **muscle** and **hormone** function and in **clotting**.

Plasma calcium (less than 1 per cent of total body calcium) is 50 per cent free and 50 per cent bound, mainly to albumin, and is maintained at a level between 2.2 and 2.6 mmol/L. Calcium is absorbed from the duodenum via **active transport**, mediated by calcium-binding protein and ATP, and regulated by 1,25-dihydroxycholecalciferol [$1,25(OH)_2$-vitamin D3] and via passive diffusion from the jejunum.

Ninety-eight per cent of the calcium filtered in the kidneys is reabsorbed, 60 per cent of this process occurring in the proximal convoluted tubules. A small amount of calcium is also excreted in stools. The three calcitropic hormones and other paracrine factors govern

13.1 Recommended daily intake of calcium

Group	Recommended intake (mg/day)
Children	600
10–25 years	1400
25–65 years	750
Lactation	2000
Postmenopausal women, fracture healing	1500

the extracellular calcium levels and the flow in and out of cells.

Table 13.1 gives the recommended daily intake of calcium in various groups.

Dietary calcium deficiency produces a progressive loss of bone mass. In elderly people, the renal hydroxylation of 25(OH)-vitamin D3 is reduced, leading to lower levels of active vitamin D3 and an increased dietary requirement for calcium.

PHOSPHATE

Phosphate is a key component of bone mineral, with 85 per cent of total body stores being found in bone. Phosphate also functions as a metabolite and as a buffer in enzyme systems. It circulates unbound in the plasma. The daily requirement of phosphate is 1–1.5 g/day. Dietary intake is usually sufficient.

REGULATORS OF CALCIUM AND PHOSPHATE METABOLISM

Vitamin D (active metabolites)

These **naturally occurring steroids** are either **ingested** in the diet from fish oils, such as cod liver oil, and plants or activated in the skin by **ultraviolet** (UV) light (see below). They **enhance calcium and phosphorus absorption** across the small intestine via promotion of synthesis of a calcium-transporting protein and **enhance osteoclastic resorption** from bone, increasing serum levels of calcium and phosphate. Vitamin D metabolites also inhibit PTH release.

The activation process occurs as follows (Figure 13.3): UV light on the skin transforms 7-dehydrocholesterol to cholecalciferol (vitamin D3). One hour of direct sunlight produces the daily requirement in people with pale skins, but the process takes longer on darker skin. Vitamin D3 is subsequently hydroxylated in the liver to 25-hydroxycholecalciferol [25(OH)-vitamin D3] (an inactive form). Serum 25(OH)-vitamin D3 is the most accurate indicator of body vitamin D stores.

Further hydroxylation of 25(OH)-vitamin D3 occurs in the mitochondria of the proximal convoluted tubular cells of the kidney to 1,25-

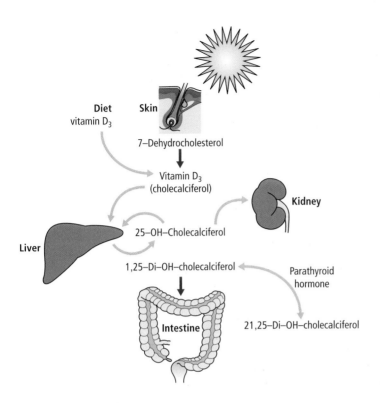

Figure 13.3 *Vitamin D metabolic pathways.*

Diet
vitamin D$_3$

Skin

7–Dehydrocholesterol

Vitamin D$_3$
(cholecalciferol)

Kidney

Liver

25–OH–Cholecalciferol

1,25–Di–OH–cholecalciferol

Parathyroid
hormone

Intestine

21,25–Di–OH–cholecalciferol

dihydroxyxholecalciferol [1,25(OH)$_2$-vitamin D3] (the active form of vitamin D). Activation is in response to raised levels of PTH or decreased levels of serum calcium or phosphate. Decreased PTH levels or raised calcium or phosphate results in conversion of the active form to the inactive 24,25(OH)$_2$-vitamin D3.

Parathyroid hormone

This is an 84-amino-acid peptide secreted by the **chief cells** of the four parathyroid glands in response to changes in extracellular calcium via a recently identified calcium-sensing receptor. PTH is secreted in response to decreased serum calcium/phosphate. Its production is inhibited by elevated serum calcium or 1,25(OH)$_2$-vitamin D3. PTH has numerous effects, including the following:

- **In the kidney:**
  - Stimulation of hydroxylation (activation) of 25(OH)-vitamin D3 in the proximal tubules, leading to indirect intestinal effects.
  - Increasing reabsorption of filtered calcium in the kidney.

- Promotion of urinary excretion of phosphate from the kidney.
- **In bone:** stimulation of osteoclasts and their precursors, producing bone resorption.
- **Overall effect:** serum calcium levels are increased and phosphate levels are decreased.

Calcitonin

Calcitonin is a 32-amino-acid peptide secreted by the **parafollicular C-cells** of the thyroid gland. Calcitonin is secreted in response to elevated serum calcium and inhibited by decreased serum calcium. Calcitonin directly inhibits osteoclasts (which have calcitonin receptors). Its effects include reduction of cellular motility, retraction of cytoplasmic extensions, and reduction in ruffled border size. This produces a transient decrease in serum calcium.

Other hormones and growth factors

- **Oestrogen:** inhibits bone resorption and therefore prevents bone loss. Also inhibits bone formation and so does not increase bone density.

- **Corticosteroids:** reduce gastrointestinal absorption and increase renal excretion of calcium, thus inhibiting bone matrix formation, causing hyperparathyroidism and leading to rapid bone loss. Patients on corticosteroids should be given calcium and vitamin D, with or without bisphosphonates.
- **Thyroid hormones:** increase bone turnover, favouring bone resorption (seen in hyperthyroidism).
- **Growth hormone:** produces a positive calcium balance by increasing gut absorption.
- **Insulin:** type I diabetes, if poorly controlled, may lead to bone loss.
- **Growth factors:**
  - IL-1, IL-6 and tumour necrosis factor alpha (TNF-α) stimulate proliferation of osteoclast precursors.
  - IGF activates osteoblasts and is produced by osteoblasts.
  - TGF activates osteoblasts; also stimulates osteoclastic precursors in vitro.

PHYSIOLOGICAL CHANGES WITH AGE

Normally, bone mass increases up to a peak between 16 and 25 years, after which there is a normal physiological loss of bone mass over time for both men and women of 0.3–0.5 per cent per year. Thus, calcium balance is positive in the first three decades of life, after which it becomes negative.

Women have an increase in bone loss (up to 2–3 per cent) at the menopause, but after the first postmenopausal decade the rate of bone loss is equivalent for both men and women.

Viva questions

1 What is the structure of bone?

2 What cells are found in bone? What are their functions?

3 What does the matrix of bone contain?

4 How does remodelling of bone occur?

5 How is calcium regulated in the body? What is the contribution of bone?

FURTHER READING

Boskey, AL, Posner, AS. Bone structure, composition, and mineralization. *Orthop Clin North Am* 1984;**15**:597–612.

Buckwalter, JA, Cooper, RR. Bone structure and function. *Instr Course Lect* 1987;**36**:27–48.

Buckwalter, JA, Glimcher, MJ, Cooper, RR, Recker, R. Bone biology: I. Structure, blood supply, cells, matrix, and mineralization. *Instr Course Lect* 1996;**45**:371–86.

Forriol, F, Shapiro, F. Bone development: interaction of molecular components and biophysical forces. *Clin Orthop Relat Res* 2005;**432**:14–33.

Posner, AS. The mineral of bone. *Clin Orthop Relat Res* 1985;**200**:87–99.

14

Bone injury, healing and grafting

PETER BATES AND MANOJ RAMACHANDRAN

INTRODUCTION

In this chapter, we review the key facts concerning fracture biomechanics and healing, and bone grafting and banking.

FRACTURE BIOMECHANICS

Fractures can be classified according to the nature of their causative force:

REPETITIVE FORCE

Stress fractures may result from cyclical loading with forces below the ultimate strength of the bone. Micro-damage may occur with each cycle of loading, with microscopic cracks forming along cement lines. The bone fails if the crack propagation moves faster than the reparative processes of internal (primary) remodelling and periosteal callus formation.

SINGLE FORCE

A single application of force produces a fracture pattern characterized by the nature of the application of force (Figure 14.1). Forces may be either **direct** or **indirect**. **Indirect forces** may act either along the length of the bone, as in spiral fractures, or via the soft tissues, as in avulsion fractures of the patella and olecranon.

Cortical bone is stiffer than cancellous bone and tolerates less strain before fracture. Cortical bone fractures at an in vitro strain of 2 per cent, while cancellous bone fractures at an in vitro strain of 75 per cent. Cortical bone is **anisotropic** and is strong in compression but relatively weak in tension and shear. Therefore, the areas where tensile and shear stresses are greatest fail first.

The rate of application of force determines the energy (E) transferred:

$$E = 1/2m \times v^2$$

where m is the mass and v is the velocity.

Thus, the energy imparted increases as the square of the velocity of the injury. Bone is **visco-elastic**, i.e. its biomechanical properties vary with the rate of application of load. Bone is stiffer, stronger and more brittle when loads are applied at a higher rate. With rapid loading, bone absorbs more energy than when loaded more slowly, and this energy is released as it fractures. Therefore, as the energy or velocity increases, the more comminuted the fracture is likely to be and the more extensive is the soft tissue injury associated with it. High-energy and high-velocity injuries and injuries associated with extensive soft-tissue damage have significantly longer times to healing and higher complication rates.

The type of fracture produced by forces acting on bone is dependent on five key factors:

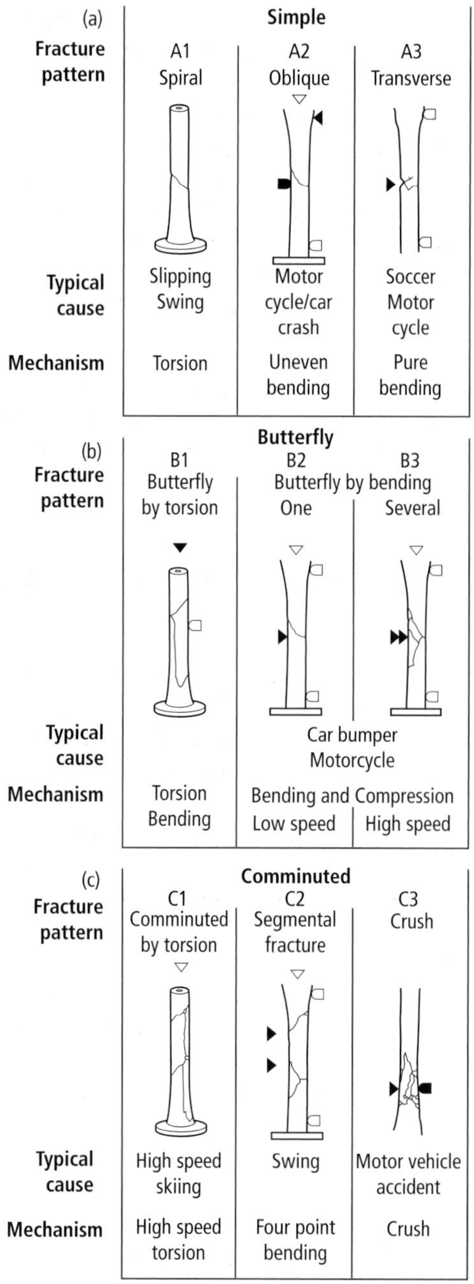

(a) Simple

Fracture pattern	A1 Spiral	A2 Oblique	A3 Transverse
Typical cause	Slipping Swing	Motor cycle/car crash	Soccer Motor cycle
Mechanism	Torsion	Uneven bending	Pure bending

(b) Butterfly

Fracture pattern	B1 Butterfly by torsion	B2 Butterfly by bending One	B3 Butterfly by bending Several
Typical cause		Car bumper Motorcycle	
Mechanism	Torsion Bending	Bending and Compression Low speed	High speed

(c) Comminuted

Fracture pattern	C1 Comminuted by torsion	C2 Segmental fracture	C3 Crush
Typical cause	High speed skiing	Swing	Motor vehicle accident
Mechanism	High speed torsion	Four point bending	Crush

Figure 14.1 *Fracture pattern is related to the nature of force applied.*

- load;
- rate;
- direction;
- bone properties, e.g. shape, anatomical area, quality of bone;
- soft-tissue forces.

Pure compression forces are rare in the skeleton but lead to shear forces, and often on to fractures at 45 degrees to the compressive load. Shear lines are formed by buckling of lamellae and oblique cracking of osteons, which occurs first at areas of stress concentration in the bone, e.g. vessels or resorption spaces, leading to **oblique fractures**. **Uneven bending forces** also create oblique fractures.

Tensile forces tend to arise at soft-tissue insertions to cancellous bone, producing **transverse fractures** due to debonding of cement lines and pulling out of osteons, e.g. olecranon, patella and medial malleolus. Note that percentage lengthening to fracture with tensile strain is 2 per cent for cortical bone and more than 75 per cent for cancellous bone, although the stress required to fracture is higher for the former.

Pure bending forces result in **transverse fractures** from tension on the convexity and compression on the convexity, with the neutral axis moving towards the fracture. A **bending wedge (butterfly) fragment** may occur on the compression (concave) side, especially with high-energy injuries. With combined **bending and compression**, the bending force causes a transverse crack in tension and the compression force causes an oblique fracture, resulting again in a **bending wedge** or **butterfly fracture**.

Torsional forces cause **spiral fractures** with two components: one spiral fracture line around the circumference of the bone at approximately 45 degrees to the horizontal caused by a failure in tension perpendicular to the crack, and a vertical line linking the proximal and distal ends of the spiral due to shear failure (the latter probably initiating the fracture). If **torsion** and **compression** are combined, then a **spiral wedge fracture** results.

Four-point bending, such as a car bumper striking a tibia, creates **segmental fractures**.

FRACTURE HEALING

PRIMARY (DIRECT CORTICAL, OSTEONAL OR HAVERSIAN) BONE HEALING

This type of healing only occurs when there has been **anatomical reduction** and **interfragmentary** compression, leading to **absolute stability** (no motion between fracture surfaces under functional load). The process is very intolerant of strain (movement) at the fracture site.

In the **first few days**, there is minimal activity in areas of direct contact (**contact healing**). New blood vessels grow into any small gaps that exist (**gap healing**), and mesenchymal cells differentiate into osteoblasts, laying down lamellar bone in small gaps and woven bone in large gaps.

Subsequently, osteoclasts form cutting cones that tunnel across the fracture site wherever there is contact between the bone ends or a minute gap. This leaves a path for blood vessels and osteoblasts to follow in their wake, laying down lamellar bone in the form of new osteons. This process of newly formed osteons bridging the gap may take many months and may be difficult to see on an X-ray. This is the same process as the **remodelling phase (stage IV)** of secondary bone healing.

SECONDARY (CALLUS) BONE HEALING

In the presence of **relative stability** (some controlled motion between fracture surfaces under functional load), strain or movement at the fracture site stimulates secondary healing by two discrete processes:

- **Periosteal bony callus (intramembranous ossification):** multipotent cells in the periosteum differentiate into osteoprogenitor cells, which produce bone directly without first forming cartilage. This hard callus forms early on at the periphery of the fracture site, providing there has not been extensive periosteal stripping.
- **Fibrocartilaginous bridging callus (endochondral ossification):** this process occurs simultaneously between the adjacent bone ends and involves the formation of fibrocartilage that becomes calcified and is then replaced by osteoid or woven bone. This process also occurs within the surrounding soft tissues.

These processes are dependent on some movement occurring at the fracture site (strain). Rigid fixation inhibits the differentiation of cells and the formation of callus. The stages of callus formation are shown in Table 14.1.

PERREN'S STRAIN THEORY OF FRACTURE HEALING

After any form of fixation or immobilization, a fracture that is loaded will undergo some degree of movement or strain. This may be compressive, tensile, bending or torsional.

Strain at a fracture site is decreased with increased fracture gap or greater surface area, such as in metaphyseal fractures (larger bone diameter) and in multifragmentary or segmental fractures (where the overall strain is shared among the individual fragments).

Fracture callus becomes increasingly stiff with time, from a gelatinous granulation tissue, to soft callus and to subsequently hard bony callus. Each of these tissues is able to tolerate a different amount of strain:

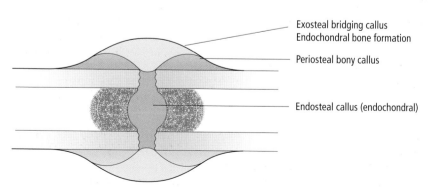

Exosteal bridging callus
Endochondral bone formation

Periosteal bony callus

Endosteal callus (endochondral)

Figure 14.2 *Macroscopic view of callus formation between stages II and III.*

Table 14.1 Stages of callus formation

Stage	Timescale	Order of events
Stage I: haematoma and inflammation	Up to 1 week	Haematoma from ruptured blood vessels forms fibrin clot. Damaged tissue and degranulated platelets release signalling molecules, growth factors and cytokines.
		Migration of inflammatory cells into the haematoma occurs, responding to local growth factors and cytokines (IL-1, IL-6, TGF-β super-family including BMPs, PDGF, FGF, IGF).
		Proliferation, differentiation and matrix synthesis as haematoma is replaced by granulation tissue. Capillary in-growth (angiogenesis) and recruitment of fibroblasts, mesenchymal cells and osteoprogenitor cells. The periosteum plays an important role in this process.
		Cell types involved include PMNs, macrophages and then fibroblasts.
		At necrotic bone ends, bone resorption is mediated by osteoclasts and removal of tissue debris by macrophages.
Stage II: soft callus	1 week– 1 month	Increased cellularity, with proliferation, differentiation and soft callus neovascularization.
		Callus is a combination of fibrous tissue, cartilage and woven bone (Figure 14.2).
		Intramembranous (bony/periosteal) callus = primary callus response: type I collagen (osteoid) laid down from periosteal osteoblasts in the cambium layer as periosteal bony callus or woven bone. This is hard callus but it does not bridge the fracture.
		Endochondral (fibrocartilaginous/bridging) callus = bridging external callus: multipotential cells differentiate to form chondroblasts and fibroblasts within the granulating callus, which produce the type II cartilaginous and fibrous elements of the matrix (chondroid). Chondroblasts then calcify the chondroid matrix they have produced, creating calcified fibrocartilage or soft callus.
		Medullary callus: this is a later process and can slowly unite the fracture if external callus fails.
Stage III: hard callus	1–4 months	Calcified soft callus is resorbed by chondroclasts and invaded by new blood vessels. These bring with them osteoblast precursors that produce the bony (type I) elements of the matrix (osteoid) and then mineralize it to form woven bone.
		Soft calcified chondroid callus becomes hard mineralized osteoid callus.
		Bony bridging continues peripherally as subperiosteal new bone formation. At this point the fracture is united, solid and pain-free to movement.
Stage IV: remodelling	Up to several years	Once the fracture has united, the hard callus is remodelled from woven bone to hard, dense lamellar bone by a process of osteoclastic resorption followed by osteoblastic bone formation. The medullary canal reforms at the end of this process.
		This is the same mechanism as for direct cortical, osteonal or primary bone healing, seen following fracture fixation with absolute stability.
		Bone assumes a configuration and shape based on stresses acting upon it (Wolff's law). Electric fields may play a role in Wolff's law, with osteoclastic activity being predominant on the electropositive tension side of bone and osteoblastic activity on the electronegative compression side.

BMP, bone morphogenic protein; FGF, fibroblast growth factor; IGF, insulin-like growth factor; IL-1, interleukin 1; IL-6, interleukin 6; PDGF, platelet-derived growth factor; PMN, polymorphonuclear neutrophil; TGF-β, transforming growth factor beta.

- **Granulation tissue:** up to 100 per cent.
- **Fibrous connective tissue:** up to 17 per cent.
- **Fibrocartilage:** 2–10 per cent.
- **Lamellar bone:** 2 per cent.

The degree of interfragmentary strain appears to govern the cellular response and therefore the type of tissue that forms between the fracture fragments. Initially the strain is high, stimulating granulation tissue formation, but as the strain decreases with time cartilage and then bone form.

In the presence of **absolute stability** (compression plating or rigid external fixation), if the fragments are in intimate contact, then the fracture site strain is so low as to inhibit callus formation and allow direct (primary) Haversian remodelling. If fragments are fixed rigidly but a gap is present, then primary bone healing (cutting cones) may not be able to bridge the gap. The lack of strain may inhibit callus formation and secondary healing, predisposing to non-union.

In the presence of **relative stability** (splint immobilization, intramedullary fixation or bridge plating), the more strain-tolerant cartilaginous callus is required to stiffen the fracture site before hard woven bony callus forming and replacing it (secondary healing). A larger strain produces a bigger callus.

In the presence of **complete instability**, callus is unable to form because the strain is too much for it to tolerate. The more strain-tolerant fibrous tissue forms, creating a hypertrophic non-union.

FACTORS INFLUENCING FRACTURE HEALING

Several factors influence fracture healing (Table 14.2).

NON-UNION

This is defined as **lack of healing** of a fracture within the expected time, which varies with the bone involved, e.g. distal radial fractures are expected to heal by 6 weeks, scaphoid fractures by 8 weeks, tibial fractures by 16 ± 4 weeks and femoral fractures by 16 ± 4 weeks. The fracture is bridged by soft tissue, the characteristics of which are defined by the local blood supply and mechanical conditions (usually cartilage and/or fibrous tissue).

Clinical union is defined by the absence of tenderness or motion at the fracture site with no pain on loading, while **radiological union** is defined as the presence of visible bridging trabeculae on three out of four cortices on X-rays.

Table 14.2 Factors affecting fracture healing

Local	Systemic
Degree of soft-tissue trauma	*Smoking (affects osteoblast function)*
Associated neurovascular injury	*Diabetes mellitus*
Degree of bone loss	*Nutrition*
Degree of immobilization	*Age*
Open fracture or presence of infection	*Drugs (steroids, NSAIDs)*
Local pathological lesion (e.g. tumour)	*Hormones*
Type of bone fractured (e.g. tibia 3–4 months, metacarpal 4–6 weeks)	*Associated head injury (enhances fracture healing)*
Site of fracture (metaphysis v. diaphysis)	
Interposition of soft tissue or inadequate reduction	

NSAID, non-steroidal anti-inflammatory drug.

Hypertrophic non-union

A good blood supply but excessive strain at the fracture site prevents progression of the callus to form bone. These usually require biomechanical stabilization to allow callus progression to bone to occur.

Atrophic non-union

A poor blood supply is caused by soft-tissue damage, periosteal stripping and/or fracture comminution, which may occur at the time of injury or during the exposure for internal fixation. A fracture fixed with rigid fixation (zero strain) and with the fragments distracted will also lack stimulation of callus formation. Atrophic non-unions require stabilization and biological enhancement in order to heal.

BONE GRAFTING

DEFINITION

Bone grafting is the use of any implanted material that alone or in combination with other materials promotes a bone-healing response by providing osteogenic, osteoconductive or osteo-inductive activity to a local site. Bone grafts have **mechanical** (providing support) and **biological** (stimulus for bone formation) functions.

INDICATIONS

- **Provision of structural stability:** massive proximal femoral grafting in revision total hip arthroplasty for the reconstruction and/or replacement of skeletal defects.
- **Stimulation of bone formation:** bone grafting in spinal fusions where the graft improves the fusion rate but does not provide any mechanical support, even in the short term.
- **Enhancement of fracture healing:**
  - **Acute:** for mechanical or biological reasons, e.g. in comminuted fractures with bone loss or during elevation of depressed joint surface.
  - **Non-union:** usually for biological reasons.

PROPERTIES OF BONE GRAFTS

Osteogenicity

The graft contains **living cells** that are capable of **differentiation** into bone. Osteogenicity occurs independent of the host bed, i.e. the graft may survive and incorporate successfully, even in a fibrotic, previously irradiated bed.

OSTEOCONDUCTION

The graft provides a **three-dimensional scaffold** that supports in-growth of capillaries, perivascular tissues and osteogenic cell precursors. The surface of the scaffold allows attachment, division and differentiation of cells and ultimately remodelling. The graft does not have to be biological in order to possess osteoconductive properties.

Osteo-induction

The graft provides a **biological stimulus** that stimulates mitosis and differentiation of undifferentiated mesenchymal cells into osteoprogenitor cells with the capacity to form new bone. The graft has the ability to promote bone formation at non-skeletal sites and may be added to osteoconductive compounds, but the condition of the host bed is critical. Note that demineralized bone graft has potent osteo-inductive properties as it contains several bone morphogenetic proteins (BMPs), insulin-like growth factors 1 (IGF-1) and 2 (IGF-2), acidic and basic fibroblast growth factors (FGFs), interleukins, granulocyte colony-stimulating factor (G-CSF) and granulocyte/macrophage colony-stimulating factor (GM-CSF).

GENETICS OF BONE GRAFTS

Autografts

Tissue is harvested from and implanted into the **same individual**. Examples include cancellous, cortical and vascularized grafts, and bone marrow.

Allografts

Tissue is harvested from one individual and implanted into **another individual of the same species**. The host mounts an immune response to the cells of a fresh allograft and, therefore, the graft is processed in order to remove immunogenic cells, decreasing the risk of both immune response and transmission of infection. Allografts can be classified according to the following:

- **Anatomy:** cortical, cancellous, corticocancellous.
- **Processing:** fresh, frozen, freeze-dried, demineralized.
- **Sterilization method:** sterile processing, irradiated, ethylene oxide.
- **Handling properties:** powder, gel, paste/putty, chips, strips/blocks, massive.

Xenografts

Tissue is harvested from one species and implanted into a **different species**. Unfortunately, a vigorous immune response precludes the use of most preparations. Some currently used xenografts include Kiel bone (defatted and deproteinated xenograft, which has a decreased immune response), processed xenograft with autologous bone marrow, and processed bovine collagen (biocompatible flexible substrate material, which is a component of several bone-graft preparations).

DANGERS OF BONE GRAFTS

- **Autografts:** donor site morbidity (scar, haematoma, infection, pain).
- **Allografts:**
  - Disease transmission: both **microbiological** (e.g. two cases of human immunodeficiency virus (HIV) per one million grafts, two cases of hepatitis C per one million grafts) and **pathological** (e.g. 8 per cent of femoral head allografts have histological evidence of disease such as malignant and benign tumours such as osteomas).
  - Immune sensitization (see below).

SPECIFIC GRAFT TYPES

The properties of common bone grafts and bone graft substitutes are shown in Table 14.3.

Table 14.3 Properties of common bone grafts and bone-graft substitutes

	Immunogenicity	Osteogenic	Osteoconductive	Osteo-inductive	Structural	Vascularized
Autograft						
Bone marrow	–	++	–	+	–	–
Cancellous	–	++	++	+	+	–
Cortical	–	+	+	+	++ *(early)*	–
Vascularized	–	++	+++	+	++	+++
Allograft						
Cancellous	+	–	++	+	+	+
Cortical	+	–	++	+	++	++
Demineralized	+	–	++	++ *(BMPs)*	–	–
Bone-graft substitutes						
Calcium phosphates	–		++	–	+	+

BMP, bone morphogenic protein; –, none; +, weak; ++, moderate; +++, strong.

Bone grafts

Cortical or cancellous bone grafts may be used. These may be:

- **Autografts:**
  - Harvested and implanted within the same individual, usually fresh and containing a living cell population and associated cytokines and growth factors.
  - Problems with donor site morbidity (scar, haematoma, infection, pain) and limited supply.
  - Vascularized autografts (e.g. fibula) have significant donor site morbidity but heal like fractures with no initial resorption (cells retain their viability). They are technically difficult to perform but allow rapid union. These grafts are best for **irradiated tissues** and for **large tissue defects**.
- **Allografts:**
  - Donor is from the same species.
  - No donor site morbidity.
  - Large amounts available.
  - High infection rate (10–12 per cent).
  - Cell population is destroyed.
- **Xenografts:**
  - Donor from a different species (porcine, bovine).
  - Seldom used.

GRAFT INCORPORATION

This is the process by which invasion of the graft by host bone occurs, such that the graft is replaced partially or completely by host bone. Initial stages of the inflammatory response (with or without a specific immune response), revascularization and osteo-induction are similar for cortical and cancellous bone, but the latter stages of osteoconduction and remodelling are different.

The process of incorporation is also different for autografts and allografts. Allograft incorporation is slower and is accompanied by a variable amount of inflammation as a result of the host immune response to the graft. As there is always some genetic disparity, the host accepts most allografts, albeit reluctantly, and incorporates them, although a few may be

rejected if there are strong genetic differences. Note that frozen allografts incorporate better than fresh allografts (due to the presence of fewer immunogenic cells) and that allografts can sensitize patients, limiting the options for subsequent organ transplants (less likely with frozen compared with fresh allograft; more likely if more than one bone donor used).

Cancellous graft incorporation

Autogenous non-vascularized cancellous grafts incorporate initially in a manner similar to that for cortical grafts, undergoing an **inflammatory response**. Subsequently, the process is similar to callus formation, with formation of an initial bony scaffold and subsequent remodelling, with all cancellous graft eventually being replaced by **creeping substitution**:

Phase 1: vascular in-growth, chemotaxis and invasion/differentiation of multipotent stem cells. As **revascularization is rapid**, surface osteocytes survive.

Phase 2: osteoblasts (whose formation is induced by factors within the graft) lay down new bone on the scaffold of dead trabeculae, with simultaneous osteoclastic resorption (**creeping substitution**). This leads to early increase in density on X-rays and an associated transient increase in strength.

Phase 3: osteoclast/osteoblast **remodelling** of the trabeculae along lines of force, with associated **decreased radiodensity**.

Allogenic grafts undergo a similar process, but with a more marked inflammatory phase and less predictable and possibly incomplete incorporation.

Since there is prompt formation of new bone on to the dead scaffold, cancellous grafts achieve early structural strength.

Cortical graft incorporation

Autogenous non-vascularized cortical grafts, after an initial but much slower process of inflammation and revascularization, incorporate in a different manner to cancellous grafts. All donor bone has to be removed before appositional bone formation occurs.

Osteoclastic resorption via cutting cones into the graft has to precede osteoblastic bone formation. Therefore, 40–60 per cent of mechanical strength is lost in the first 3–6 months and returns fully only over 1–2 years. Initial incorporation occurs at the **host–graft junction** via endochondral bone formation. Subsequently, there is new **appositional bone formation** by ingrowth of new osteons, following the new blood vessels. In contrast to cancellous grafting, the entire graft is not incorporated and there is no remodelling phase.

Allogenic grafts undergo a similar process, but more slowly and with less overall ingrowth. Rarely, allografts may undergo immunogenic destruction following a massive inflammatory response.

Vascularized grafts are autogenous and incorporate in a manner analogous to fracture repair, as similar biological and mechanical conditions prevail. The cells retain their viability.

Factors affecting incorporation

- **Modification of inflammatory response:** use of indomethacin delays response.
- **Mechanical environment of graft:** inadequate mechanical stability of graft leads to formation of granulation tissue and fibrosis.
- **Quality of host bed:** abundance and competence of progenitor cells affects incorporation. Host bed may be deficient in cells if:
  - previous infection;
  - poor vascularity;
  - previous irradiation;
  - immunocompromised host.

OSTEOCHONDRAL ALLOGRAFT

The cartilage component also induces an **immune response** and, therefore, tissue typing is required. Survival of cartilage may be improved by immersion in glycerol or dimethyl sulphoxide. These grafts are used increasingly in tumour surgery.

AUTOGENOUS BONE MARROW

Bone marrow aspirates contain osteogenic precursors. These may be incorporated into osteoconductive grafts.

BONE GRAFT SUBSTITUTES

- **Calcium phosphates:**
  - **Bulk**, e.g. tricalcium phosphate (which undergoes partial conversion to hydroxyapatite in vivo), hydroxyapatite and combinations of the two. These materials degrade at a very slow rate.
  - **Injectable**, e.g. Norian SRS: injectable paste of inorganic calcium and phosphate used to fill bone voids after acute fractures, which hardens in minutes and is osteoconductive. Eventually resorbed and replaced by host bone.
- **Calcium carbonates**, e.g. Biocora: chemically unaltered marine coral that is resorbed and replaced by bone.
- **Coralline hydroxyapatite**, e.g. Pro-Osteon: calcium carbonate skeleton undergoes a thermo-exchange process to convert this into calcium phosphate.
- **Calcium sulphate**, e.g. Osteoset: osteoconductive calcium sulphate pellets.
- **Silicon-based**, e.g. bioactive glasses, glass-ionomer cement: used as delivery systems for osteo-inductive compounds.
- **Synthetic polymers**, e.g. polylactic acid and polyglycolic acid: problems include the production of acidic degradation products.
- **Ceramic composites**, e.g. Collagraft: calcium-collagen graft material – an osteoconductive composite of hydroxyapatite, tricalcium phosphate and collagen used as a bone graft substitute or expander mixed with autologous bone marrow to provide cells and growth factors.

OSTEO-INDUCTIVE AGENTS

Growth factors act as osteo-inductive signalling molecules but may have other effects, as detailed below. Some, such as BMPs, are gaining popularity in the clinical arena.

Transforming growth factor beta

- Super-family of growth factors found in platelets and many cell types.
- Broad range of activity within bone and fracture callus.

- Induces synthesis of type II collagen and proteoglycans.
- Stimulates proliferation/differentiation of osteoblasts and other cell types.
- Stored in bone matrix and released during resorption.

Bone morphogenetic proteins

- Family of at least 17 glycoproteins able to stimulate ectopic bone formation.
- BMP-2, -3 and -7 appear to be the most important.
- Induce differentiation of mesenchymal cells to osteogenic lineages.
- One example is OP-1 (BMP-7), shown to be of benefit in various clinical situations such as tibial non-union.

Fibroblast growth factor

- Mitogenic for many cell types.
- Released from endothelial cells.
- Stimulates angiogenesis and callus formation.

Platelet–derived growth factor

- Potent chemotactic activity following fracture.
- Released from platelets and monocytes after trauma.
- Stimulates deoxyribonucleic acid (DNA) synthesis.

BONE BANKING

As human bone grafts are available in only limited quantities, bone banks have been set up to provide bone to institutions that require it. The following principles apply to the process of bone banking:

DONOR CONSENT

- **Living donors:** consent is needed in order to cover retrieval, testing and access to medical records.
- **Cadavers:** the prerequisite is lack of objection from the next of kin.

DONOR SCREENING

- **Medical and behavioural history:** this helps to pick up certain donors that may need to be excluded, e.g. intravenous drug abuse. The history is usually obtained from the next of kin for living donors and from general practitioner notes for cadavers.
- **Blood tests:** performed for hepatitis B and C, HIV, syphilis and Rhesus status.

A dedicated nurse is required to counsel patients who are to be donors.

EXCLUSION CRITERIA

- HIV.
- Hepatitis B and C.
- Malignancy.
- Systemic disorders that may compromise biological or biomechanical integrity of graft, e.g. rheumatoid arthritis, autoimmune disease, long-term steroid treatment.
- Diseases of unknown origin, e.g. Alzheimer's disease, Creutzfeldt–Jakob disease, multiple sclerosis.

ALLOGRAFT PROCESSING

Allografts are processed to remove superfluous proteins, cells and tissues in order to decrease immune sensitization and disease transmission. Processing also allows better graft preservation. Techniques may include:

- **physical debridement** of unwanted tissue;
- **ultrasonic processing** with or without pulsatile washes to remove remaining cells and blood;
- **ethanol treatment** to denature cell proteins and reduce bacterial and viral load;
- **antibiotic soak** to kill bacteria;
- **irradiation** to sterilize tissue, particularly if contaminated or if not processed in a sterile manner (but this affects collagen and alters mechanical strength);
- **demineralization**.

ALLOGRAFT PRESERVATION

Preservation techniques include the following:

- **Fresh:** immunogenic.

- **Fresh-frozen** at −70°C:
  - has least impact on mechanical strength;
  - decreases immunogenicity;
  - preserves BMPs.
- **Lyophilized** (freeze-dried):
  - least immunogenic;
  - lowest likelihood of disease transmission;
  - BMP depleted;
  - may structurally weaken during rehydration.

EXAMPLES OF PRODUCTS AVAILABLE FROM BONE BANKS

- **Fresh-frozen femoral head:** a whole femoral head, retrieved from a living donor, which is unprocessed and greater than 50 g in weight. Available only frozen, and supplied only to hospitals that collect fresh-frozen femoral heads for tissue services when limited stock available.

- **Cancellous cubes:** approximately 1 cm^3 in volume. Available freeze-dried and irradiated in packs of five.
- **Cortical struts:** struts of cortical bone from femoral shafts that are cut to various lengths from 2 cm to 22 cm. Available as freeze-dried or frozen and sterilized by gamma-irradiation.
- **Massive bone allografts:** grafts prepared with articular cartilage and soft tissue removed. Available frozen and irradiated. A small stock of proximal and distal femora and proximal tibiae is normally maintained.

AUGMENTING FRACTURE HEALING

In addition to the use of bone grafts, bone-graft substitutes and osteo-inductive agents, other techniques used to enhance fracture healing include the following:

Table 14.4 Advantages and disadvantages of bone graft and bone-graft substitutes

	Advantages	Disadvantages
Autograft	Non-immunogenic No disease transmission Rapid incorporation	Donor site morbidity Limited amounts available
Allograft	More available No donor site morbidity	Immunogenic (fresh < frozen < freeze-dried) Disease transmission Slow incorporation
Fresh	No preservation required	Availability and need may not coincide
Frozen	Simple technique Reduced immunogenicity	Expensive Needs to be transported frozen
Freeze-dried	Easily transported Stored at room temperature	Expensive Structurally weak Less completely incorporated
Xenograft	Unlimited amounts	Immunogenic No osteogenesis unless autograft added
Kiel bone	Reduced immunogenicity	
Bone-graft substitutes	Unlimited amounts Biocompatible No disease transmission Osteoconductive Biodegrades No donor site morbidity	Brittle No osteo-induction

SYSTEMIC ENHANCEMENT

Several systemic approaches have been hypothesized, but none is in wide usage. Examples include IGF-1 and IGF-2, growth hormone, parathyroid hormone, vitamin D3 and prostaglandins.

DISTANT SKELETAL INJURY

Injury to bone marrow enhances bone healing at distant sites. Corticotomy in a long bone has a stimulatory affect on fracture healing elsewhere in the same bone.

ELECTROMAGNETIC FIELDS

Piezoelectric currents are produced within bone as the collagen fibres are deformed. **Streaming potentials** (electrokinetic currents) are produced as charged constituents of extracellular matrix flow past the mineral phase of bone as it is deformed. The endogenous electric fields produced from these processes are integral to bone homeostasis, influencing normal bone modelling and remodelling. Clinical devices use electromagnetic induction waveforms to try to reproduce these potentials and so speed up or augment fracture healing.

ULTRASOUND

There is good evidence that low-intensity ultrasound can affect gene expression, stimulate chondroblast and osteoblast activity, enhance blood flow, and accelerate or augment fracture healing in animal models. Pressure waves from ultrasound may also stimulate differentiating bone lining cells along the edges of a fracture.

MECHANICAL METHODS

Controlled axial micromotion has been shown to enhance the healing of tibial fractures.

SUMMARY

Table 14.4 summarizes the advantages and disadvantages of different types of bone grafts and bone-graft substitutes.

Viva questions

1 How do fractures heal?

2 What factors affect fracture healing?

3 What are the indications for the use of bone allografts? Are there any precautions to consider?

4 What types of bone graft do you know of? What are their pros and cons?

5 How are allografts processed?

FURTHER READING

Aaron, RK, Ciombor, DM, Simon, BJ. Treatment of nonunions with electric and electromagnetic fields. *Clin Orthop Relat Res* 2004;**419**:21–9.

Einhorn, TA. Enhancement of fracture healing. *J Bone Joint Surg Am* 1995;**77**:940–56.

Khan, SN, Cammisa, FP, Jr, Sandhu, HS, *et al.* The biology of bone grafting. *J Am Acad Orthop Surg* 2005;**131**:77–86.

Stevenson, S, Emery, SE, Goldberg, VM. Factors affecting bone graft incorporation. *Clin Orthop Relat Res* 1996;**324**:66–74.

Termaat, MF, Den Boer, FC, Bakker, FC, Patka, P, Haarman, HJ. Bone morphogenetic proteins: development and clinical efficacy in the treatment of fractures and bone defects. *J Bone Joint Surg Am* 2005;**87**:1367–78.

15

Intervertebral disc

WILLIAM ASTON AND RAJIV BAJEKAL

INTRODUCTION

Knowledge of the structure of the intervertebral disc and how this relates to its biomechanical function is essential in order to gain an understanding of the injury mechanisms and healing potential of the disc. This chapter details the level of knowledge appropriate to the general orthopaedic surgeon.

STRUCTURE

Embryological development of the vertebral column and associated discs occurs at approximately week 4 of gestation. Each vertebra is formed from two adjacent **sclerotomes** (derived from the mesodermal cell layer), the caudal portion of each sclerotome segment binding to the cephalic half of the subjacent sclerotome, forming the precartilaginous vertebral body. Mesenchymal cells, which go on to form part of the intervertebral disc, are located between the vertebral bodies. The **notochord** (a structure derived early in gestation from the endothelial germ layer), which regresses in the region of the vertebral bodies, enlarges in the region of the disc and forms the **nucleus pulposus**, which then becomes surrounded by the circular fibres of the **anulus fibrosus**. The intervertebral disc becomes a constituent of a secondary cartilaginous joint between the two vertebral bodies (also known as an **intervertebral symphysis**).

Macroscopically, the disc is made up of two components – the **outer anulus fibrosus** and the **inner nucleus pulposus**. The anatomy of the 23 discs changes throughout the spine. In general, they become larger caudally, but they also have regional characteristics. In the **cervical** region, the discs are thicker in their anterior portion, contributing to the lordosis. **Thoracic** discs are uniform in height and thicken caudally (possibly allowing increased mobility), with the spinal curvature being due to the shape of the vertebral bodies. In the **lumbar** region, the discs are again thicker in their anterior portion, maximally at L5/S1. This, in combination with the vertebral body shape, contributes to the lumbosacral angulation. The largest disc is at the level of L4/5; this is also the most avascular disc.

The **microscopic** arrangement of the disc is essential to its function. The fibrocartilaginous **anulus fibrosus** is attached to both the anterior and the posterior longitudinal ligaments of the spine as well as the vertebrae on either side. In the thoracic spine, the annulus also has ligamentous attachments to the head of the articulating ribs laterally. The **outer anulus fibrosus** consists of a number of densely packed layers of predominantly type I collagen called **lamellae**, giving it form and tensile strength, along with fibroblast or fibrocyte-like cells. The layered fibres are oriented at about 30 degrees to the horizontal, the direction alternating with each layer, enabling the disc to resist both distractive and shear forces (Figure 15.1).

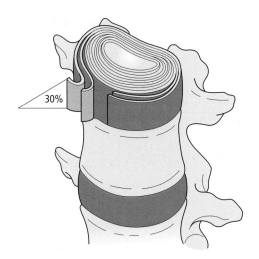

Figure 15.1 *Collagen fibre arrangement in intervertebral disc.*

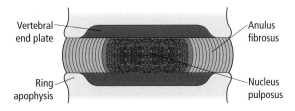

Figure 15.2 *Detailed structure of vertebral end plate.*

A larger fibrocartilaginous **inner anulus fibrosus** layer is found more centrally, containing chondrocytes and a less dense predominantly type II collagenous matrix lacking lamellar organization.

The **nucleus pulposus** lies most centrally, containing a mass of interconnected notochordal cells at birth (**chorda reticulum**) from which individual cells separate during growth. With age, notochordal cells disappear completely, with chondrocyte-like cells being present only in adults. The nucleus is made up of predominantly **type II collagen** in a mucoprotein gel rich in polysaccharides and a **proteoglycan** matrix (consisting of central hyaluronan filaments and multiple aggrecan molecules, stabilized by link proteins) that gives it visco-elasticity, stiffness and resistance to compression through its interaction with water.

The disc can be divided into two regions – the outer third and the inner two-thirds. In the **outer third**, the disc is anchored to the vertebrae on either side by Sharpey's fibres, forming a **ring apophysis**. The layers of the **inner two-thirds** curve into and form the fibrocartilaginous component of the **vertebral end plate** covering the superior and inferior surfaces of the disc (Figure 15.2).

The **end plate** consists of hyaline cartilage in children and young adults and calcified cartilage and bone in elderly people. The end plate has

no fibrillar connection with the collagen of the vertebral subchondral bone, making it susceptible to horizontal shear forces.

The proportion of type II collagen increases towards the nucleus pulposus. Other types of fibril-forming collagen are also present, notably collagens V and XI. In addition, short-helix collagens that do not form fibrils are also present, such as collagens VI (unique to discs), IX and XII. In the disc, a high proportion of collagens I and II is cross-linked with pyridinoline residues, which are vital for maintenance of tissue cohesiveness (as seen in other tissues that bear high mechanical loads).

Nerve fibres are found in the outer rings of the annulus only, dorsally from the sinuvertebral nerve (a branch of the spinal nerve as soon as it is formed in the intervertebral foramen) and ventrally from the sympathetic chain.

The intervertebral disc is relatively avascular in the adult, with vessels lying only on the surface of the annulus; some vessels may penetrate the outer layers. The disc is sustained by diffusion and convection of nutrients through the porous central concavity of the end plate and the porous-permeable solid matrix.

Age-related changes within the nucleus are due to the gradual loss of cells and proteoglycans, leading to a decreased water and proteoglycan content and fibrous replacement of the nucleus from the third decade. Specifically, the proportion of non-aggregated proteoglycans and non-collagenous proteins increases, and the size of aggrecan molecules and the concentration of functional link protein decrease. The anulus becomes fibrotic (appearing firm and white macroscopically as opposed to soft and translucent) and is eventually microscopically indistinct from the fibrous nucleus. Fissures and cracks appear in the annulus, with concomitant myxomatous degeneration and loss of the orientation of collagen fibres. The resultant loss of volume, shape and microstructure adversely affects spinal biomechanics, e.g. loss of disc height leads to abnormal loading, causes facet joint degeneration and weakens the disc, increasing the risk of herniation. This process is complete by the sixth to seventh decades, by which time the entire disc, apart from the fibrotic outer annulus, has become stiff fibrocartilage.

FUNCTION

The physiological function of the disc is to **redistribute compressive load** and **resist tensile**, **rotational** and **shear forces**, while facilitating smooth motion in an otherwise rigid spine. Each part of the disc has a specific make-up in order to achieve this. Consequently, if one of these parts is damaged, the biomechanical properties of the entire disc are altered. The microscopic fibre arrangement of the annulus fibrosus enables it to resist tensile, rotational and shear forces. The visco-elastic properties of the nucleus allow it to absorb load and maintain height by a combination of the hydrostatic pressure in the interstitial fluid, the Donnan osmotic pressure (repulsive forces between fixed negative charges on proteoglycans and also forces arising from freely mobile interstitial counter-ions such as sodium and calcium), and the loose framework of the porous-permeable collagen–proteoglycan matrix. These properties are also present in the inner annulus and permit large deformations in response to load, creating intradiscal fluid flows that dissipate energy and visco-elastic creep. This is the basis for the **biphasic theory** for soft-hydrated biological materials and is equally applicable to meniscus, articular cartilage, tendon and ligament. Note that the **biphasic phenomenon** for discs relates to the hoop stresses generated during compression in the outer layers of the annulus, in comparison with the inner layers, which deform and act as shock absorbers.

During prolonged periods of axial loading, interstitial water is squeezed out of the discs, causing a decrease in height and therefore bulging of the annulus. When loading is ceased, e.g. during sleep, the disc height is restored by the in-flow of water back into the discs. The latter phenomenon explains why most disc herniations occur in the morning when the disc is loaded on upright posturing.

INJURY AND HEALING

The symptoms of an **anular tear** are thought to be due to the contents of the nucleus irritating the innervated outer layers of the annulus, secondary to a tear in the inner layers. The initial tear is thought to be due to a sudden increase in intradiscal pressure. Subsequent indefinite symptoms are related to fluctuations in pressure. **Herniation** of the nucleus pulposus through a defect in the annulus fibrosus most often occurs at the insertion of the outer annulus into the vertebral body in the cervical and lumbar regions, where the stresses and motion are greatest. This leads to either bulging of the annulus or herniation of nuclear material, causing spinal-cord, thecal or nerve-root compression. Herniation has the capacity to resolve with time (90 per cent of patients with painful disc herniations are pain-free by 3 months), although the ability of the annulus to self-repair is limited.

Degeneration of the disc is thought to be the result of a number of factors, the most important of which is a decrease in the amount of nutrition reaching the cells and the removal of waste products. This occurs with ageing, as the blood supply of the periphery of the disc gradually declines with the onset of adulthood, and is compounded by calcification of the cartilaginous end plates, accumulation of degraded matrix macromolecules and decrease in matrix water concentration, all of which serve to interfere with nutrient convection and diffusion. Factors thought to accelerate degeneration include physical activity causing increased loading, immobilization, scoliosis and vibration. Factors that may additionally compromise the blood supply include diabetes, smoking and arterial disease. The age-related changes outlined above are also thought to contribute to this process, although degeneration may be a process distinct from ageing. Further degenerative changes in the disc include disruption of collagen fibrils (due to impaired formation, increased cross-linking and increased denaturation) and anulus delamination (at its weakest area, through the interlamellar ground substance), decreasing the ability of the disc to recover from deformation and resulting in more solid-like behaviour. The end plate is also damaged, with thinning and micro-fractures preventing the disc from maintaining its hydrostatic pressure and leading to increased fluid exudation on loading.

Pain due to disc degeneration has been explained by a number of theories, including nerve and blood-vessel in-growth, altered biomechanical loading of surrounding structures, and cell necrosis stimulating the inflammatory cascade, with subsequent cytokine and free-radical release, which may sensitize nerve endings.

Viva questions

1 What type of joint is present between two vertebrae?

2 What is the function of an intervertebral disc?

3 How does the microscopic anatomy of the disc relate to its function?

4 What is an anular tear, and how does it differ from herniation?

5 Disc degeneration inevitably occurs with age. What changes occur during this process?

FURTHER READING

Boos, N, Weissbach, S, Rohrbach, H, *et al.* Classification of age-related changes in lumbar intervertebral discs: 2002 Volvo Award in basic science. *Spine* 2002;**27**:2631–44.

Buckwalter, JA. Aging and degeneration of the human intervertebral disc. *Spine* 1995;**20**:1307–14.

Gruber, HE, Hanley, EN, Jr. Recent advances in disc cell biology. *Spine* 2003;**28**:186–93.

Kaplan, KM, Spivak, JM, Bendo, JA. Embryology of the spine and associated congenital abnormalities. *Spine J* 2005;**5**:564–76.

Roberts, S. Disc morphology in health and disease. *Biomed Soc Trans* 2002;**30**:864–9.

16

Basic concepts in biomechanics

MANOJ RAMACHANDRAN

INTRODUCTION

The workings of the musculoskeletal system, although complex, can be understood using basic laws of mechanics. A working knowledge of biomechanics is essential for the orthopaedic surgeon. Material and fluid mechanics are dealt with in Chapters 17 and 25, respectively.

Biomechanics is the branch of science dealing with the action and effects of internal and external forces on living biological systems using the principles and techniques of engineering and mechanics.

Biomechanics involves the study of:

- **Statics:** study of forces acting on rigid bodies in equilibrium, either at rest or moving at a constant velocity.
- **Dynamics:** study of forces acting on rigid bodies in motion, of which there are three subtypes:
  - **Kinetics:** relates the forces acting on a rigid body to its resulting motion.
  - **Kinematics:** study of motion with respect to the relationships between displacement, velocity and acceleration, without concern for the cause of the motion.
  - **Kinesiology:** study of human movement.

BACKGROUND

HISTORY

In early civilizations (e.g. Babylonian, Egyptian, Greek), humans used parts of their body and elements in their environment to define measurements. Standard units were defined for time (periods of the sun), length (cubit = distance from the elbow to the tip of the middle finger; span = distance from the tip of the thumb to the tip of the little finger, with the hand spread fully; digit = width of the thumb) and weight (Babylonians used standard, well-polished stones; the Egyptians and Greeks used the wheat seed, which evolved into the unit of the grain; the Arabs used a small bean called the carob, which evolved into the unit of the carat).

The British (imperial) system evolved from the above measuring systems and initially involved the use of body measurements, such as foot (from the Roman *pes*), inch (from the 12 Roman divisions of *pes* known as *unciae*) and yard (originally from the Saxon word *gird*, which was the circumference of a person's waist, but later the yard was measured on King Henry I as the distance from his nose to the end of his thumb, with his arm extended). With time, standard references were employed primarily through royal decrees, such as yard (measured as the length of a permanent measuring stick made of iron in the time of King Edward I), foot (one-third of the length of the stick) and inch (one-thirty-sixth of the length of the stick). A brass bar with a gold button at each end was legalized by the British Parliament as the standard yard in 1824.

In 1790, in the era of the French Revolution, the French Academy of Sciences established the metric system. The metre was defined as one-ten-millionth of the distance from the North Pole to the equator on a line passing through Paris, with other linear measurements being decimal fractions of the metre. Although Napoleon renounced the metric system in 1812, the system was later adopted as the international standard and formalized as le Systéme International d'Unitès (SI units) in 1960. Definitions of base units are now sophisticated, e.g. the metre was defined as the wavelength of radiation emitted from the krypton-86 atom and then redefined in 1983 as the distance travelled by light in a vacuum in 1/299 792 458 of a second.

SI UNITS

SI units consist of three groups:

- **Base units**, e.g.
  - metre (m) for length;
  - kilogram (kg) for mass;
  - second (s) for time.
- **Derived units**, e.g.
  - area (m^2);
  - volume (m^3);
  - speed (m/s);
  - acceleration (m/s^2).
- **Derived units with special names**, e.g.
  - force $(kg\ m/s^2)$ = newton (N);
  - moment (Nm).

Note that there are two broad types of unit: scalar and vector. **Scalar units** have magnitude but no direction, e.g. length, mass, time, area, volume, speed. **Vector units** have both magnitude and direction, e.g. acceleration, force, moment. Velocity is a vector as it has both magnitude (speed) and direction. Vectors, in addition to **magnitude** (length of the vector) and **direction** (head of the vector in degrees), are also characterized by their **point of**

application (tail of the vector) and **line of action** (orientation of the vector).

NEWTON'S LAWS

The unit of force was named after the English scientist Sir Isaac Newton (1642–1727), whose work on gravitation was allegedly inspired by an apple falling from a tree on to his head (interestingly, 1 N is approximately equivalent to the weight of a medium-sized apple, i.e. approximately 0.1 kg, and is defined as a force magnitude capable of producing an acceleration of $1\ m/s^2$ to a rigid body with 1 kg of mass). Newton's fundamental equations of physical laws are key to understanding biomechanics as related to human movement:

Newton's first law (inertia)

A body at rest will remain at rest, and a body in motion will remain in motion at a constant velocity in a straight line. This requires the sum of the external forces acting on the body to be zero (i.e. the body is in equilibrium), and so static analysis can be performed with the help of the equations $\Sigma F = 0$ (sum of forces is zero) and $\Sigma M = 0$ (sum of moments is zero).

Newton's second law (action)

A body with a non-zero net force will accelerate in the direction of the force, the magnitude of the acceleration being proportional to the magnitude of the force ($F = ma$). This is useful for dynamic analysis.

Newton's third law (reaction)

For every action, there is an **equal and opposite reaction**. The forces of action and reaction are equal in magnitude but in the opposite direction. This law is important for free-body analysis and understanding ground-reaction forces.

TRIGONOMETRY

A basic knowledge of trigonometry is helpful in biomechanical analysis. The mnemonic

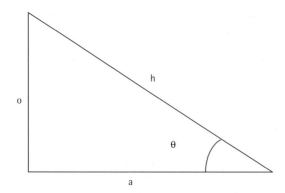

Figure 16.1 *Basic trigonometry.*

sohcahtoa is helpful in remembering that for the angle θ in Figure 16.1:

- $\sin \theta$ = opposite/hypotenuse;
- $\cos \theta$ = adjacent/hypotenuse;
- $\tan \theta$ = opposite/adjacent.

It also helps to remember the following approximations:

- $\sin 30° = \cos 60° \approx 0.5$;
- $\sin 45° = \cos 45° \approx 0.7$;
- $\sin 60° = \cos 30° \approx 0.9$.

MOMENT OF FORCE

FORCE

A **force** is a **mechanical disturbance** or **load** that acts on a body. In its most basic form, a force can either be a push or a pull. Forces can be **external** to the human body (e.g. gravity, ground reaction, air resistance) or **internal** to the human body (e.g. joint contact and shear forces, muscle contraction forces, tendon forces, capsuloligamentous constraint forces). As forces are vectors, they are usually represented by a **boldface** letter or a letter with an arrow, $\rightarrow$, or bar, —, over it. Vectors can be resolved into their component vectors in the x, y and z planes, which are mutually perpendicular Cartesian coordinate axes:

$$\mathbf{F} = \mathbf{F}_x + \mathbf{F}_y + \mathbf{F}_z$$

Use of the Pythagorean theorem allows the magnitude of the force $\mathbf{F}$, denoted by $|\mathbf{F}|$, to be calculated:

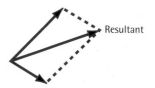

Figure 16.2 *Parallelogram method of vector addition.*

$$|\mathbf{F}|^2 = |\mathbf{F}_x|^2 + |\mathbf{F}_y|^2 + |\mathbf{F}_z|^2$$

Two forces can be added using the parallelogram method (or graphic) of vector addition, where the two vectors are represented pictorially as two sides of a parallelogram and a third arrow is drawn along the diagonal (Figure 16.2).

We can also add vectors by connecting the tail of one vector to the tip of the other (tail-to-tip method).

When three forces act upon a body, and the body is in equilibrium, the three forces can be drawn to scale in their correct directions to form a closed triangle. This is useful, because when the magnitude and direction of two of the forces are known and the triangle is drawn to scale, the third force can be calculated with ease.

MOMENT

The moment of force is the **effect** of a force at a perpendicular distance from an axis, which results in rotational movement and angular acceleration:

$$M_o = Fd$$

where M_o is the moment of force about axis O, F is the magnitude of the force and d is the moment arm or perpendicular distance from the axis of rotation to the line of force.

The **magnitude** of a moment is known as **torque**. Torques generated by the body translate skeletal flexor and extensor muscle contraction into rotational movements of limbs about joints.

LEVERS

In essence, the musculoskeletal system is a collection of lever systems linked together. There are three types of lever systems in the

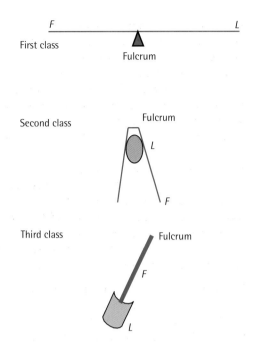

Figure 16.3 *Three classes of lever.*

body. The difference lies in where the **fulcrum** (i.e. the **joint**) and applied **forces** (*F*) are in relation to the load (*L*) (Figure 16.3):

- **First-class lever:** the fulcrum lies in **between the applied force and the load**. Mechanical advantage is gained by increasing the force arm length in relation to the load arm length. An example is the atlanto-occipital joint as the fulcrum, with the weight of the head as the load and the counter-force being applied by the erector spinae muscles. An everyday example is the use of a pair of scissors.
- **Second-class lever:** the fulcrum is at **one end of the lever**, with the applied load force at the other end and the load in between. The force arm length is always greater than the load arm length. An example is the act of standing on one's toes, with the toes as the fulcrum, the weight of the ankle offering resistance being the load, and the counter-force being applied by the calf muscles. An everyday example is the use of a nutcracker.
- **Third-class lever:** the fulcrum is at **one end of the lever**, but the **load is at the other end**, with the applied force in between. The

load arm length is always greater than the force arm length, and so a greater force is needed to move the load. This is the most common type of lever found in the human body. An example is the elbow joint as the fulcrum, with the load being any object held in the hand and the elbow flexors providing the counterforce. An everyday example is a shovel.

COUPLES

The final basic concept is that of a **couple**, which is a moment created by **equal, non-colinear, parallel** and an **oppositely directed pair of forces**, e.g. the effect of two hands on a steering wheel or two fingers twisting off a bottle cap. Note that colinear forces act along the same line. A couple is a free pure moment vector with no resultant force. Couples are useful for understanding the effects of muscle action about joints.

STATICS

STATIC EQUILIBRIUM

From Newton's first law (inertia), an object is in **static equilibrium** if the sum of all the forces acting on it is balanced (i.e. no linear acceleration occurs, as $\Sigma F = 0$) and all the moments acting on it are balanced separately from the forces (i.e. no angular acceleration occurs, as $\Sigma M = 0$). Balance of forces is termed **translational equilibrium**, since forces will translate the object, while balance of moments is termed **rotational equilibrium**, since moments will rotate the body. The best way to state the required balance of forces and moments is to break down the force balance equations into their *x*, *y* and *z* components. The resulting equations for forces ($\Sigma F_x = 0$, $\Sigma F_y = 0$, $\Sigma F_z = 0$) and moments ($\Sigma M_x = 0$, $\Sigma M_y = 0$, $\Sigma M_z = 0$) can be used to solve for unknown forces and moments in a given plane. Biological systems are rarely in equilibrium, but static analysis is a useful tool in estimating unknown musculoskeletal forces that balance the known forces in a system at rest.

In **statically determinate** systems, the number of unknown forces and moments is equal to the number of equations available (six equations in three dimensions – force equilibrium in the x, y and z directions and moment equilibrium in the x, y and z axes), thus allowing the unknown forces to be calculated. In **statically indeterminate** systems, there are more unknowns than available equations, and therefore there are no unique solutions. Unfortunately, in orthopaedic biomechanics, the latter situation is prevalent when determining muscle and joint forces, as a large number of muscles span each joint. Approaches to this problem include reduction and optimization methods, the former being used more commonly in order to reduce the number of unknowns to equal the number of equations, e.g. the concept of a **single equivalent muscle** allows forces around a joint to be calculated. A group of muscles, e.g. elbow flexors, is first represented by a common line of action, the moment arm and angle of pull are estimated, and finally, assuming that a single equivalent muscle generates the net joint moment, the muscle force can be calculated as:

$$\text{Muscle force } (F) = \text{net moment } (M_o)/\text{moment arm } (d)$$

STATIC ANALYSIS

Static analysis by **free-body diagram** is a method of determining the forces and moments acting on a body by isolating that body part and ensuring that it is in static equilibrium. As forces and moments are vectors, they must sum up to zero in each of three perpendicular directions. Therefore, in the x, y and z dimensions, there are six equations of equilibrium (see above), allowing a maximum of six unknowns to be solved.

A number of assumptions are involved in free-body analysis in order to estimate important joint or muscle forces:

- The musculoskeletal system model assumes that the **bones are rigid rods** (they do not stretch, compress or deform, regardless of the forces and moments acting on them) and the **joints are rigid frictionless hinges**.

- There is **no antagonistic muscle action**.
- The **weight** of the body is concentrated at the exact **centre of the body mass**.
- Only external forces and moments acting on the free body are usually considered. **Internal forces** are assumed to **cancel** each other out.
- Muscles are assumed not to exert compressive forces and, therefore, **act only in tension**.
- The line of action of the muscle is along the centre of **cross-sectional area of muscle mass**.
- Joint reaction forces are assumed to be only **compressive**, as tensile forces would lead to loss of contact of the joint surfaces.
- The joint acts as only a **hinge**, ignoring other possible axes of rotation and translation.

Examples of free-body diagram analysis can be found in the relevant chapters on the biomechanics of individual joints.

For rigid bodies subjected to concurrent forces (where all forces intersect at one point), when these forces are joined from tip to tail in any sequence all the force vectors must form a closed polygon. This **static analysis by graphical method** can be used to solve for unknown forces within a concurrent force system.

DYNAMICS: KINETICS

BASIC CONCEPTS

Work (W) is the product of force acting along the direction of displacement (only components parallel to the displacement) and the displacement of a rigid body in motion. The unit of work is the newton-metre (Nm) or joule (J), i.e. work = force × distance. **Energy** is the ability to perform work and is measured in joules or newton-metres. Using the law of conservation of energy, energy is neither created nor destroyed but instead is transferred from one type to another (i.e. the sum of all energies is constant). It is important to understand the following:

- **Potential energy** (E_p): the potential of a body to do work due to its position (e.g. height) or configuration (strain energy), i.e. stored energy.

- **Kinetic energy (E_k):** the amount of work required in order to stop a body moving at velocity v or to move a body from rest to velocity v. For a rigid body with mass m, $E_k = 1/2mv^2$. It is assumed that no energy is dissipated through friction (f), which is the opposing force created by two bodies as they slide over each other.

Power (P) is the work done per unit time and is measured in joules per second, or watts. **Momentum** (L) is equal to the product of a body's mass and velocity, i.e. $L = mv$. **Mass moment of inertia** (I) is the tendency of a rigid body to resist rotation (as opposed to pure mass, which tends to resist translation). The mass moment of inertia depends on the magnitude of the mass and its geometric distribution. The further the mass is distributed from its centre of rotation, the larger the mass moment of inertia.

KINETIC ANALYSIS

In general, **direct dynamic problems** (DDP) predict motion of rigid bodies from known forces, while **inverse dynamic problems** (IDP) involve the calculation of forces from known motions.

In a dynamic (non-equilibrium) situation, the forces acting on a rigid body will accelerate the body (i.e. increase its velocity). **Linear forces** cause linear acceleration ($\sigma F = ma$), while **moments about an axis of rotation** cause angular acceleration ($\sigma M = I\alpha$, where α is the angular acceleration). These equations can be used to solve for unknown forces and moments acting on rigid bodies in motion, similar to equations of equilibrium in static analysis.

In reality, calculating forces and moments for the human body is far more difficult, as the accelerations of different parts of the body must be taken into account. The body is usually divided into segments linked together (**link-segment model**), and the forces, moments and accelerations of each segment are calculated separately from distal to proximal, either using mathematical equations (**indirect method**) or using devices such as accelerometers, magnetic tracking systems and optoelectronic motion analysis systems (**direct method**).

DYNAMICS: KINEMATICS

JOINT KINEMATICS

Degrees of freedom (DOF) are defined as the number of independent modes of motion in a joint. In two dimensions, a free joint has three DOF: translation in x direction, translation in y direction and rotation in z direction. A free joint in three dimensions would have six DOF: three in translation and three in rotation along the x, y and z axes. Closely packed hinge joints (e.g. the ulno-humeral joint) have one DOF, universal joints have two DOF, and ball-and-socket joints (e.g. the hip) have three DOF, all in rotation.

There is a direct relationship between DOF and joint constraint forces. In two dimensions, the total number of DOF and constraint forces is three (i.e. one DOF has two associated joint constraint forces); for example, in the sagittal plane, the proximal interphalangeal joint has one DOF (flexion-extension) and two constraint forces (axial compression and palmar-dorsal shear). In three dimensions, the total number of DOF and constraint forces is six; for example, the wrist joint has two DOF (flexion-extension and radial-ulnar deviation) and four constraint forces (axial compression, medial-lateral shear, volar-dorsal shear and axial rotational torque).

Joint kinematics are even more complex, as joints undergo two kinds of motion:

- **Gross joint motion:** used to study joint function and to calculate forces and moments passing through the joint centre under dynamic conditions.
- **Articulating surface motion:** of three types, although a combination of all three is found in most anatomic joints (Figure 16.4):
  - **Rotation:** the circular body rotates on a flatter surface.
  - **Rolling:** contact points on circular and flat surfaces constantly change but remain at a constant zero velocity, i.e. no slip occurs. The circular surface undergoes a relative motion of translation and rotation on the flat surface. As the contact point changes constantly, this type of motion leads to the least amount of wear.

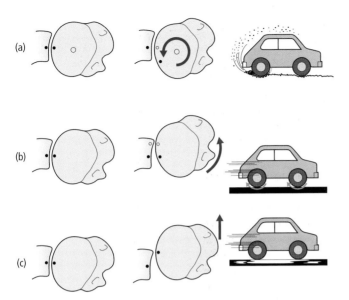

Figure 16.4 *Three types of articulating surface motion: (a) rotation, (b) rolling and (c) translation (gliding).*

- **Gliding:** pure translation, in which one surface is flat and the contact point on the circular surface does not change (like it does on the flat surface).

RIGID-BODY KINEMATICS

The position of a moving object (again assumed to be a rigid body) can be defined relative to a reference frame, usually in the x–y plane. Two reference points are sufficient to define an object's position in the x–y plane at a given time (three points are needed for a three-dimensional position). If these two points are moving in the same direction, translation occurs. If the two points are moving in two different directions, both translation and rotation occur. **Linear velocity** is denoted v (units of m/s), while **angular velocity** (i.e. rotational velocity) is denoted by ω (units of radians/s). The motion of any rigid body can be defined by a combination of translation and rotation. Further knowledge of rigid-body kinematics is beyond the level expected for the practising orthopaedic surgeon.

Viva questions

1 What are the three Newton's physical laws relevant to orthopaedics?

2 What is a force?

3 What is a moment?

4 Draw a free-body diagram of the x joint (where x can be any large joint in the human body).

5 What are the assumptions made when performing free-body analysis?

FURTHER READING

Burstein, AH, Wright, TM (eds). *Fundamentals of Orthopaedic Biomechanics*. Baltimore, MD: Williams & Wilkins, 1994.

Cochrane, GVB. *A Primer of Orthopaedic Biomechanics*. New York, NY: Churchill Livingston, 1982.

Fung, YC (ed.). *Biomechanics: Mechanical Properties of Living Tissues*, 2nd edn. New York, NY: Springer-Verlag, 1993.

Mow, VC, Hayes, WC (eds). *Basic Orthopaedic Biomechanics*, 2nd edn. New York, NY: Lippincott-Raven, 1997.

Nordin, M, Frankel, VH (eds). *Basic Biomechanics of the Musculoskeletal System*, 2nd edn. Philadelphia, PA: Lea and Febiger, 1989.

17

Biomaterial behaviour

SUBHAMOY CHATTERJEE AND GORDON BLUNN

INTRODUCTION

In order to describe biomaterials accurately, it is necessary to understand the basic concepts of material behaviour. In this chapter, the basic concepts of stress, strain, strength, deformation and failure as applied to biomaterials are described. For the purposes of any orthopaedic examination, one should be able to reproduce a stress–strain curve and explain its salient features. One should also be able to explain the mechanics of bending and torsional forces on simple constructs such as plates and nails. The concepts of tribology (friction, lubrication, corrosion, wear) are covered in Chapter 25.

BASIC DEFINITIONS

All materials can be described by their stress–strain behaviour. The force applied can be compressive, tensile, bending or shear, and in many cases the mechanical properties can vary according to the direction in which forces are applied. For example, cortical bone, due to the columnar structure of its osteons, is extremely strong in axial loading (compression) but is not as strong against transverse forces (bending).

Stress = force applied to a material per unit area

Materials that behave identically, irrespective of the direction of the applied force, such as most orthopaedic metals, alloys, polymers and woven bone, are termed **isotropic**. However, almost all living tissues, including cortical bone and some composite biomaterials, display directionally dependent behaviour and are termed **anisotropic**.

Tensile stresses occur when two forces pull away from each other along the same line, while **compressive stresses** occur when two forces push towards each other along the same line.

When a material is subjected to a force, strain is the change in length of a material with respect to its original length. Technically, strain has no units, as it is normalized with respect to the original length. Commonly, however, stress is referred to in either in millimetres per millimetre or as a percentage. Strain is a relative measure of the deformation of a body as a result of loading.

Strain = change in length/original length

However, strain does not take into account the cross-sectional area of the material being tested. So, in order to characterize a material more completely, we combine the properties of stress and strain in terms of a stress–strain curve that eliminates the variables of initial material length and material cross-sectional area. Stress–strain curves, however, are still different for anisotropic materials, as the curve varies according to the direction of the force applied. **Young's modulus** (Thomas Young was a physician before turning his mind toward physics), or the **elastic modulus**, is found by dividing the stress by the strain over the linear portion of the stress–strain curve. As a result, the Young's modulus for an isotropic material is constant. Note that the units of Young's modulus are newtons per square metre and in Systéme International (SI) units 1 N/m^2 is equal to 1 pascal (Pa).

Summary

Stress = force per unit area applied (N/m^2)

Strain = change in length with respect to original length

Young's (elastic) modulus (σ) = stress/strain (N/m^2)

Isotropy: material behaves similarly in all directions of application of force.

The Young's modulus for common materials is shown in Table 17.1. A useful approximation is shown next to the true figures. The modulus is the constant, which quantifies the linear relationship between stress and strain over the linear portion of the graph. This relationship is known as **Hooke's law**.

STRESS–STRAIN CURVE

A typical stress–strain curve is shown in Figure 17.1. Key features are described below.

TOE REGION (NOT ALWAYS PRESENT – SEE CHAPTER 8)

This refers to the initial portion of the curve where there is a non-linear relationship. Here, there is low stiffness. A classical example of this is the crimping of collagen fibres in tendons (see Chapter 8). As tendons are initially stretched, the collagen fibres unfurl readily until they are straightened, and then the stiffness increases quickly. The stress–strain relationship therefore becomes linear.

ELASTIC PORTION

Here, the stress–strain relationship is linear and Hooke's law is obeyed. The Young's modulus can be determined from the gradient of the line in this region of the graph. All the deformation present in this portion of the graph is **elastic**,

Table 17.1 Young's modulus of common orthopaedic materials

Material	Young's modulus (GPa)	Approximate values
Cartilage	0.02	0.02
Tendon	0.4	0.5
Cancellous bone	0.5–1.5	1
UHMWPE	1.2	1
PMMA bone cement	2.2	2
Cortical bone	10–30	20
Titanium alloy	110	100
Stainless steel	190	200
Cobalt chrome	210	200

PMMA, polymethylmethacrylate; UHMWPE, ultra-high molecular weight polyethylene.

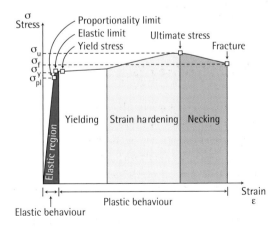

Figure 17.1 *Typical stress–strain curve.* σ_f, *fracture stress;* σ_{pl}, *proportionality limit;* σ_u, *ultimate stress;* σ_y, *yield stress.*

i.e. recoverable. The stiffness of the material increases as the gradient of the line becomes steeper. Note that a linear elastic material is insensitive to the rate of loading.

PLASTIC PORTION

At this point in the graph, further deformity is no longer recoverable, i.e. it is **plastic**. This commences at the **yield point** (where there is a dramatic increase in strain with little increase in stress) and is followed by a **perfectly plastic** region and then a region where **strain hardening** occurs. Strain hardening refers to the phenomenon where the plastic deformation actually increases the material's resistance to further deformity. An example of this is cold working of metal alloys (see Chapter 18). The **yield stress** is defined as the stress necessary to produce a specific amount of permanent deformation, i.e. 0.002 (0.2 per cent). Note that in orthopaedics, the proportionality limit, the elastic limit (where Hooke's law is not obeyed but the deformation is recoverable) and the **yield stress** are so close that they are taken to be the same point and it is termed the yield point.

Where the graph ends abruptly, the material's integrity is breached and it is therefore fractured. The stress level at which this happens is termed the **fracture stress**. Sometimes, this almost coincides with the maximum amount of stress the material can withstand before which fracture is imminent, termed the **ultimate tensile stress**.

OTHER TERMS

- **Ductility:** ductile materials undergo a large amount of plastic deformation before failure, e.g. metals.
- **Brittleness:** brittle materials do not deform plastically but display elastic behaviour right up to failure, e.g. ceramics. In brittle materials, the yield stress is almost equivalent to the fracture stress.
- **Stiffness:** deflection under a given load. The steeper the stress–strain curve, the stiffer the material. The less steep the curve, the more flexible the material.

- **Strain energy:** area under the stress–strain curve. Combines recoverable strain energy (elastic region of the curve) and absorbed strain energy (plastic region of the curve).
- **Toughness:** amount of energy per unit volume that a material can absorb before failure. This value is also related to the area under the stress–strain curve. When comparing brittle and ductile materials with the same ultimate tensile strengths, the brittle material is less tough, as it has less area under its stress–strain curve.
- **Strength:** a somewhat imprecise term that can be said to represent the degree of resistance to deformation of a material. A material is strong if it has a high ultimate tensile strength.
- **Hardness:** surface property of a material; ability of a material to resist scratching and indentation on the surface. Its value is not determined from the stress–strain curve, but it does influence the durability and machinability of the material.

Stress–strain curve lexicon

- **Gradient of elastic region:** stiff if steep, flexible if shallow.

- **Extent of plastic deformation:** ductile if long, brittle if short.

- **Ultimate tensile strength:** strong if high, weak if low.

- **Area under the curve:** tough if large, not tough if small.

FATIGUE FAILURE AND NOTCH SENSITIVITY

Fatigue failure refers to failure of a material with repetitive loading at stress levels below the ultimate tensile strength. It is worth knowing the *S–n* curve (Figure 17.2), where stress (*S*) on the *y*-axis is plotted against number (*n*) of cycles (millions) on the *x*-axis.

The **endurance limit** is defined as the stress at which the material can withstand 10 million

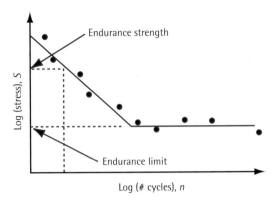

Figure 17.2 *Typical S–n curve.*

cycles without experiencing fatigue failure. Clinically, total hip replacements operate above the endurance limit, while total knee replacements operate at the endurance limit, especially the polyethylene component, predisposing the latter to fatigue failure.

Notch sensitivity is the extent to which the sensitivity of a material to fracture is increased by the presence of a surface inhomogeneity, e.g. cracks and scratches. Ductile materials such as stainless steel have low notch sensitivity, while brittle materials such as ceramic and titanium have high notch sensitivity.

The above discussion is aimed at material properties. When discussing a structure, one must also consider the shape of the structure, along with forces applied and material properties. For example, **stiffness** refers to a material's ability to resist deformation, while **rigidity** refers to a structure's ability to resist deformation.

TIME–DEPENDENT BEHAVIOUR

The elastic behaviour discussed above does not always occur. Sometimes, there is time-dependent behaviour, termed **visco-elasticity**. Materials and structures such as cartilage, ligaments and intervertebral discs display such behaviour. **Viscous** properties are time-dependent and involve **non-recoverable deformation**; elastic properties are time-independent and involve **recoverable**

deformation. Several phenomena characterize visco-elasticity, namely **creep, stress relaxation, time-dependent strain behaviour** and **hysteresis**.

When a material is loaded with a constant force there is an initial elongation (the elastic component), but in visco-elastic materials there is further continuous deformation over time (viscous component). This is termed **creep** (time-dependent deformation in response to a constant load) (Figure 17.3a).

If the material, after being loaded, is held at a specific strain (i.e. at a certain length), then the stress level required to maintain this strain decreases over time until equilibrium is reached. This is termed **stress relaxation** (time-dependent decrease in load required to maintain a material at a constant strain) (Figure 17.3b).

Time-dependent strain behaviour can be illustrated by the behaviour of plasticine. If we gradually pull apart a blob of plasticine, we create a long thin thread of plasticine before it eventually breaks into two. However, if we pull the blob apart quickly, then the plasticine breaks quickly. Note that the strength required to break the plasticine is higher when pulling it apart quickly and less when trying to break the long thread after slowly pulling the plasticine apart. Translating this into mechanical terms, the rate of change of length of the plasticine (the strain rate) affects the behaviour. The faster the strain rate, the higher the stress at a given level of strain. Conversely, a low strain rate requires more time but less stress to fracture the material. This is shown graphically in Figure 17.3c.

Hysteresis refers to the stress–strain curve differing during loading and unloading (Figure 17.3d). Strain energy is lost between loading and unloading as heat due to the internal friction within the material.

The underlying mechanisms responsible for visco-elastic behaviour are, first, **friction** internally, as micro-elements in the structure move against each other as a material is stretched, as described previously in the unfurling of collagen fibres. Second, the movement of interstitial fluid through a material that is a semi-porous matrix creates a

(a)

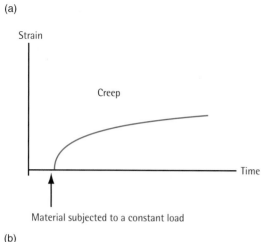

Material subjected to a constant load

(b)

(c)

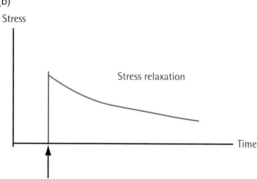

(d)

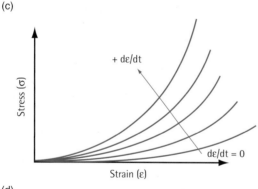

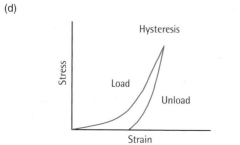

Figure 17.3 *Graphs of visco-elastic behaviour.*

drag, which produces visco-elastic behaviour. The femur exhibits features of visco-elastic behaviour in terms of stress relaxation. When implanting an uncemented femoral prosthesis in hip replacements, one is advised to tap down the prosthesis, wait a few seconds, tap it down again, wait a few seconds, and so on. As one taps down the prosthesis, circumferential hoop stresses are generated in the femur. If one now waits a few seconds, the femur exhibits stress relaxation and the hoop stresses diminish, so that one can continue tapping the prosthesis down. This technique reduces the risk of femoral fracture, as it limits the level of stresses generated during implantation.

SHEAR FORCES

A **shearing force** is a force applied parallel to or in line with the surface of an object. **Shear stresses** occur when two forces are directed parallel to each other but not along the same line or in the same direction. Shear stresses and strains can be evaluated in the same way as compressive and tensile forces, but it is necessary to take into account the entire cross-sectional area of the material, as the shear forces act over the whole area. As with linear forces, there is a relationship between shear stress and shear strain, and we can calculate a shear modulus, which gives an idea of a material's resistance to shearing forces:

Shear modulus = shear stress/shear strain

A useful rule of thumb is that the shear modulus is between 30 per cent and 50 per cent of the elastic modulus for most materials. It is worth noting that bone is weakest against shear forces (and also tensile forces), while it is strong in compression. When analysing forces acting on bone, note that in reality almost all the forces to which a bone may be subjected are a combination of tension, compression, bending, torsion and shear. As a result, bone tends to fail (fracture) in the shear component first. Analysing the forces on bone in a given situation is complex, and computed analysis is essential for calculating accurately the various force components.

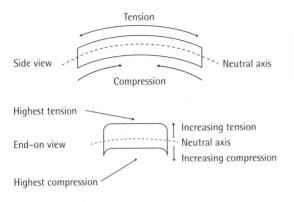

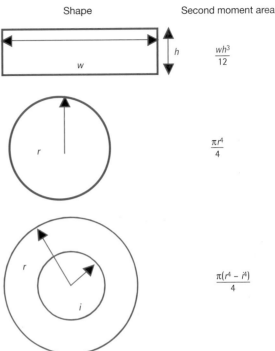

Figure 17.4 *Bending forces applied to a beam (longitudinal and cross-sectional views).*

Figure 17.5 *Common geometric shapes and their second moment areas.*

BENDING FORCES

Having introduced the concepts above, it is clear that in the body most forces are not pure tension or compression but a combination of the two. Bending forces are common in the skeleton, e.g. loading of the femur causes it to bend. In the case of the femur, it is bowed anteriorly. The shape is the result of the femur being subjected to loading forces, which cause the anterior surface to be put in tension and the posterior surface into compression. A simplified model of this is shown in Figure 17.4.

If we examine a cross-section of the beam, there is a graduation of stresses from extreme edges of the beam, where the compressive and tensile forces are the largest respectively, towards the centre of the beam (the mid-point of the cross-section), where there is no resulting force. The line of no force throughout the beam is termed the **neutral axis**.

In order to calculate the bending stress at any given point, we apply the following equation:

$$\text{Bending stress} =$$

$$\frac{(\text{applied force} \times \text{distance from neutral axis})}{\text{second moment area of material}}$$

The **second moment area** (SMA) is a variable that describes the spatial distribution of a material within a structure. The type of material does not affect the SMA. The SMA is affected by the organization and shape of the material. Some basic shape types and formulae for SMAs are shown in Figure 17.5.

Note the following:

- For materials with rectangular cross-sections, the perpendicular distance away from the neutral axis (h) has a third power effect on the SMA.
- For materials with a solid circular cross-section, the radius (which is the distance from the neutral axis) has a fourth power effect on the SMA.
- For materials with a hollow circular cross-section, the total SMA equals the SMA of the solid outer portion minus the SMA of the missing inner hollow portion.

Using the formula to compare a pipe and a solid rod, it can be seen that for identical cross-sectional areas, the SMA is actually larger for the hollow pipe. As a result, the hollow pipe deforms less (is stronger) than the solid pipe of the same cross-sectional area. An example of this is that as bone ages, outward appositional growth enlarges the medullary canal and increases the overall girth of the whole bone. This increases the SMA and consequently the bone strength and resistance to fracture. This probably helps to offset the loss of bone strength from osteoporosis.

It is worth noting that the calculation of forces in bending does not take into account the nature of the material being tested but considers only its shape and size. However, once bending moments have been calculated, we can think about relevant materials that can withstand the forces applied.

Rigidity in bending is a particularly important concept when choosing metal plates for fracture fixation:

Bending rigidity = SMA × Young's modulus

When defined in this way, rigidity incorporates both the nature of a material and its shape, size and structure. From this equation, some important conclusions can be derived. Choosing a material that is twice as stiff (i.e. double the Young's modulus), such as cobalt chrome over titanium, makes a plate of a given shape, size and structure twice as rigid. More importantly, working through the equations for a rectangular shaped plate, then doubling the thickness of the plate results in an increased SMA and consequently increased rigidity by the third power of the multiplying factor; i.e. doubling the plate thickness increases rigidity by 2^3 (= 8).

TORSIONAL FORCES

Equal and opposite shear forces, as applied to a cylinder constrained in space, cause the cylinder to twist. This is known as a **torsional** or **torque force**. If we substitute the cylinder for a tibia, then the following discussion can be applied to understanding how a skier sustains a spiral fracture in the tibia when the skis twist around. The twisting of the skis applies a torsional force.

Similar to bending forces, graduations of the torque force apply through the cylinder, from the surfaces edges, where the torque is

maximal, to the centre of the cylinder, where the resultant force of the two opposite shearing forces is zero. A line connecting areas of zero net force throughout a structure is termed the **axis of twist**. The formula for calculating the shear stress force generated by the torque forces at any given point is:

Shear stress =

$$\frac{(\text{applied torque} \times \text{distance from axis of twist})}{\text{polar moment of inertia}}$$

The **polar moment of inertia**, or **polar moment area** (PMA), similar to the SMA, is a variable parameter related to the size and shape of a structure but not the material from which it is constructed. Figure 17.6 shows the formulae for calculating the PMA for cylindrical shapes.

Returning to the skiing example, the ski tip is a long distance from the tibia of the skier. As a result of the long moment arm, the force applied to the tibia is high. Using the formula below for a hollow cylinder, we can calculate the order of magnitude of forces required to fracture the tibia. Again, it is clear from the formulae that in terms of the dimensions of the

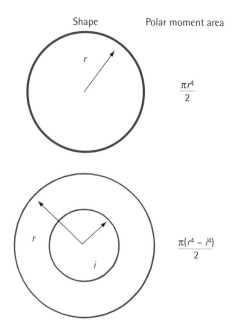

Figure 17.6 *Cylindrical shapes and their polar moment areas.*

cylinder, the radius (i.e. the distance from the axis of twist) affects the PMA to the fourth power.

The rigidity of materials to torsion is calculated in a similar way to that of bending rigidity:

Torsional rigidity = PMA × shear modulus

Torsional rigidity is a measure of the resistance of a material in a particular size and shape to torsional forces. From Figure 17.6, we see that for a cylinder, the polar moment varies to the fourth power of the radius. Therefore, an intramedullary rod that is twice as thick has 2^4 (= 16) times the rigidity. Considering intramedullary nail types, note that when comparing nails of the same diameter and length, cannulation or slotting of the nail decreases the polar moment area according to the earlier formula. As a result, torsional rigidity of slotted or cannulated nails is lessened, although bending rigidity is affected only minimally.

Viva questions

1 Draw a stress strain curve and describe how to calculate the Young's modulus.

2 What do you understand by the term 'fatigue failure'? Draw an *S–n* curve.

3 Explain how increasing the thickness of metal plates affects their rigidity.

4 Explain how your choice of solid or slotted nails affects the rigidity of the construct.

5 How does the phenomenon of creep govern your surgical technique of implanting uncemented femoral prostheses?

FURTHER READING

Burstein, AH, Wright, TM (eds). *Fundamentals of Orthopaedic Biomechanics*. Baltimore, MD: Williams & Wilkins, 1994.

Cochrane, GVB. *A Primer of Orthopaedic Biomechanics*. New York, NY: Churchill Livingston, 1982.

Mow, VC, Hayes, WC (eds). *Basic Orthopaedic Biomechanics*, 2nd edn. New York, NY: Lippincott-Raven, 1997.

Nordin, M, Frankel, VH (eds). *Basic Biomechanics of the Musculoskeletal System*, 2nd edn. Philadelphia, PA: Lea and Febiger, 1989.

Radin, EL. *Practical Biomechanics for the Orthopedic Surgeon*, 2nd edn. New York, NY: Churchill Livingstone, 1992.

18
Biomaterials

SUBHAMOY CHATTERJEE AND GORDON BLUNN

INTRODUCTION

Biomaterials are essential in the practice of orthopaedic surgery. The choice available to the surgeon is diverse. Therefore, one must be aware of the properties of the commonly used metal alloys, ceramics and polymers so that one can evaluate the suitability of a given material for a specific purpose. In orthopaedic examinations, one will be expected to discuss these properties, including the advantages and disadvantages of their use in orthopaedics.

A biomaterial is any substance or combination of substances (other than a drug), synthetic or natural in origin, that can be used for any period of time as a whole or part of a system that treats, augments or replaces any tissue, organ or function of the body.

GENERAL PROPERTIES OF METAL ALLOYS

Metal alloys are constituted from metallic and non-metallic elements. The three most common metal alloys used in orthopaedics are stainless steel, titanium alloy and cobalt chrome. Orthopaedic-grade **stainless steel** is comprised mainly of iron and chromium. **Titanium alloys** come in several forms, but the form used most in orthopaedics is titanium 64, where the alloying elements are aluminium and vanadium. **Cobalt chrome alloys**, as the name suggests, are constituted primarily from cobalt, with the addition of varying amounts of chromium; there are a number of commonly used cobalt-based alloys. All the metal alloys share some properties in terms of microstructure, mechanical properties and chemical reactivity.

MICROSTRUCTURE

Metal elements in pure form have a **crystalline lattice microstructure**. This structure involves a repeating three-dimensional unit that favours a closely packed high-density arrangement of the metal atoms. Most metals fall into one of three crystalline arrangements: body-centred cubic (**BCC**), face-centred cubic (**FCC**) and hexagonal close-packed (**HCP**) (Figure 18.1).

Densities vary, depending on how many atoms are in contact with each other. As a result, the FCC and HCP forms have higher densities, as 12 atoms surround each atom. Note that for clarity, the atoms are not shown in direct contact in Figure 18.1.

Plastic deformation is easiest in the FCC arrangement, as the three-dimensional packing of this unit allows easy movement of the crystalline units against each other. As a metal cools and solidifies from a liquid (molten) state, the crystalline units described above amalgamate. The units do not combine perfectly in a geometric sense but tend to form clusters of perfectly formed crystal units (**grains**), imperfectly aligned with other clusters. The areas between adjoining grains are termed

(a)

(b)

(c)

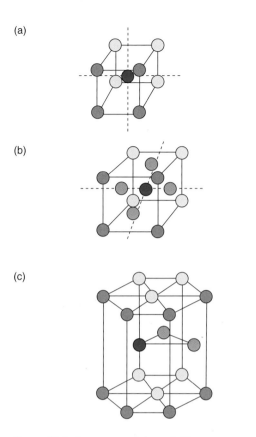

Figure 18.1 *Common metal crystalline arrangements. (a) Body-centred cubic: each atom is in contact with eight atoms. (b) Face-centred cubic: each atom is in contact with 12 atoms. (c) Hexagonal close-packed: each atom is in contact with 12 atoms.*

grain boundaries, and these represent imperfections in the solid structure. There may also be defects known as **vacancies** and **dislocations** within the grain microstructure. Note that defects in the macrostructure of metals include **scratches** and **voids**.

Grain size is an important attribute of the microstructure: the smaller the grain size, the more uniform the material. This confers the mechanical properties of **strength** and **isotropy** on the material. During manufacture, the grain size of materials is examined, as high grain sizes are associated with earlier fatigue and failure of the material.

Alloys are usually formed by adding molten alloying metal elements to the principal metal element in its molten state. As this mixture solidifies, the alloying elements, such as

chromium and nickel in the case of stainless steel, substitute for iron atoms in the FCC arrangement. This can occur because the sizes of the metal atoms involved are similar. If non-metallic alloying elements are added, then they often try to fit in the free spaces in the crystal structure among the metal atoms because the atoms are considerably smaller.

If there is a high concentration of added elements, then as the mixture of molten elements solidifies, an initial precipitate may form with the usual crystalline structure (the **alpha phase**); then a second precipitate forms (the **beta phase**), which has a high concentration of the added elements, which causes it to form a different crystalline structure. This beta phase, being of a different crystalline structure, can weaken the strength of the material and make it more brittle; however, depending on the type of beta phase, this phase can provide resistance to fatigue.

MECHANICAL PROPERTIES

Almost all metal alloys are **stiff**, **ductile** and **hard**. However, during the manufacturing process, several options can be employed to alter the mechanical properties of the alloy. For example, the concentration of smaller non-metallic alloying elements (**solutes**), such as carbon, oxygen, hydrogen and nitrogen, added to the base metal (**solvent**) can be increased. In such instances, initially, these elements try to fill the spaces available between the metal atoms in the crystal structure, but their atoms do not fit into these spaces perfectly. As a result, there is some deformation of the crystal structure. This in turn causes resistance to the flow of the crystal units against each other when the material is subject to tension, in particular preventing dislocations. This translates as an increase in the resistance to plastic deformation of the material, which implies an increase in the yield stress. As an example, increasing the content of carbon in stainless steel strengthens the stainless steel against plastic deformation.

Work hardening is a process that involves repeatedly tensile loading a metal alloy until it plastically deforms and reduces its cross-sectional area and then removing the load before the material fails. In reality, the alloy is squeezed between rollers; when performed at room temperature, this is termed **cold working**. This has the effect of making strains (dislocations) in the microstructure of the material that build during cold working permanent, which confers strength to the material by increasing its yield stress. However, the ductility is decreased, as the local strains (dislocations) induced in cold working become permanent. Biomechanically, this phenomenon is termed strain hardening. This process is commonly used in the manufacture of stainless steel, as the stainless steel can be made stronger with only a small amount of ductility being sacrificed.

Cold working followed by annealing can cause grain-size alterations. **Annealing** is a process whereby the metal is heated to a certain level at which the mechanical properties revert to the original characteristics before cold working was performed. A combination of cold working followed by annealing decreases the grain size. As described earlier, the effect of a finer grain size is an increase in the strength of the material. Annealing also relieves internal stress and increases ductility.

As an aside, note that in the long term, metals may undergo **fatigue failure**, defined as the growth of cracks in a structure subjected to repetitive loading below the failure load of that structure. Crack initiation and propagation are important processes leading to ultimate failure of the metal. The higher the intensity of loading, the lower the number of loading cycles required for failure. The endurance limit is defined as the stress at which the metal (or material) can withstand 10 million cycles without experiencing fatigue failure (see Chapter 17).

CHEMICAL PROPERTIES

Metallic bonds are strong interatomic bonds that form between metal ions. The metal atoms in the lattice lose their electrons (all are electron donors) and become metal ions in the crystal structure. The electrons are free to circulate about the ions in the crystal structure (**free electron model**). This confers the chemical properties of **electrical** and **thermal conductivity** on metals. It also explains the **high chemical reactivity** of metals. Naturally, metals usually occur in their oxide form, and energy is required to release them into their pure state. As a result, metals are highly susceptible to react again to form their oxides. **Corrosion** (see Chapter 25) is the term used when this occurs at room temperature in an aqueous solution. Fortunately, due to the process of **passivation**, metals form a thin oxide layer as a film protecting the metal from the atmosphere. Metals can be passivated by immersion in, for example, a strong nitric oxide bath during the manufacturing process in order to ensure creation of the oxide layer.

Summary of metal alloy properties

- **Microstructure:** metal ions in a crystalline lattice structure with free circulating electrons.

- **Grain size:** strength and fatigue resistance increase with decreasing grain size.

- **Mechanical properties:** stiff, ductile, hard.

- **Work hardening:**
  - Cold working increases strength and decreases ductility.
  - Annealing decreases grain size and increases strength.

- **Chemical properties:** conduct electricity and heat; highly reactive; prone to corrosion.

COMMON ORTHOPAEDIC METAL ALLOYS

STAINLESS STEEL

Steel is normally comprised of **carbon** and **iron**. If **chromium** (18 per cent) is added, it forms an oxide layer on the outer surface that protects from corrosion – these alloys are **stainless steels**. Stainless steels vary in the proportions of the various elements described above, but the form of stainless steel used most commonly in orthopaedics is 316L. The number '316' refers to the 3 per cent molybdenum and 16 per cent nickel added to the normal alloy of iron, carbon and chromium. The letter 'L' indicates a low (less than 0.03 per cent) carbon content, which improves corrosion resistance further. Increasing the carbon content has the effect of weakening the material: carbon reacts with the chromium to form brittle carbides, thereby exposing the metal to corrosion and subsequent failure. This process, known as **sensitization**, has been responsible for the failure of stainless-steel implants in clinical scenarios, when the carbon content has been too high during manufacture.

Stainless steels have a variety of crystalline structures, including BCC and FCC (also known as **austenite**). The FCC structure tends to form at higher temperatures, but the addition of nickel to stainless steels stabilizes the FCC structure at room temperatures. Therefore, 316L stainless steel is sometimes referred to as **austenitic steel**.

The stabilization of the FCC structure means that 316L stainless steel is more ductile than other stainless steels and has a low yield stress level. As this form of stainless steel is cooled from the molten state, there is only one precipitate, as the concentrations of the additives are relatively low. Stainless steel is usually cold worked by about 30 per cent to improve its yield and ultimate stress. This can double its yield stress as compared with annealed stainless steel, although ductility is decreased.

Properties of stainless steel 316L

Contains:

- iron (62.97 per cent);
- chromium (18 per cent);
- nickel (16 per cent);
- molybdenum (3 per cent);
- carbon (0.03 per cent).

Advantages:

- strength (after cold working);
- ductility (only marginally sacrificed with cold working);
- reasonable resistance to corrosion (due to addition of chromium and carbon);
- reasonable biocompatibility;
- relatively cheap.

Disadvantages:

- susceptibility to crevice corrosion;
- susceptibility to stress corrosion.

Stainless steel is susceptible to both **stress** and **crevice corrosion** (see Chapter 25). Stress corrosion involves application of a low-level constant stress in a corrosive environment not normally associated with metal failure. The combination leads to a higher susceptibility of crack initiation and propagation. Crevice corrosion occurs in oxygen-depleted regions, e.g. under the head of a screw or under a bone plate. The pH of these regions decreases, which favours more rapid metal oxidation.

TITANIUM ALLOYS

Titanium alloys are available in several forms. The most commonly used orthopaedic titanium alloy is **titanium 64**. The numerical suffix refers to the proportions of the alloying elements **aluminium** (6 per cent) and **vanadium** (4 per cent). As titanium alloys precipitate from the molten state, two phases are formed. The **alpha phase** is an HCP arrangement, and the **beta phase** is arranged in a BCC fashion. This **biphasic structure** confers the advantage of improved fatigue resistance on titanium. In addition to this property, the other advantages of titanium are a remarkable resistance to corrosion (far greater than that of stainless steel) and excellent biocompatibility. Titanium forms an oxide layer (TiO_2) by **passivation**, which protects the material from corrosion, even in adverse environments. As a result, titanium alloy does not suffer from the same failings as stainless steel. The **biocompatibility** in long-term implant studies is excellent, with the oxide layer becoming incorporated into bone. The Young's modulus of titanium is roughly half that of stainless steel (100 compared with 200). This implies that a bone plate constructed from titanium alloy will be half as rigid as that made from stainless steel. Thus, simply altering the material of construct can lessen the phenomenon of stress shielding.

The disadvantages of titanium include **notch sensitivity**, whereby scratches or notching of the titanium surface predispose to fatigue failure. Other disadvantages include the fact that titanium is **less resistant to wear** (softer) than stainless steel and cobalt chrome alloys and so cannot be used as a bearing surface. Hip prostheses manufactured from titanium show early pitting, scratching and wear, presumably as a consequence of the material softness. There is also some concern regarding the long-term biocompatibility of titanium alloy: the release of vanadium ions into the system may be cytotoxic, and the phenomenon of particle-induced wear is prevalent in a material that is soft. This has led to concerns regarding the use of titanium for long-term prostheses, despite the excellent biocompatibility. A possible solution to this shortcoming is the development of a new titanium alloy (**Ti-6Al-4N**), where the more inert niobium is substituted for vanadium (to combat systemic cytotoxic metal ion release) and other elements such as molybdenum and zirconium are added. This alloy is reported to have even better ductility and biocompatibility than Ti 64 alloy. Most importantly, however, its wear-resistant properties are much improved. Long-term studies with this alloy are under way at the time of writing.

Titanium alloy (Ti-6Al-4V)

Contains:

- titanium (89 per cent);
- aluminium (6 per cent);
- vanadium (4 per cent);
- others (1 per cent).

Advantages:

- excellent resistance to corrosion (better than stainless steel);
- excellent biocompatibility (oxide layer TiO_2) – integrates with bone well;
- ductility;
- lower Young's modulus (cf. stainless steel) – prevents stress shielding;
- excellent fatigue resistance (biphasic HCP alpha/BCC beta structure);

- new alloy may confer better properties (no vanadium/add molybdenum).

Disadvantages:

- notch sensitivity (scratching reduces fatigue resistance);
- susceptible to wear;
- systemic cytotoxic vanadium ion release;
- accelerated particle-induced wear from titanium prostheses;
- relatively expensive.

COBALT CHROME ALLOYS

Cobalt chrome alloys contain primarily **cobalt**, but with significant amounts of added **chromium** to improve corrosion resistance. Minor amounts of **carbon**, **nickel** and **molybdenum** are also added (Table 18.1). Cobalt chrome alloys are commercially available in several different forms, as the techniques used to manufacture the alloy have improved over recent years.

Originally, cobalt chrome alloys were **cast wrought**. This involves pouring molten cobalt chrome into prefabricated ceramic moulds. The alloy cools and then the mould is broken away, leaving the alloy in the desired shape. The difficulty with this method is that as the molten alloy cools slowly, large grain sizes tend to form; also, if the added carbon (needed to improve strength) is in too high a concentration, it precipitates as carbides. This has the overall effect of limiting strength and reducing resistance to corrosion.

Forging (**cold working** and **annealing**) cobalt chrome is an improvement on this technique. The alloy is cast as a bar, and then the bar is forged in order to improve its strength and reduce the grain size. This produces a far superior alloy in terms of suitability for orthopaedic purposes. The disadvantage of this process is that the bars require **further machining** in order to achieve the desired shape, which is expensive.

The most recent manufacturing method is **powder metallurgy**. This involves sieving fine powder of the alloy, with the smallest particles being compressed together into a die cast of the

Table 18.1 Cobalt chrome alloys (values are approximate and variable)

Alloy	Composition	Manufacture method	Young's modulus (GPa)	Yield strength (MPa)	Ultimate tensile strength (MPa)
F75	Co (61%), Cr (30%), Mo (6%), Ni (2.5%), Ca (0.35%)	Cast wrought	210	500	800
F799	Co (61%), Cr (30%), Mo (6%), Ni (2.5%), Ca (0.35%)	Forged	210	1050	1500
F562	Co (34%), Cr (20%), Mo (10%), Ni (35%), Ca (0.020%)	Powder metallurgy	230	1000	1200

desired final shape. This produces an even finer grain size, with much less carbide formation.

All of these alloys tend to adopt the FCC structure at room temperature, although they are actually **biphasic materials** with FCC (alpha phase) and HCP (beta phase).

The main advantage of cobalt chrome alloys is their excellent resistance to corrosion, especially **crevice corrosion** (superior to stainless steel). Other advantages include their good long-term biocompatibility and the fact that they are extremely strong. Given their varied methods of manufacture, cobalt chrome alloys can also be adapted to meet the mechanical requirements of a variety of situations. They have few mechanical disadvantages, although their cost of manufacture must be considered. A comparison of the properties of the common metal alloys is shown in Table 18.2.

Cobalt chrome alloy

Contains (for relative proportions, see Table 18.1):

- cobalt;
- chrome;
- molybdenum;
- nickel;
- carbon;
- tungsten.

Advantages:

- excellent resistance to corrosion (especially crevice corrosion);
- excellent biocompatibility in long-term studies;
- strength (can be the strongest of the alloys, depending on treatment);

Table 18.2 Comparison of metal alloys

Alloy	Elastic modulus (GPa)	Yield strength (MPa)	Ultimate tensile strength (MPa)	Advantages	Disadvantages
Stainless steel 316 (cold worked)	190	500	750	Cheap, ductile, strong	Stress/crevice corrosion
Titanium (6Al 4V)	110	800	900	Fatigue-resistant, corrosion-resistant, lower elastic modulus Biocompatible	Notch sensitivity, wear, metal toxicity
Cobalt chrome F562	230	1000	1200	Very strong, biocompatible, variety of properties	Expensive

- mechanical properties can be altered by manufacturing methods.

Disadvantages:

- expensive.

CERAMICS AND GLASSES

Ceramics are compounds of metallic elements, such as **aluminium**, **zirconium** and **silicon**, bound ionically and/or covalently with non-metallic elements. Common ceramics include aluminium oxide (**alumina**), silicon oxide (**silica**), zirconium oxide (**zirconia**) and hydroxyapatite (**HA**).

MICROSTRUCTURE AND MANUFACTURE

Most ceramics are structured with an **ionic bond**, whereby there is free electron transfer from the metal to the non-metallic element. Some ceramics are **covalently bonded**, with a sharing of electrons between the elements. Both bond types are strong. However, similarly to metals, ceramics have a **granular** structure, and their properties are dependent on grain size and phases. These factors are affected by the manufacturing methods used. Ceramics are made by mixing powdered ceramic and water and pressing them into **prefabricated casts**. The casts are then removed and the ceramic is heated to a high temperature (**sintered**) in order to achieve a higher density in the granular structure. The porosity is affected by sintering times (increased sintering time leads to increased porosity, which decreases the strength). The grain size of the structure is set predominantly by the initial size of the particles. The smaller the particle size, the smaller the resulting grain size and, consequently, the higher the strength.

CHEMICAL AND MECHANICAL PROPERTIES

Ceramics are **chemically inert**, as the metal has reacted with oxygen to return to a lower energy state. Ceramics are also **insoluble**, and this combination means that they possess the best biocompatibility of all the biomaterials. They are **hard** materials and consequently very resistant to wear. They have a **high elastic modulus** (high stiffness) and are similar in strength to cold-worked stainless steel. These properties would seem to make ceramics ideal as orthopaedic biomaterials, but their great failing is that they display almost no plastic deformation before failure; this is termed **brittleness**. This makes it difficult to predict the behaviour of ceramics, as they can fail dramatically.

These mechanical properties have limited the use of ceramics to two main regions. First, ceramics are used for the **femoral head component** of total hip replacements. Here, their hardwearing properties can be used to their full potential by placing the ceramic head on a metal stem. The stem component of a total hip replacement is not suitable for construction from ceramic materials, due to its brittleness. Second, ceramics are used as a **coating for metal implants** to increase their biocompatibility. Ceramics are osteoconductive substances, i.e. they act as a scaffold for the in-growth of blood vessels and osteoprogenitor cells and, as a result, will bond to bone. Alumina and zirconia are commonly used for femoral head manufacture (see Chapter 25), whilst HA is commonly used for coating metallic implants.

HYDROXYAPATITE

Calcium hydroxyapatite ($Ca_{10}[PO_4]_6[OH]_2$) is the mineral phase of bone. HA coatings are good osteoconductors and bond to bone. However, as HA is brittle, there are difficulties with coating metal implants, as the HA coating tends to strip off the implant. HA in combination with cement can also be used as a bone filler when injected into defects. The HA cures into a hard substance with properties similar to those of cancellous bone. More recently, bioactive glasses, which generally are weak and brittle, have found some favour as a coating for metal implants. When implanted in the body, the glasses partially dissolve and form a calcium-rich gel, which crystallizes into an apatite and subsequently bonds to bone.

POLYMERS

Polymers are used extensively in orthopaedics. The most commonly used are polymethylmethacrylate (**PMMA**) bone cement and ultra-high-molecular-weight polyethylene (**UHMWPE**) for acetabular cups.

MICROSTRUCTURE AND MANUFACTURE

Polymers consist of many repeating units of a basic sequence (**monomer**). A monomer consists of a long-backbone carbon chain linked by covalent bonds. Each carbon atom has four bonding sites available. One or two bonding sites may be taken up by other carbon atoms; the remaining bonds form side chains. The basic units for PMMA and UHMWPE are shown in Figure 18.2. Polymers are formed together by adding many repeating sequences; this can be performed by **addition** or **condensation polymerization**. Addition polymerization occurs when a free radical is added to a monomer that contains a double carbon bond. The free radical breaks the carbon bond and occupies one of the bonding sites. This results in one carbon having a free bonding site, which then proceeds to react with another free radical, and the reaction progresses. This is how high-density polyethylene (HDP) is manufactured. Condensation polymerization occurs when monomers with symmetrical end groups react, losing a water (condensation) or carbon dioxide molecule and then bonding together.

These reactions form long chains with little or **no cross-linking** between them. In this state,

only weak van der Waals forces stop movement of polymer chains relative to each other. Cross-linking (cross-bond formation) or entanglement of chains increases their overall strength.

The other main structural factor affecting strength is the **length** and consequent **molecular weight** of the chain. As the molecular weight of any polymer increases, shear strength, tensile strength and wear resistance also increase. There are two modes of structural development as molecular weight increases. **Crystallinity** occurs where there is organized arrangement of the chains in a three-dimensional pattern. This results in a high-density structure with close proximity of the elements and higher van der Waals forces, which strengthens the overall construct; this is the case with high-density polyethylene (as compared with UHMWPE). The second mode of structural development is the random entanglement of chains (**amorphous**) and induction of further cross-linking of the polymer chains. The longer the chains, the more this occurs; this is the case with UHMWPE. This provides greater strength than the crystalline formation.

PMMA BONE CEMENT

Bone cement is used to fix in place orthopaedic prostheses. Clinically, bone cement is available as a liquid and a powder. The liquid contains the monomer N,N-dimethyltoluidine (the **accelerator**) and hydroquinone (the **inhibitor**). The powder contains the PMMA copolymer, barium or zirconium dioxide (the **radio-opacifier**) and benzoyl peroxide (the **polymerization initiator**). As the liquid and powder are mixed together, addition polymerization commences. There are several macroscopic stages of the reaction. The first stage is the sandy stage, in which the liquid and powder appear to be separate. In the second stage, the mixture appears stringy. In the third stage, the cement is doughy and does not stick to the glove; this stage coincides with the start of the working time of the cement. In the final stage, the cement is hard and warm from the exothermic reaction. Many variables affect the stages of the polymerization, but the clinically relevant variables are described in the box below.

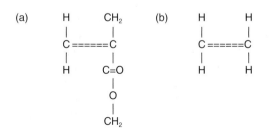

Figure 18.2 *Structure of common orthopaedic monomers: (a) methylmethacrylate; (b) ethylene.*

Working with PMMA bone cement

- **Environmental temperature and humidity:** increasing the temperature or humidity leads to a decrease in working time.

- **Powder (P)/liquid (L) ratio:**
  - normally 2 mL/1 mg;
  - decreased P/L ratio (i.e. more liquid added) leads to increased setting time.

- **Insertion time:** as soon as the cement starts setting, it becomes pseudo-plastic, i.e. the viscosity lowers as flow rate increases. This is the rationale for pressurization of the cement into the medullary canal.

- **Cement mantle temperatures:** polymerization is an exothermic reaction. The amount of heat generated depends on the surface area and thickness of the mantle: increased thickness or decreased surface area leads to an increase in the temperature generated. This is the rationale for a uniform cement mantle of a thickness of a few millimetres in order to prevent heat-induced tissue necrosis.

- **Vacuum mixing:** reduces voids and so decreases the porosity of the cement. This increases the strength of the cement.

- **Antibiotics:** do not usually affect cement properties.

UHMWPE

UHMWPE is by definition a **polyethylene polymer** with at least 3 million units. UHMWPE is formed by **condensation polymerization** and **sintering** (fusing) of the polyethylene fine granular powder into a prefabricated cast in a low-pressure (4–6 bar) and low-temperature (66–88°C) environment, with the addition of **calcium stearate** to prevent yellowing. This is clinically relevant, because when the particles are not sintered together well there may be fusion defects. There are reports in the literature of early failure of UHMWPE due to high wear, and this is thought to be due to fusion defects from the manufacturing process. UHMWPE does not crystallize fully (i.e. it is a **semi-crystalline polymer**), it but tends to form an **amorphous structure**, with random arrangement and entangling of polymer chains. This structural feature gives UHMWPE unparalleled strength and resistance to wear, compared with the HDP used previously.

The sterilization of UHMWPE gives rise to some difficulties. It cannot be sterilized by autoclave, as it softens at about 70°C and melts at 135°C, and so it needs to be irradiated. This is advantageous, because **gamma radiation** promotes cross-linking of the polyethylene, which increases the tensile strength and wear resistance. Normally gamma irradiation is performed in an oxygen atmosphere, but this tends to cause some degree of oxidation of the polyethylene, which damages the polyethylene by breaking down the carbon—carbon bonds, resulting in the formation of free radicals. By various methods, this leads to a decrease in molecular weight and a resultant deterioration of the mechanical properties.

Considerable research has been performed to find an acceptable method of sterilization that does not oxidize the polyethylene. Currently, irradiation in an inert argon or nitrogen atmosphere followed by vacuum packing appears promising, although post-irradiation oxidation of UHMWPE does occur.

Viva questions

1 What are the advantages and disadvantages of titanium alloy for the manufacture of orthopaedic plates?

2 What are the concerns regarding the use of ceramics for manufacturing hip prosthesis?

3 How is stainless steel manufactured, and how can its mechanical properties be improved?

4 What factors affect the characteristics of polymethylmethacrylate (PMMA) bone cement?

5 What are the structural differences between high-density polyethylene (HDP) and ultra-high-molecular-weight polyethylene (UHMWPE), and how do their mechanical properties differ?

FURTHER READING

Ducheyne, P. *Functional Behavior of Orthopedic Biomaterials*, Vols 1 and 2. Boca Raton, FL: CRC Press, 1984.

Hamadouche, M, Sedel, L. Ceramics in orthopaedics. *J Bone Joint Surg Br* 2000;**82**:1095–9.

Radin, EL. *Practical Biomechanics for the Orthopedic Surgeon*, 2nd edn. New York, NY: Churchill Livingstone, 1992.

Simon, JP, Fabry, G. An overview of implant materials. *Acta Orthop Belg* 1991;**57**:1–5.

19

Biomechanics and joint replacement of the hip

MARK MULLINS AND JOHN SKINNER

INTRODUCTION

The hip joint is the most common site of arthroplasty, with over 43 000 hip replacements performed annually in the UK. The success or failure of management of hip problems is dependent on a sound understanding of the biomechanics of the hip joint and how the various components of this may be modified. In addition, it is important to appreciate the factors that affect implant survival in order to be optimally informed when selecting an implant for a particular patient.

BIOMECHANICAL FACTORS IN HIP PATHOLOGY

The basis of free-body analysis is covered in Chapter 16. The dynamic forces on the hip joint are enormous. Normal walking exerts a force of three times the body weight through the hip joint, increasing to seven times the body weight in fast walking. Even the seemingly innocuous activity of straight-leg raising puts a force in excess of the twice body weight across the joint.

Free-body analysis of the hip joint makes certain assumptions. These include a single leg stance and that the weight of the leg is one-sixth of the total body weight. Figure 19.1 shows the free-body analysis for the hip joint.

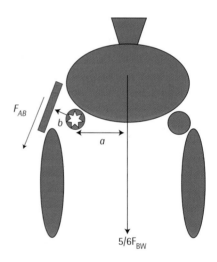

Figure 19.1 *Free-body analysis of the hip joint.* $a = 0.15\,m$; $b = 0.05\,m$; *body weight (BW) = 600 N.*

It is important to note the direction of action of the abductor muscle force, as the primary role of this group of muscles is to stabilize the pelvis in single-leg stance. Resolving the moments:

$$F_{ab} \times b = a \times 5/6F_{bw}$$

$$F_{ab} \times 0.05 = 0.15 \times 500$$

$$F_{ab} = 1500\ \text{N}$$

The hip joint reaction force is calculated by resolving the vector triangle shown in Figure 19.2.

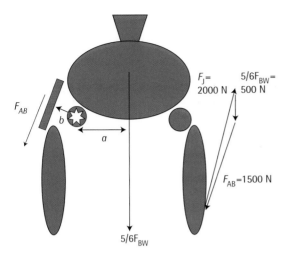

Figure 19.2 *Resolving the hip joint reaction force. a = 0.15 m; b = 0.05 m; body weight (BW) = 600 N.*

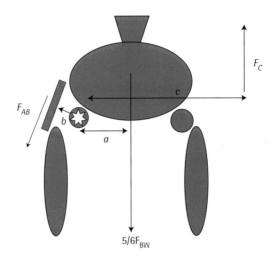

Figure 19.3 *Effect on joint reaction force of a walking stick in the contralateral hand. a = 0.15 m; b = 0.05 m; c = 0.50 m; body weight (BW) = 600 N; F_c = 100 N.*

The major determinant of joint pathology is the joint reaction force, which is the resultant of the abductor force F_{ab} and 5/6 body weight F_{bw}. Of these two factors, the abductor force predominates, but a reduction in either will reduce the joint reaction force and, thus, symptoms at the hip joint. In osteoarthritis, the near-frictionless articular cartilage is worn away and the resultant increased frictional forces exert a resistant moment. To overcome this, an increased abductor force is required.

Strategies to reduce joint reaction force

- **Reduce body–weight moment:**
  - Reduce body weight.
  - Decrease lever arm:
    - medialize the axis of rotation;
    - Trendelenburg gait.
- **Help the abductors:**
  - Provide additional moments:
    - walking stick in opposite hand;
    - suitcase in ipsilateral hand.
  - Increase abductor lever arm:
    - increase offset;
    - osteotomy;
    - lateral transfer of greater trochanter;
    - varus angulation of stem of total hip replacement (THR).
  - Improve abductor line of function.

In a **Trendelenburg gait**, the patient sways the body weight over, towards the affected side. This lateral motion decreases the body-weight moment arm and, hence, the joint reaction force. The effect of using a walking stick in the contralateral hand is shown in Figure 19.3. Resolving the moments clockwise:

$$500 \times 0.15 = (F_{ab} \times 0.05) + (100 \times 0.5)$$

Therefore, F_{ab} is 500 N, a reduction of 67 per cent when using a walking stick.

Carrying a suitcase in the ipsilateral hand provides another anticlockwise moment, thereby reducing the abductor force.

FEMORAL OSTEOTOMIES

The **varus osteotomy** has obvious advantages in **increasing the abductor lever arm** as well as providing a **more horizontal line of action** of the abductors. It may also increase congruency and displace the joint reaction force medially.

In a **valgus osteotomy**, the main effect is to **make the capital drop osteophyte weight-bearing**, thus increasing the size and quality of the surface available for weight-bearing. Other effects are possible, depending on the precise pattern of abnormality in the proximal femur; these effects may include **lengthening the abductor lever arm** and making the **abductor**

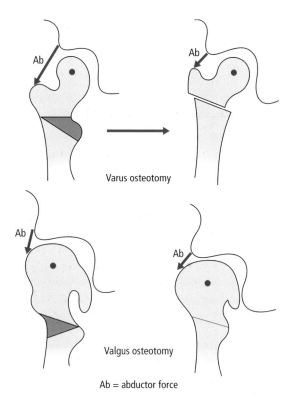

Figure 19.4 *Effects on the hip of valgus and varus osteotomies. Ab, abductor force*

action more horizontal. These effects are summarized in Figure 19.4.

TOTAL HIP ARTHROPLASTY

Sir John Charnley applied the basic principles listed above to his low-friction arthroplasty. He advocated routine lateralization of the abductors and medialization of the centre of rotation by deepening the socket and using a small head size. Although these principles are well founded in biomechanical terms, they are not universally

---

Frictional torque of hip arthroplasty depends on:

- materials bearing surface made from (ceramics < cobalt chrome < steel);
- femoral head size;
- polyethylene (if used) thickness;
- peripheral or equatorial versus polar contact.

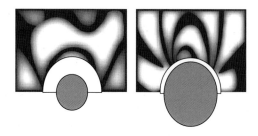

Figure 19.5 *Effect of polyethylene thickness and head size on dissipation of stress within bone.*

applied today, for the reasons discussed in this section.

Greater force is required to initiate than to maintain movement. At low speed and with poor lubrication, **stick-slip** movement (also known as **stiction-friction**) may occur. This produces torques some 40 times higher than in unaffected arthroplasties and may cause acetabular loosening.

In addition, the combination of thick polyethylene and small head size diffuses load more than thin polyethylene, leading to lower frictional torque and decreased stress at the cup interface, with widening of stress dissipation within the bone (and therefore less loosening) (Figure 19.5).

ACETABULAR COMPONENT

Deepening the socket by removing the subchondral bone plate results in plastic deformation of the softer cancellous bone, which undergoes necrosis, with formation of a fibrous membrane. There is subsequent bone resorption, leading to decreased stiffness and, ultimately, failure of the construct. Because of this and in order to preserve bone, sockets are no longer routinely medialized but are placed in the **correct anatomical location**, with a smaller head size effectively medializing the centre of rotation.

Laboratory tests have demonstrated that the acetabular preparation that gives the strongest fixation in cemented cups is the use of **three large keyholes** with preservation of the subchondral plate. However, even the weakest combinations have a lowest turning moment to failure some four times higher than the greatest frictional moments.

Modern cemented acetabular cups often have **flanges** to compress the cement, **grooves** to increase the surface area and improve bonding, and **pods** to prevent bottoming out. However, deep grooves reduce polyethylene thickness, which may result in stress risers predisposing to creep, fatigue and failure.

Uncemented cups rely on an initial press-fit or screw fixation before bone on-growth. As yet, there are no long-term data to support their increased popularity.

FEMORAL COMPONENT

A stylized femoral component is shown in Figure 19.6. As discussed above, increasing the offset of a hip joint – in this case, using a stem design with a large medial offset – results in an increased abductor lever arm. Although this may be advantageous with weakened postoperative abductor function, if it is achieved by increasing the neck length this leads to an increase in stress transfer at the tip of the component and an increase in strain on the medial cement mantle, which can lead to implant failure.

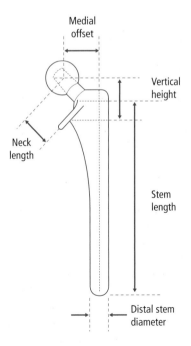

Figure 19.6 *Key elements of a femoral prosthesis.*

There are three commonly used modes of femoral stem fixation:

- **cementless** fixation;
- **cemented** – all interfaces fixed (**composite beam**);
- **cemented** – bone interface fixed, stem cement interface free of slip (**taper slip**)

A well-bonded cementless implant and a cemented implant with all interfaces fixed produce similar stresses at the interface between the implant (including cement) and bone. These are high shear stresses, low compressive stresses and medium tensile stresses.

By contrast, implants using cemented taper fit exhibit low shear stresses, high compressive stresses and almost no tensile stresses. The ability of bone cement to undergo creep and stress relaxation is primarily responsible for the conversion of tensile stress to compressive stress at the cement–bone interface.

A constant source of interest in hip arthroplasty is the optimal bearing surface for young high-demand patients. The place of metal/polyethylene bearing surface is well established in lower-demand patients, but in more challenging cases the option of hard-on-hard bearing surfaces such as ceramics now exists. As yet, although there are attractive possible benefits in terms of wear debris and its nature, there are few long-term clinical studies to support its use. In addition, ceramic bearings have the additional potential complication of head or liner fracture, which presents extreme difficulties in revision surgery due to third-body particles. At present, the surgeon should have good reasons for departing from well-proven technology.

Hip resurfacing with metal-on-metal bearings is an attractive concept, as it is bone-conserving, allows normal femoral loading, avoids stress shielding, improves functional results, restores anatomy (although it may not restore offset as well as once thought) and reduces the risk of dislocation. In addition, lubrication at the interface is likely to be fluid-film in nature. However, there are no long-term results from non-inventor surgeons, the surgery is not conservative on the acetabulum, and the long-term effect of raised plasma metal ion levels is unclear (possible risks of sensitivity, teratogenicity, carcinogenicity and lymphocyte activation) (see Chapter 25).

OSTEOLYSIS AND WEAR IN HIP ARTHROPLASTY

The most common mode of failure for established implants is osteolysis from wear debris. This debris is generated from all surfaces where contact and movement occur, and it is important to consider that this may arise from modular components, at the prosthesis–cement and cement–bone interfaces and at bearing surfaces.

Radiolucent zones have been characterized in the femur by Gruen *et al.* and in the

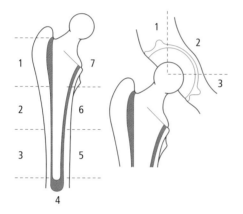

Figure 19.7 *Radiolucent zones of (a) the femur and (b) the acetabulum.*

acetabulum by Delee and Charnley (Figure 19.7). The subsequent **modes of femoral component failure** have also been characterized by Gruen *et al.* (Figure 19.8).

Since the turn of the twenty-first century, there has become a vogue for 'mini-incision' THR. The exact definition of this term is unclear, with wound sizes of less than 10 cm or 12 cm being suggested as well as the use of alternative approaches such as the two-incision technique. Some of the factors driving this change have undoubtedly been the potential commercial gains together with the goal of shorter inpatient stay. As yet, only the proponents of these techniques have demonstrated markedly improved results in terms of inpatient stay; how much of this has been due to improved anaesthesia, rehabilitation programmes and social support is unclear. It is vital to stress that any decrease in inpatient stay should not be at the expense of the long-term survivorship of the prosthesis. These moves have, however, encouraged all arthroplasty surgeons to consider ways of optimizing the surgical procedure and associated patient care.

In conclusion, knowledge of the biomechanics of the hip is essential in order for informed decisions about patient management and implant design to be undertaken. Published long-term data on differing implants must also be considered in the light of previous experiences, such as the Capital hip replacement, and meta-analyses such as the Swedish Hip Register are particularly valuable.

1	1a	Pistoning: stem within cement	
	1b	Pistoning: stem within bone	
	I	Medial midstem pivot	
	III	Calcar pivot	
	IV	Bending cantilever (fatigue)	

Figure 19.8 *Modes of failure of femoral components.*

Viva questions

1 Which total hip prosthesis would you use, and what is the evidence to support this choice?

2 Describe the modes of failure of different types of total hip replacement (THR).

3 When planning a THR, which are the important factors to consider?

4 When reviewing a THR in a follow-up clinic, what clinical symptoms and radiological signs are of particular concern?

5 Which approach do you prefer for THR, and what are its relative merits and weaknesses?

FURTHER READING

Barrack, RL, Mulroy, RD, Jr, Harris, WH. Improved cementing techniques and femoral component loosening in young patients with hip arthroplasty: a 12-year radiographic review. *J Bone Joint Surg Br* 1992;**74**:385–9.

DeLee, JG, Charnley, J. Radiological demarcation of cemented sockets in total hip replacement. *Clin Orthop Relat Res* 1976;**121**:20–32.

Gruen, TA, McNiece, GM, Amstutz, HC. Modes of failure of cemented stem-type femoral components: a radiographic analysis of loosening. *Clin Orthop Relat Res* 1979;**141**:17–27.

Murray, DW, Carr, AJ, Bulstrode, C. Survival analysis of joint replacements. *J Bone Joint Surg Br* 1993;**75**:697–704.

Murray, DW, Carr, AJ, Bulstrode, C. Which primary total hip replacement? *J Bone Joint Surg Br* 1995;**77**:520–7.

20

Biomechanics and joint replacement of the knee

ALISTER HART, RICHARD CARRINGTON AND PAUL ALLEN

BIOMECHANICS OF THE NORMAL KNEE

RELEVANT BONE GEOMETRY

Femur

The **medial femoral condyle** is larger and extends more distally in comparison to the lateral condyle.

Tibia

There is **asymmetry** of the **tibial plateaus**, which is made more congruent to the femoral condyle by the presence of the menisci. Both compartments have a **posterior tilt** of the articular surface of approximately seven degrees. This tilt is usually one degree greater on the lateral side. The asymmetry of the tibial plateaus allows for rotation of the tibia about its anatomical long axis during knee flexion.

TIBIOFEMORAL ALIGNMENT AND MALALIGNMENT

Normal alignment is described in the frontal and lateral planes. The normal frontal alignment is described by the **weight-bearing axis** (from the centre of the hip to the centre of the ankle) of the limb passing through the centre of the knee (Figure 20.1). In **varus malalignment**, the centre of the knee is lateral to the weight-bearing axis; in **valgus malalignment**, the centre of the knee is medial to the weight-bearing axis.

The normal weight bearing axis of the knee lies just anterior to the centre of the knee. This creates an extension force which is balanced by passive resistance of the posterior capsule and ligaments with minimal muscular action. If the centre of the knee is located well behind the weight-bearing axis, then there will be **hyperextension malalignment**. If the centre of the knee is located in front of the weight-bearing axis, then **flexion malalignment** exists.

HOW DOES THE KNEE MOVE?

Flexion–extension and femoral rollback

Initially, it was thought that the femur rolled across the tibia with flexion because the cruciate ligaments, in conjunction with the femur and tibia, provided a rigid four-bar linkage. This mechanism produces a mixture of femoral rollback and slide, which allows the high degree of flexion seen in the normal knee (Figure 20.2). This simplistic mechanism has been used to design successful knee replacements.

More recently, magnetic resonance imaging (MRI) of cadaveric knees has revealed that the lateral femoral condyle does rollback across the tibia during flexion, but the medial femoral

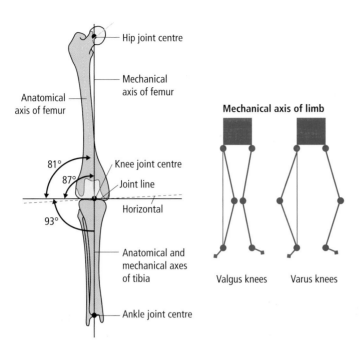

Figure 20.1 *Anatomical and mechanical axes of the femur and tibia, and abnormalities of coronal mechanical axis alignment.*

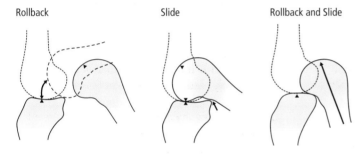

Figure 20.2 *Femoral rollback allowing deep flexion.*

condyle rolls back to a much lesser extent. In other words, there is **internal rotation** of the tibia with **flexion**.

The **biomechanical functions** of femoral rollback are two-fold: to **increase the lever arm** of the quadriceps and to allow **clearance** of the femur from the tibia in deep flexion (see Figure 20.2). During knee extension, the femur rolls forwards, increasing the lever arm of the hamstrings to act as a brake on hyperextension.

The rigid four-bar linkage mechanism is disputed. Anatomically, one visualizes the four linked bars of two cruciate ligaments and the two areas of bone that lie between the insertions of the cruciates, but in practice the ligaments are not rigid and do not have a single isometric point at all positions of flexion. The result is variable tension in different bundles of

fibres of the same ligament at different degrees of flexion.

The **flexion–extension axis** for the knee is reasonably approximated to the **transepicondylar line** (TEL). A lateral view of the femur reveals that the posterior projections of the condyles are defined by two concentric circles centred on the TEL.

Rotation during flexion–extension

The **medial compartment** is deeply dished by the concave tibial plateau and a relatively fixed meniscus. The result is an **anteroposterior excursion** of the tibiofemoral contact point of only 1 cm. The **lateral compartment** with its convex tibial plateau and more mobile lateral meniscus has a much greater excursion of the tibiofemoral contact point. The asymmetry allows axial rotation of the lateral compartment around the medial compartment by up to 30 degrees over the whole of flexion range.

From extension to full flexion, the tibia internally rotates with respect to the femur. From full flexion to extension, the tibia externally rotates with respect to the femur. The external rotation of the tibia on the femur that occurs during the terminal degrees of knee extension is termed the **screw-home mechanism** and results in tightening of both the cruciate ligaments, locking the knee such that the tibia is in the position of maximal stability with respect to the femur. Contraction of the popliteus, causing internal rotation of the tibia, is responsible for the unlocking of the knee when the knee moves from full extension to initiation of flexion.

The geometry and alignment of the bony anatomy creates articular surfaces with a constant flexion–extension gap, so that the tension is maintained in the supporting ligaments throughout flexion and extension.

FUNCTIONAL BIOMECHANICS

There are **static** and **dynamic** elements to the biomechanics of the knee. The static elements include the **alignment** of the articulating bones, the **geometry** of their weight-bearing surfaces, and the **laxity** of the connecting ligaments. The dynamic elements are the **coordinated activity** of the muscles. Proprioception helps to optimize knee function within the static limits.

THE PATELLOFEMORAL JOINT

The biomechanical function of the patella is to act as a pulley for the quadriceps and increase the power of the quadriceps by increasing the moment arm. Patellectomy reduces quadriceps strength by at least 20 per cent.

Patellofemoral joint alignment

The **Q angle** is defined by the intersection of lines joining the centre of the patella with the anterior superior iliac spine and the tibial

tubercle. The normal Q angle varies between 5 and 20 degrees. Women have an increased Q angle compared with men. Angles greater than 20 degrees are associated with patellofemoral instability and pain.

Patellar geometry

Patella geometry is variable and can be grouped into three types according to **Wiberg**. Type 1 has equal medial and lateral facets, which are both concave. Type 2 has a concave lateral facet and a smaller concave medial facet. Type 3 has an even smaller medial facet, which is convex. Wiberg proposed that the patella with a deficient medial facet is more likely to develop patellofemoral osteoarthritis (OA).

In fact, susceptibility to OA is a result of uneven pressures on the patella as it tracks through the femoral sulcus. The common denominator for the development of OA in most joints is the failure to distribute load evenly, resulting in the creation of areas of **high contact stress**. The variables that determine patella tracking are patella geometry (the Wiberg type 3 patella tracking laterally due to its deficient medial facet), flattening of the femoral sulcus angle, and a laterally placed tibial tubercle.

Measurement of the tibial tuberocity – trochlear groove (TT-TG) distance by superimposing two CT images (through TT and through trochlear) indicates laterally placed tibial tuberocity when the TT-TG is greater than 20 mm. In such cases a medial transfer of the tibial tuberocity may be indicated.

Patellofemoral joint motion

The patella first engages the femoral sulcus at 20 degrees of knee flexion and tracks along a conforming groove. At 20 degrees of flexion, the distal part of the patella makes contact first. As the knee flexes, the contact area of the patella shifts proximally. Beyond 90 degrees, the patella rotates externally and only the medial facet articulates. At extreme flexion, the patella lies in the intercondylar groove.

Patellofemoral contact pressure is 0.5 times body weight during walking, increasing to between 2.5 and 3.3 times body weight when ascending and descending stairs.

HOW IS STABLE MOVEMENT OF THE KNEE ACHIEVED?

There are **primary** and **secondary restraints** to all degrees of freedom of movement of the knee. Sectioning studies have quantified the contribution of the secondary restraints. Individual ligaments have primary and secondary functions.

Anterior translation

The **primary restraint** to anterior translation of the tibia on the femur is the **anterior cruciate ligament** (ACL). The ACL is composed of two bundles – the anteromedial (tight in flexion) and the posterolateral (tight in extension). When the knee is flexed to 30 degrees, the ACL provides 87 per cent of the restraint against anterior translation.

The remaining anterior restraint is provided by the following structures whose function as secondary anterior restraints has been quantified as:

- Iliotibial band: 24 per cent.
- Mid-medial capsule: 22 per cent.
- Mid-lateral capsule: 20 per cent.
- Medial collateral ligament (MCL): 16 per cent.
- Lateral collateral ligament (LCL): 12 per cent.
- Menisci.

In addition, the hamstrings are dynamic stabilizers of anterior translation.

The ACL is important in controlling the anteroposterior tibiofemoral contact point at all positions of flexion. The function of the ACL to resist varus, valgus and rotational forces is most relevant in combined ligament injuries.

Posterior translation

The **primary restraint** to posterior translation of the tibia is the **posterior cruciate ligament** (PCL). The **secondary restraint** is the LCL.

The primary function of the PCL is to resist posterior tibial translation on the fixed femur.

The PCL is also a secondary restraint to external rotation, varus and valgus joint space opening, and hyperextension. The PCL contributes 95 per cent of the restraining force to posterior translation at 90 degrees of knee flexion. The posterolateral corner (LCL, arcuate ligament, popliteal muscle/tendon complex, posterolateral capsule, fabellofibular ligament) provides 59 per cent of additional restraining force after the PCL has been sectioned, and the MCL supplies an additional 16 per cent restraint.

Internal rotation

The **primary restraint** is the **ACL**. The **secondary restraint** is the **popliteal oblique ligaments** (POL) and posteromedial complex (PMC).

External rotation

The **primary restraints** to external rotation are the **popliteofibular ligament**, and the LCL and the posterolateral complex at 30 degrees of flexion. The MCL is important also at all degrees of flexion.

Valgus

The **superficial MCL** is the **primary restraint** to valgus stress at all angles, with its least effect at full extension. The PMC is tight at full extension but slackens with flexion greater than 30 degrees. The deep MCL has little resistance to valgus load. The ACL acts as a secondary restraint to valgus force.

Varus

The **LCL** is the **primary restraint** to varus stress in all positions of flexion. Its greatest effect is at 30 degrees, and its least effect is at full extension. The ACL and posterolateral structures are the secondary restraints to varus stress.

THE POSTEROLATERAL STRUCTURES

The posterolateral corner of the knee is composed of the iliotibial band, biceps femoris

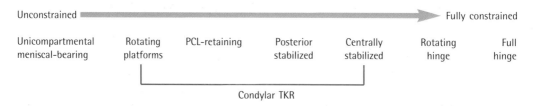

Figure 20.3 *Spectrum of constraint in knee arthroplasty. TKR, total knee replacement.*

tendon, LCL, popliteus tendon, fabellofibular ligament, popliteofibular ligament (PFL), arcuate ligament, coronary ligament, posterior horn of the lateral meniscus, middle third of the lateral capsular ligament, and posterolateral joint capsule.

There are three distinct layers within the lateral structures of the knee:

- **Superficial layer:** iliotibial tract and biceps.
- **Middle layer:** quadriceps retinaculum anteriorly and the two patellofemoral ligaments posteriorly.
- **Deep layer:** superficial and deep capsular lamina. The superficial lamina includes the LCL and the fabellofibular ligament. The deep lamina consists of the coronary ligament, popliteus hiatus, arcuate ligament and PFL.

The LCL is a primary restraint to varus rotation at 30 degrees of knee flexion and a secondary restraint against external rotation and posterior displacement. The PFL prevents excessive posterior translation and varus angulation, and restricts excessive primary and coupled external rotation (greater effect at 30 degrees than at 90 degrees).

Isolated PCL sectioning results in increased posterior translation that is maximal at 70–90 degrees of knee flexion. Combined sectioning of the LCL and PFL results in increased varus rotation, external rotation and posterior translation that is maximal at 30 degrees of flexion. Combined LCL, PFL and PCL injury results in increased varus rotation, external rotation and posterior translation at all angles of knee flexion. Additionally, isolated sectioning of the popliteus muscle belly does not cause significant posterolateral instability of the knee.

BIOMECHANICS OF KNEE ARTHROPLASTY

INTRODUCTION

Before the modern designs of condylar total knee replacement (TKR), TKR was performed using fixed hinges with poor medium- and long-term survival. Condylar TKRs were conceived by three groups (Insall *et al.*, Freeman and Samuelson, and Walker and Sledge) between 1969 and 1974. This enabled resurfacing of the distal femur and proximal tibia with implants whose shape resembled the natural knee.

The design of TKRs can be classified into **surface replacement** (condylar) and **constrained**. Surface replacements can be subdivided further into **cruciate-sacrificing**, **PCL-retaining** and **PCL-substituting** prostheses. There is a spectrum of constraint within condylar knee replacements (Figure 20.3). The least constrained TKRs are the PCL-substituting and PCL-retaining designs.

Natural knee motion is complex, involving six degrees of freedom (translation and rotation about each of the axes x, y and z). Rigid-hinge TKR allows only one degree of freedom (rotation about the x axis), resulting in flexion and extension. This provides a stable articulation, but it also increases the force transmitted to the implant–cement–bone interface and thus increases the risk of loosening. Modern hinge designs use **sloppy hinges**, by incorporating metal on polyethylene bushings and rotating platforms. The development of the non-hinged TKR reflects the evolution of the understanding of knee kinematics, stability, constraint and conformity.

The first **condylar TKRs** were cruciate-sacrificing. Stability in the sagittal plane (resisting anteroposterior translation) was achieved by a curved tibial articulating surface. The surface is therefore **conforming** because the radii of the tibial and femoral surfaces are similar. Importantly, this does not imply that the knee is constrained, since constraint is a function of the surface contours together with the periarticular soft tissues. Stability in the coronal plane (resisting varus/valgus forces) was achieved with the median intercondylar eminence. To reiterate, **conformity** is a purely **static mechanical** concept, whereas **constraint** is a **dynamic kinematic** concept.

The **PCL-retaining** TKR is thought to replicate knee kinematics more closely because the native PCL causes femoral rollback and increased stability. This is controversial. These implants have low conformity with a **round-on-flat design** to allow femoral rollback. In the coronal plane, the disadvantage of a round-on-flat design is that **lift-off** can occur, followed by **slam-down** and **edge-loading** of the polyethylene, resulting in increased contact stress and wear.

The **PCL-substituting** (or **posterior-stabilized**) TKRs have increased tibial contouring (conformity) in both the sagittal and the coronal planes. Sagittal plane stability is achieved with the femoral cam and tibial post. Coronal plane stability is achieved with the conforming surfaces and collateral ligaments.

Revision condylar prostheses have increased constraint provided by an intimately fitting cam and spine mechanism that is broader and more elevated than the posterior stablised TKR. Some allow only 1.25 degrees of varus and valgus motion. Its use is restricted to partial collateral ligament insufficiency or bone loss requiring augments to recreate an equal flexion–extension gap. The greater constraint of such devices increases the forces transmitted to the implant–cement–bone interface and therefore, intramedullary stems are used to distribute the forces over a larger area.

The rest of this chapter focuses on the condylar TKR.

CONDYLAR TKR DESIGN

A successful TKR is well fixed to the supporting bone, is durable and allows good knee function with near-normal knee kinematics. This requires a compromise of competing objectives. For example, replication of the sliding and rolling back of the normal femur during deep flexion requires low conformity, such as that seen with a flat polyethylene tibial tray in the sagittal plane. The disadvantage is reduced contact area and high contact stress, resulting in increased wear. Higher conformity increases contact area, but higher constraint transmits greater force to the bone–cement–implant interface to increase the risk of loosening.

Kinematics of TKR

Flexion–extension is controlled by the geometry of the femoral condyles and the polyethylene insert. The natural femoral condyles have two radii of curvature – a large **anterior radius** in contact with the tibia during extension and a small **posterior radius** in contact during flexion. Most condylar TKRs approximate this natural geometry. However, some, condylar TKRs, such as the Scorpion TKR, have a single femoral radius. Most TKRs match medial and lateral condylar geometry. An exception is seen with the medial pivot knee, which has a more conforming medial compartment and a less conforming lateral compartment capable of sliding.

Condylar design compromise

The ideal TKR minimizes contact stress but allows near normal knee kinematics and provides sufficient constraint to ensure stability throughout functional use. Unfortunately, constraint is defined by its limitation of degrees of freedom.

If a TKR is designed such that it is completely conforming in the coronal and sagittal planes, then contact stress would be low but kinematics would be similar to a simple hinge with virtually only one degree of freedom, i.e. flexion and extension. This would increase the torsional stress across the joint, causing loosening (unless the stress was dissipated through a rotating platform).

The condylar compromise

- Contact stress inversely proportional to constraint.
- Normal kinematics inversely proportional to constraint.
- High contact stress causes wear.
- Increased constraint increases loosening.

Solution: compromise constraint to allow low contact stress and reduce loosening.

Thus, the femoral and polyethylene radii determine both the rotation and the flexion–extension constraint. In terms of **coronal plane geometry**, a relatively **flat-on-flat** design can result in edge-loading and consequent slam-down during varus–valgus loading, whereas a **curved-on-curved** design reduces edge-loading, spreading the load over a wider area during varus–valgus loading (Figure 20.4).

Polyethylene thickness

Polyethylene inserts with a thickness greater than 8 mm reduce the variability in contact

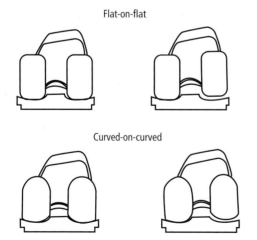

Figure 20.4 *Coronal plane geometry and the effect of flat-on-flat versus curved-on-curved design.*

stress, resulting in less polyethylene wear. However, the manufacture, sterilization and storage of polyethylene are also important in reducing wear. For more detail, see Chapter 25.

BIOMECHANICAL GOALS OF TKR

From a purely anatomical perspective, the following goals allow optimal biomechanical performance of a condylar TKR:

- Restore the mechanical axis so that it passes through the centres of the hip, knee and ankle.
- Make the bone cuts perpendicular to the mechanical axis.
- Preserve the level of the joint line.
- Balance the ligaments.
- Ensure rigid durable fixation.

These goals are achieved through design and surgical technique.

Mechanical alignment

Restoring the mechanical alignment prevents a net varus or valgus force, which causes uneven contact pressure on the polyethylene and early failure. It also prevents instability and pain through unbalanced ligaments. In the case of incompletely correctable deformities, additional soft-tissue releases are required for ligament balance.

Mechanical alignment is determined by the femoral and tibial bone cuts. The femur and tibia are cut in order to allow the thickness of the prosthesis to re-create the original thickness of the bone and cartilage in both flexion and extension.

Tibial bone cuts

The natural tibial plateau is three degrees varus to the mechanical axis; however, it is recommended that the tibia is cut perpendicular to the mechanical axis to allow even loading of the medial and lateral sides of the tibia. Tibial component rotation is a critical variable. The extensor mechanism aligns the rotation according to the position of the tibial tubercle, i.e. in the normal knee and a rotating hinge TKR, the extensor mechanism dictates the rotation of the tibia.

Femoral bone cuts

The valgus cut angle is the angle between the femoral anatomical axis and the mechanical axis. It is between five and seven degrees and should be calculated with full-length lower-limb X-rays in certain patients, e.g. very tall/very small patients, history of previous trauma, or congenital deformity.

The valgus cut angle aims to cut the femur perpendicular to the mechanical axis. The femoral component is three degrees externally rotated with respect to the femoral neutral axis in order to create a rectangular flexion gap with the tibia. The natural tibia is in three degrees of varus, but the recommended tibial cut is perpendicular to the mechanical axis, therefore placing the tibial component in three degrees of valgus with reference to the natural tibia. To create a rectangular flexion gap in this situation, the femur must be cut with three degrees of external rotation. If, after the femoral and tibial cuts, the flexion gap is not equal, then the tight ligaments on the concave side of the deformity usually require release.

There are several methods used to judge femoral component rotation (Figure 20.5). The **epicondylar axis** is actually one to three degrees externally rotated to the neutral axis, and therefore a femoral component that is parallel to this axis is in optimum position. Note that this line is almost universally present at revision surgery. **Whiteside's line** is a vertical line joining the roof of the notch with the deepest point of the trochlear. A perpendicular line to Whiteside's line is the neutral femoral axis. The **posterior condylar axis** is parallel to the neutral axis when the posterior condyles are not worn or hypoplastic.

Ligament balancing

Ligament balancing in both the coronal and the sagittal planes is essential in order to create a stable knee, reduce wear and maintain function. The degenerate knee has either contracted or stretched ligaments. A degenerate knee with a **preoperative varus deformity** that has non-parallel bone cuts usually has a contracted MCL, which must be released. A degenerate knee with a **preoperative valgus deformity** that has non-parallel bone cuts usually has contracted lateral structures (popliteus, LCL, iliotibial band). A degenerate knee with a **preoperative fixed flexion deformity** that is tighter posteriorly after bone cuts are made has tight posterior structures (capsule and PCL).

The release is therefore performed on the concave side of the deformity. A preoperative correctable deformity is likely to be balanced using the bone cuts alone and removal of osteophytes.

The order of structures to be released for a **varus knee** is as follows: deep MCL, posteromedial corner with attachment of semi-membranosus, superficial MCL and PCL.

The order of structures to be released for a **valgus knee** is as follows: lateral capsule, iliotibial band (tight in extension), popliteus (tight in flexion), LCL, intermuscular septum and lateral head of gastrocnemius.

How does the PCL affect TKR function?

The normal PCL is taut in knee flexion, preventing posterior translation of the tibia and

Femoral component
External rotation

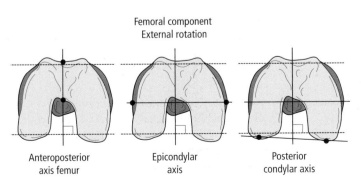

Anteroposterior
axis femur

Epicondylar
axis

Posterior
condylar axis

Figure 20.5 *Axes used to judge femoral component rotation.*

allowing femoral rollback to occur in deep flexion, enabling a greater degree of flexion by preventing impingement. An unconstrained TKR sacrificing the ACL and PCL risks flexion instability and, without femoral rollback, may limit flexion to 95 degrees. Preserving the PCL should reduce flexion instability and allow femoral rollback. However, in a degenerate knee, the PCL is contracted and unlikely to function normally.

PCL resection combined with a cam-and-post mechanism to mimic the femoral rollback was developed in the 1970s as the solution to this problem. Modern designs of PCL-sacrificing TKR use, first, a relatively **high tibiofemoral congruency** to reduce contact stress and increase anteroposterior stability and, second, a **cam-and-post mechanism** to control femoral rollback. Some surgeons cite biomechanical reasons for choosing a posterior-stabilized TKR, such as previous patellectomy (weakens the extensor mechanism, which increases anteroposterior instability), inflammatory arthritis (which can cause late rupture of the PCL) and previous trauma to the PCL.

PATELLOFEMORAL JOINT IN TKR

There are three design solutions for patellar implants: **dome** (eliminates rotational alignment problems), **anatomical** (increases conformity but requires accurate alignment of components and soft tissue balancing) and **mobile bearing** (the need for metal backing here reduces the thickness of the polyethylene).

What is the importance of the Q angle in TKR?

The Q angle (defined earlier) is formed between the intersection of the line describing the direction of pull of the quadriceps superior to the patella and the line describing the direction of the patella tendon. Increasing the Q angle increases the force acting in a lateral direction at the patellofemoral joint, which causes patella mal-tracking and subluxation.

Optimizing patella tracking in TKR

The key to optimal patellar tracking is correct rotational alignment of the femoral and tibial components. Tracking can be improved further by aligning the femoral component with the lateral cortex of the lateral femoral condyle and by slight medialization of the patella.

What is the effect of patella baja in TKR?

A short patellar tendon causes patella baja. If the patient has patellar baja preoperatively, then one should consider re-creating the correct patellar height by lowering the joint line by under-resecting the distal femur, over-resecting the tibia, or upsizing the femur to balance the flexion gap and placing the patella dome superiorly.

If the joint line is inadvertently raised as a consequence of TKR, then the patellar tendon becomes functionally short. This can result in impingement of the inferior patella pole on the polyethylene insert during flexion.

BIOMECHANICS OF TKR FAILURE

What are the factors that cause polyethylene wear in TKR?

- **Thickness of polyethylene:** if the polyethylene used is less than 8 mm thick, then the contact stress is greater than the yield strength of the polyethylene. Note that polyethylene insert thickness is usually expressed as the thickness of the tibial base plate and polyethylene together, so that an 8-mm insert may be approximately 6 mm thick at its lowest point.
- **Articular geometry:** flat polyethylene reduces the contact surface area and maximizes the contact load. Conforming polyethylene has the opposite effect.

Other factors include the method of **polyethylene sterilization, increased conformity** leading to increased backside wear, and the use of **all polyethylene components** (see Chapter 25).

What is backside wear?

Backside wear is wear of the non-articulating surface of the tibial insert. This has been observed in all designs of knee prostheses, independent of the capture mechanism of the polyethylene insert. New designs of modular tibial components are needed in order to prevent the generation of polyethylene wear debris through backside wear of TKRs.

What factors in TKR design increase the probability of loosening?

Factors that affect load transfer and increase the probability of implant loosening are as follows:

- flexible implant (low thickness/length ratio);
- small contact area;
- load transfer at the edges of contact (e.g. caused by a large varus–valgus movement, or anteroposterior or medial-lateral instability) in an unbalanced knee;
- features that concentrate stress, e.g. peripheral tibial tray pegs.

A NOTE ON MOBILE BEARING TKR

These are a result of design attempts to reduce wear by using bearings with less constraint. Examples include the meniscal type and the rotating platform. They aim to allow muscles and ligaments more control over the kinematics and constraint of a TKR. However, no study has shown an objective increase in range of motion, and it is too early to determine whether wear is reduced by use of these bearing surfaces. Further information on mobile bearing TKRs may be found in the list of further reading below.

Viva questions

1 Which total knee replacement (TKR) would you use, and what is the evidence to support this choice?

2 When planning a TKR, which are the important factors to consider?

3 When reviewing a TKR in a follow-up clinic, what clinical symptoms and radiological signs are of particular concern?

4 How would you correct a varus/valgus/fixed-flexion knee deformity during TKR?

5 What factors contribute to failure of TKRs?

FURTHER READING

Conditt, MA, Stein, JA, Noble, PC. Factors affecting the severity of backside wear of modular tibial inserts. *J Bone Joint Surg Am* 2004;**86**:305–11.

Davies, H, Unwin, A, Aichroth, P. The posterolateral corner of the knee: anatomy, biomechanics and management of injuries. *Injury* 2005;**35**:68–75.

Freeman, MA, Pinskerova, V. The movement of the normal tibio-femoral joint. *J Biomech* 2005;**38**:197–208.

Jones, RE. Mobile bearings in revision total knee arthroplasty. *Instr Course Lect* 2005;**54**:225–31.

Morgan, H, Battista, V, Leopold, SS. Constraint in primary total knee arthroplasty. *J Am Acad Orthop Surg* 2005;**13**:515–24.

21

Biomechanics of the spine

AMIR ALI NARVANI, BRIAN HSU AND LESTER WILSON

INTRODUCTION

The three main functions of the spine are to **allow movement**, to **carry loads** and to **protect neural structures**. The components responsible for the structure and function of the spine can be regarded as the **spinal system**. Movement in the spine is determined by the shape of the structures, i.e. the anatomy, and by neurological control. This movement is restricted in order to avoid neurological damage and to prevent deformity. In other words, the spine must be **stable**, as defined as follows by White and Panjabi (1990):

> Clinical stability of the spine is the ability of the spine under physiological loads to limit patterns of displacement so as not to damage or irritate the spinal cord or nerve roots, and in addition to prevent incapacitating deformity or pain due to structural changes.

How is this stability provided? A number of models and theories exist, but the one offered by Panjabi (1992) is logical and integrates the different components of the spinal system well. In this model, the spinal system consists of three subsystems:

- **passive musculoskeletal subsystem;**
- **active musculoskeletal subsystem;**
- **neural subsystem.**

These three subsystems work together to provide the overall stability of the spinal system. Note that a motion segment in the spine is defined as two vertebrae and their intervening soft tissues.

PASSIVE MUSCULOSKELETAL SUBSYSTEM

The passive system consists of the **vertebrae, facet joints, intervertebral discs, spinal ligaments** and **joint capsules** (Figure 21.1).

Generally speaking, flexion is resisted by posterior structures, which are the ligaments, facet joints, capsules and the posterior part of the intervertebral discs. In the thoracic spine, the ribs and their associated musculature add considerable mechanical stiffness and stability, especially in flexion. Extension is restricted by the anterior longitudinal ligament, the anterior part of the annulus fibrosus and the facet joints. The facet joints and intervertebral discs limit rotation. Each individual component of the passive system confers different biomechanical properties on the spinal system.

VERTEBRAE

There are 33 vertebrae: 7 cervical, 12 thoracic, 5 lumbar, 5 sacral and 4 coccygeal. The sacral and coccygeal vertebrae are fused. Each **vertebra** consists of an **anterior body** and a **posterior neural arch**.

The **vertebral body** is rectangular in shape in both sagittal and coronal section and consists of

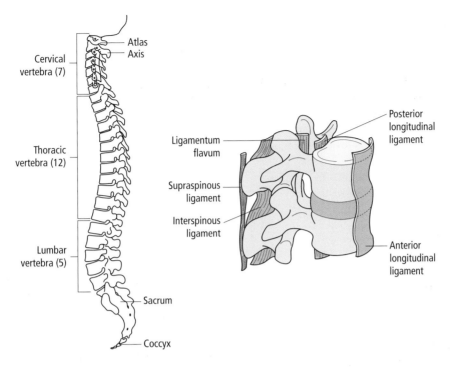

Figure 21.1 *Anatomy of the spine.*

a thin shell of cortical bone surrounding a mass of cancellous bone. This cancellous bone comprises both vertical and horizontal trabeculae. The **neural arch** consists of two pedicles, two laminae, two transverse processes and a single spinous process.

Important biomechanical features of the vertebrae contribute to the stability of the spine. These features include the following:

- The **width** and **depth** of the vertebral bodies increase in size as one moves caudally, and these changes are paralleled by an increase in strength and in loading. The changes in size appear to be a mechanical adaptation. Strength is also related to the bone mineral content in the spine.
- The internal architecture of cancellous vertebral body bone is in the form of both **horizontal** and **vertical trabeculae**. The horizontal trabeculae prevent the side walls from collapsing when the body is subjected to large compressive forces (note that loss of horizontal trabeculae in osteoporosis leads to decreased vertebral body stiffness). The

vertical trabeculae aid the transmission of the force from the superior surface to the inferior surface of the body (note that compression fractures occur at the end plate).

- In the sagittal plane, the spine is **S-shaped**. The cervical and the lumbar spine are concave posteriorly (**lordosis**), whereas the thoracic spine is concave anteriorly (**kyphosis**). These curvatures provide certain biomechanical advantages. First, the S-shape ensures that the body mass is distributed away from the central axis of rotation. Maintaining balance is therefore easier (this has been compared to the process of tightrope walking). Second, the curvatures provide shock-absorbing qualities, as they change with each strike during walking and running. Third, combined lumbar bending and pelvic rotation in each cycle aid walking. To some extent, the rotation of the pelvis is dependent on the rotation of the lumbar spine during the gait cycle. Coupling of the lumbar spine allows rotation of the lumbar spine to occur whenever there is lateral bending of the lumbar spine. This coupling is in turn dependent on the orientation of the facet joints and the lordosis of the lumbar spine.

- The **spinous process**, which is part of the neural arch, provides an insertion site for interspinous ligaments and paraspinal muscles. By providing a **long moment arm** for the muscles and ligaments, they reduce the forces that are required to resist flexion deformities. Note that the axis of rotation in the normal spine is positioned in the posterior part of the vertebral body.

Coupling

Coupling occurs when movement in one plane causes an associated movement in another plane. This occurs in both the cervical and the lumbar spine. In the cervical spine, lateral bending is associated with rotation of the spinous processes towards the convexity of the curve; in the lumbar spine, lateral bending is associated with the rotation of the spinous processes towards the concavity of the curve.

FACET JOINTS

The facet joints are synovial joints between the superior articular facet of one vertebra and the inferior articular facets of the vertebra above. The direction of possible movements between adjacent vertebrae is dependent on the orientation of the facet joints, which varies in the different regions of the spine. In the **cervical region**, the facet joints are orientated at 45 degrees to the sagittal plane and parallel to the coronal plane. Because of this orientation, anteroposterior translation is resisted, but there is less resistance to flexion/extension, lateral bending and rotation.

In the **thoracic spine**, the facet joints are oriented at 60 degrees to the sagittal plane and at 20 degrees to the coronal plane.

In the **lumbar region**, the facet joints are oriented in the sagittal plane proximally but become more oriented coronally towards the lumbosacral junction. In addition, the joints are

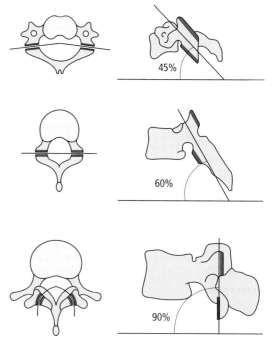

Figure 21.2 *Facet joint orientation in the spine: (a) cervical vertebra, (b) thoracic vertebra and (c) lumbar vertebra.*

tilted in the coronal plane by up to 45 degrees. This orientation permits flexion and translation, but rotation is resisted.

In summary, the **facet joints progressively tilt up** (45–60–90 degrees) **and in** (neutral–20–45) **as one moves caudally** (Figure 21.2).

The percentage of the compressive load on the spine supported by the facet joints is dependent on the posture and is increased in extension. The facet joints also play an important role in torsional stability, contributing 40 per cent of torsional load resistance in the lumbar spine (with a further 40 per cent contribution from the disc and 20 per cent from the ligamentous structures). In the cervical spine, the facet joints also provide stability in flexion in addition to torsion (cervical facetectomy of more than 50 per cent leads to loss of stability with these movements).

SPINAL LIGAMENTS

The spinal ligaments include the ligamentum flavum, intertransverse ligaments, interspinous ligaments, supraspinous ligaments, anterior and posterior longitudinal ligaments and (in the lumbar region) the iliolumbar ligaments.

Important biomechanical points about the spinal ligaments include the following:

- The **ligamentum flavum** contains a high proportion of elastin fibres, which allow it to stretch under tension and recoil and shorten when relaxed, preventing it from buckling into the spinal canal when it is healthy. In a degenerate motion segment, the disc height is lost, allowing the facet joints to override and the ligamentum flavum to buckle into the spinal canal – two contributory factors in the development of spinal stenosis.
- Two factors determine the degree of support provided for the spinal column by the spinal ligaments:
  - the **intrinsic strength** of the ligament;
  - the **length of lever arm** (moment) through which the ligament acts (the perpendicular distance from the axis of rotation, which as discussed above lies in the posterior part of the vertebral body). Therefore, a weak ligament might still be effective as it is attached further away from the axis of rotation.
- The anterior and posterior longitudinal ligaments **resist excessive extension** and **flexion** of the spinal column, and the posterior longitudinal ligament also has an important role in protecting the neural structures from bony fragments when large compressive forces are applied to the vertebral body.
- Biomechanical analyses performed on the spinal ligaments confirm that these ligaments provide **significant resistance** only beyond the physiological range of motion.

INTERVERTEBRAL DISCS

The intervertebral discs are important structures with a crucial biomechanical role, which deteriorates with degeneration. They are discussed in detail in Chapter 15, but here we summarize their important biomechanical factors:

- Their main biomechanical function is to **distribute compressive forces evenly** from one vertebral body to the next while permitting a small degree of movement. They also provide some degree of shock absorption.
- They are composed of a peripheral ring of fibrous tissue, the **anulus fibrosus**, and a central bubble of semi-liquid gelatinous material, the **nucleus pulposus**.
- The anulus fibrosus is composed of concentric laminae of collagen, with alternate layers of fibres being positioned at right-angles to each other. This arrangement allows the anulus to provide some resistance to forces applied in any direction, in addition to the hoop stresses generated by physiological loading of the nucleus.
- The nucleus pulposus consists of hydrophilic proteoglycans; the water content is as high as 90 per cent in newborns, decreasing to 70 per cent in old age. The **high water content** enables the nucleus to deform like fluid when compressive forces are applied, spreading hydraulically to equalize these forces and keeping the disc anulus under balanced tension during axial loading. As the water content of the nucleus decreases with age or with prolonged compressive loading, the ability of the disc to behave hydraulically is impaired. The anulus is less able to tolerate the compressive loads and may deform, leading with time to fissure formation and disc degeneration.

ACTIVE MUSCULOSKELETAL SUBSYSTEM

According to Panjabi's model, the active musculoskeletal subsystem consists of muscles and tendons that generate forces and thereby contribute significantly to spinal stability. In vitro experiments have demonstrated spinal column buckling with loads as small as 9 kg (90 N) in the absence of any force generated by muscles. Physiological loads on the spinal column are much greater than this value – when standing upright, the load on the column is two to three times body weight.

The muscles involved are extensor spinal muscles, intercostal muscles, abdominal-wall muscles and lower-trunk muscles. The extensor muscles can be divided into three layers – deep, intermediate and superficial:

- The **deep layer** consists of interspinalis and intertransversalis.
- A group of muscles that run between the transverse processes and the spine (sometimes referred to as transversospinalis) form the **intermediate level**. Muscles included in this layer are the thoracic spine rotators, multifidus and semispinalis.
- The erector spinae muscles make up the powerful **superficial layer**. From lateral to medial, the erector spinae on each side consists of the iliocostalis, longissimus, spinalis and (in the neck) splenius.

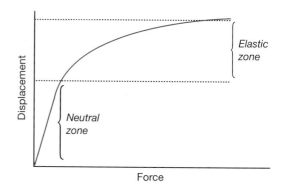

Figure 21.3 *Force–displacement curve for spine, demonstrating the neutral and the elastic zones. The complete range of movement is the neutral zone and the elastic zone.*

NEURAL SUBSYSTEM

The neural subsystem activates and controls muscle force generation. Components and pathways of this subsystem are beyond the remit of this chapter. This subsystem receives information and feedback from force and motion transducers, which are located in ligaments, tendons and muscles. The control system compares this feedback with the values required for stability and adjusts its commands to the muscles accordingly. Therefore, the pattern and the degree of force generation vary with different postures, movements and loads.

INTEGRATION OF THE SUBSYSTEMS

How do the three different subsystems interact, and what is the relative importance of each? In order to answer these questions, we need to consider another of Panjabi's concepts: the **neutral zone**.

Studies that have addressed the load–displacement behaviour of a typical spinal motion segment have demonstrated a non-linear load–displacement curve. As force is applied to the spine, initially there is a large deformation. As the force is increased, the system stiffens and the displacement reduces. This adaptation allows free movement near the neutral position

and increased resistance to movement near the end ranges of spinal motion. The **initial zone of high flexibility** is referred to as the **neutral zone**, and the **zone of increased resistance to motion** is referred to as the **elastic zone**. These zones are demonstrated in the load–displacement curve shown in Figure 21.3.

Studies suggest that in the neutral zone, the passive subsystem applies very little resistance to movement, with most of the resistance in this zone coming from the active and the neural subsystems. In the elastic zone, the passive subsystem significantly resists motion.

The passive system does, however, play an important role in the neutral zone. It is thought that in this zone, the passive system functions as a **force transducer**, supplying feedback information to the neural subsystem. Intervertebral discs, facet joint capsules and the interspinous and supraspinous ligaments all contain afferent nerve fibres that provide proprioception information to the neural subsystem.

The active subsystem provides most of the stability in the neutral zone; the lumbar spine without any musculature is highly unstable when very small loads are applied to it. Furthermore, it has been demonstrated that with most demanding tasks, when large compressive forces are applied, the spinal stability is increased as a result of high muscular activity. Conversely, during activities with low loads, muscles are under reduced tension and sudden movements may lead to instability. Appropriate activation of the small intersegmental muscles of the spine, such as the multifidi, is likely to be of significant importance with small-load activities. The neural subsystem becomes crucial here, because it has to coordinate the precise recruitment of the appropriate muscles. A suboptimized neural subsystem may allow uncoordinated muscle activity, which can lead to instability and damage.

As well as determining stability in the neutral zone, it has been proposed that **muscle activation reduces the size of the neutral zone**. This becomes particularly significant in situations where the neutral zone is initially increased. This increase is seen in pathological conditions where displacement under physiological loads causes symptoms. These conditions include disc degeneration, spinal injuries, compression and burst fractures. The increase in the neutral zone in these conditions is greater than the increase in total range of movement. The size of the neutral zone therefore appears to be a better indicator of clinical problems in these conditions than the total range of movement.

Based on these observations, Panjabi has redefined instability as follows:

> A significant decrease in the capacity of the stabilizing system of the spine to maintain the intervertebral neutral zones within physiological limits so that there is no neurological dysfunction, no major deformity, and no incapacitating pain.

Instability occurs when the neutral zone increases beyond the physiological range of movement, and therefore the stabilizing systems do not reach the stiffening phase of the force–displacement curve within the physiological range of movement.

In those pathological processes where the elastic zone is increased, muscular activity, with coordination of the active and the neural subsystem, will attempt to decrease the neutral zone. The active and the neural subsystems are then compensating for a fault in the passive subsystem, which has occurred as a result of

disc degeneration or damage to the spinal column.

Conversely, there are situations where the passive subsystem compensates for suboptimal active and neural subsystems. Ageing may be an example where the decreased muscular activity is compensated for by osteophyte formation and facet joint hypertrophy, which stiffen the passive subsystem.

SUMMARY

The functions of the spinal system are to allow movement, to carry load and to protect the neural structures. In order to fulfil its function, the spinal system must be stable. Stability is a consequence of the coordinated activity of the three different subsystems (passive, active, neural). Each subsystem possesses specific mechanical and biological properties, which allow it to play its role. When one subsystem breaks down, the others attempt to compensate. Stability is linked to the size of the neutral zone. Disc degeneration and injury increase the size of this zone, whereas muscle activation decreases it.

Viva questions

1 What is spinal stability?

2 What unique features of the spine contribute to stability?

3 What do you know about the subsystems of the spine?

4 What is coupling as related to the spine?

5 How does vertebral anatomy change as one proceeds caudally in the spine?

FURTHER READING

Benzel, EC. The essentials of spine biomechanics for the general neurosurgeon. *Clin Neurosurg* 2003;**50**:86–177.

Panjabi, MM. The stabilizing system of the

spine: part I. Function, dysfunction, adaptation and enhancement. *J Spin Disord* 1992;**5**:383–9.

Panjabi, MM. The stabilizing system of the spine: part II. Neutral zone and instability hypothesis. *J Spin Disord* 1992;**5**:390–6.

Resnick, DK, Weller, SJ, Benzel, EC. Biomechanics of the thoracolumbar spine. *Neurosurg Clin North Am* 1997;**8**:455–69.

White, AA, Panjabi, MM. *Clinical Biomechanics of the Spine*, 2nd edn. Philadelphia, PA: Lippincott, 1990.

22

Biomechanics and joint replacement of the shoulder and elbow

MARK FALWORTH AND SIMON LAMBERT

SHOULDER

The shoulder demonstrates a range of motion greater than any other joint in the body. Its movement is governed by complex biomechanical principles in order to allow a multiplanar range of motion. This flexibility does, however, necessitate less constraint, and hence the risk of developing certain pathological conditions is high and the design and technicalities of prosthetic joint replacement challenging.

ANATOMY

The shoulder complex is made up of a number of joints. There are three articular joints: the **glenohumeral**, **acromioclavicular**, and **sternoclavicular** joints. There are also two physiological joints – the **scapulothoracic** joint and the **subacromial** joint – the latter being formed between the rotator cuff and the overlying acromion.

Humerus

The **humeral head** is **inclined superiorly** with respect to the humeral shaft, with a neck–shaft angle of between 130 and 140 degrees. In addition, the humeral head is **retroverted** by approximately 30 degrees, as measured against the transepicondylar axis. The humeral head is **eccentrically placed on the shaft**, approximately 9 mm posterior to the neutral axis of the shaft. Failure to replicate this version and posterior offset during prosthetic replacement results in poor biomechanics and may end in early failure.

Glenoid and scapula

The anatomy of the glenoid is much less variable. The glenoid demonstrates approximately five degrees of **superior tilt** with reference to the vertical plane. It is also **retroverted** approximately seven degrees from the plane perpendicular to the scapular plane, which in turn is 30–40 degrees **anteverted** to the coronal plane (Figure 22.1).

Joint congruency is also important, particularly as the surface area of the glenoid fossa is only approximately one-third that of the humeral head. The distribution of cartilage on the glenoid fossa and the presence of the glenoid labrum increases congruency and, hence, stability of the shoulder.

Clavicle

The clavicle is an important strut off which the glenohumeral joint is suspended. It acts as an osseous antagonist to the combined actions of the pectoralis major muscle and the trapezium and maintains the lateral position of the shoulder. During shoulder movement, the clavicle circumducts around the sternoclavicular

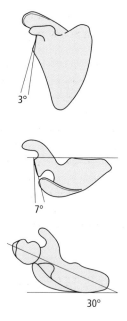

Figure 22.1 *Glenoid and scapular orientation.*

JOINT MOVEMENT

Normal shoulder function is dependent on both glenohumeral and scapulothoracic movement. Failure of normal movement at either of these joints results in abnormal kinetics and increases the risk of pathology, such as impingement and instability.

A large number of muscles are responsible for shoulder movement. These can be divided into **glenohumeral, scapulothoracic** and **thoracohumeral** muscles (Table 22.1). The role of each of these muscles in shoulder movement is dependent upon the position of the arm in space and can be investigated individually with electromyography (EMG).

During **forward elevation** in the **scapular plane**, the **deltoid** and **supraspinatus muscle** work together, creating a **vertical shear force**, which, if performed in a cuff-deficient shoulder, would result in superior migration of the humeral head. The **subscapularis, teres minor** and **infraspinatus**, along with the **supraspinatus muscles**, must therefore force the humeral head firmly into the glenoid fossa in order to minimize humeral head translation (Figure 22.2a).

Although both the supraspinatus and the deltoid muscles are active during forward elevation of the arm, at the initiation of abduction the supraspinatus plays a much larger

joint, leading to a change in orientation of the clavicle. Its relationship to the acromion is, however, maintained by the integrity of the coracoclavicular ligaments. Disruption of these would, therefore, result in the loss of skeletal stabilization of the scapula, with subsequent protraction of the shoulder and scapulothoracic dyskinesia.

Table 22.1 Muscles controlling shoulder movement

Glenohumeral muscles	Scapulothoracic muscles	Thoracohumeral muscles
Deltoid	Trapezius	Pectoralis major
Supraspinatus	Levator scapulae	Latissimus dorsi
Infraspinatus	Rhomboid major	
Subscapularis	Rhomboid minor	
Teres minor	Serratus anterior	
Teres major	Pectoralis minor	
Biceps brachii		
Coracobrachialis		
Triceps		

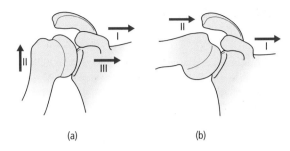

(a)   (b)

Figure 22.2 *(a) Muscle forces across the glenohumeral joint at initiation of abduction. (b) Muscle forces in 90 degrees of abduction. (I) Supraspinatus; (II) deltoid; (III) remainder of cuff.*

role. However, as the arm is elevated, the deltoid muscle becomes more active and at 90 degrees the vectors of each muscle are almost equal (Figure 22.2b). This explains why patients with a supraspinatus cuff tear may have pain and weakness at 30 degrees of elevation but good power at 90 degrees.

SCAPULOTHORACIC MOTION

The humeral head both rolls and translates during shoulder movement. Humeral head translation is variable, with the greatest amount – approximately 11 mm – in an inferior direction.

If the glenoid was fixed in a rigid position, then the range of possible shoulder movement would be far less. The glenoid must therefore move in order to minimize the degree of humeral head translation; this is achieved by scapulothoracic motion. However, the scapula must be mobile enough to facilitate a wide arc of motion while still acting as a stable base for glenohumeral movement, such that the net joint reaction force passes through the glenoid fossa. Failure to position the glenoid accurately to receive these forces may result in instability.

Scapular rotation therefore serves three important roles: it permits the glenoid to function as a **stable base** during arm elevation, it **minimizes the risk of mechanical impingement** of the rotator cuff, and it enables the **deltoid muscle fibre length to be preserved**. Scapulothoracic dynamics are therefore an important factor in the assessment of the

painful shoulder, and failure to recognize a scapulothoracic dyskinesia may result in missed pathology.

The relationship between glenohumeral and scapulothoracic movement is variable, depending on the degree of arm elevation. The first 30 degrees of abduction and 60 degrees of forward flexion are achieved largely at the exclusion of scapulothoracic movement. Thereafter, scapulothoracic motion has an increasing role, with a ratio of 2 : 1 of scapulothoracic to glenohumeral movement from 30 degrees onwards. In the final 60 degrees of movement, however, the ratio may change again to 1 : 1.

GLENOHUMERAL STABILITY: CLINICAL APPLICATIONS

Unlike in the hip joint, which is stabilized primarily by its osseous geometry, the glenohumeral joint is reliant on the synchronous function of both static and dynamic stabilizing factors, with no one structure stabilizing the glenohumeral joint throughout its entire range of motion.

Static factors

HUMERAL HEAD AND GLENOID VERSION

The importance of version and offset has already been discussed, and these factors are of particular importance in instability surgery. It is possible that **anterior instability** may occur if there is significantly less than 30 degrees retroversion of the humeral head. If this is found to be the case, then a humeral shaft rotation osteotomy can be considered. Similarly, scapular neck osteotomies can be performed in order to correct excessive retroversion of the glenoid.

CONFORMITY

The greater the congruency of an articulating joint, the greater the stability. Although it is reported that the glenoid radius is approximately 2 mm greater than that of the humeral head, the glenohumeral joint can still be regarded as congruent. Lack of congruency would result in greater translation and instability. Increasing the concavity of the glenoid by having a thicker layer of cartilage at its periphery, as compared with the centre of the glenoid, also increases the conformity. Furthermore, congruence is increased following the cartilage deformation that occurs when the joint is loaded.

LABRUM

The **labrum** is a fibrocartilage structure that is triangular in cross-section superiorly but becomes more rounded inferiorly. Superiorly and anterosuperiorly, the labrum is meniscal in appearance and fairly mobile compared with inferiorly, where it is attached more firmly, thereby helping to **prevent translation**. The weakest part of the capsule and labral complex is at the 4 o'clock position, which is the standard position of the Bankart lesion. The labrum also acts as an area of **attachment** for the **glenohumeral ligaments** and therefore has influence on this aspect of stability.

The height also varies, such that the combined effect of the labrum and glenoid concavity results in the glenoid fossa being 9 mm deep supero-inferiorly compared with 5 mm deep in the anteroposterior direction. The labrum accounts for approximately 3 mm of this height and is responsible for increasing humeral head coverage as well as the contact surface area of the glenohumeral joint. It is thought that the effect of the labrum is **responsible for 20 per cent of shoulder stability**.

GLENOHUMERAL LIGAMENTS AND CAPSULE

The capsuloligamentous complex consists of the **superior**, **middle** and **inferior glenohumeral ligaments**, all of which blend with the capsule. These do not act like true ligaments but instead became taut at varying degrees of humeral rotation and abduction.

The **inferior glenohumeral ligament** (IGHL) consists of an anterior and a posterior band, with the portion of ligament between the two bands being referred to as the axillary pouch, which supports the humeral head. The majority of the IGHL takes its origin form the labrum, with only approximately 15 per cent coming directly from the glenoid rim. It inserts just inferior to the greater and lesser tuberosities.

The axillary pouch extends from the inferior two-thirds of the glenoid rim to the inferior one-third of the humeral head, creating a hammock-like structure. It is the most consistent of the three glenohumeral ligaments with respect to its insertion and orientation; however, the quality of the ligament varies, with only one-third forming a distinct band. The remainder blends with the capsule. The anterior band of the IGHL tightens in 90 degrees of abduction and external rotation, thus spanning the mid portion of the glenohumeral joint and preventing anterior and inferior translation of the humeral head. Stability is enhanced further in flexion and internal rotation, when the posterior band tightens. The IGHL is the primary stabilizer of the abducted glenohumeral joint and is the most frequently injured portion of the capsule, resulting in instability.

The **middle glenohumeral ligament** (MGHL) originates from the supraglenoid tubercle and the anterosuperior labrum between the 1 o'clock and 3 o'clock positions. The MGHL inserts into the lesser tuberosity, blending with the subscapularis at its insertion. The MGHL provides anterior stability between 0 and 90 degrees of abduction; however, it provides the most restraint to anterior displacement between 45 and 60 degrees of abduction, with the inferior ligament becoming the more dominant anterior restraint thereafter.

The **superior glenohumeral ligament** (SGHL) arises from the supraglenoid tubercle just anterior to the long head of biceps and inserts into the humerus near the lesser tuberosity. The SGHL forms an anterior cover to the long head of biceps and with the coracohumeral ligament constitutes the rotator interval, which has an important role in shoulder stability, acting as an inferior stabilizer and limiter of internal rotation in the adducted arm.

CORACOHUMERAL LIGAMENT

The coracohumeral ligament is part of a capsuloligamentous complex. It inserts into the dorsolateral coracoid and is comprised of a thickening of the anterosuperior capsule. Its fibres then extend laterally, blending with the superficial fibres of the supraspinatus and subscapularis. It has both an anterior and a posterior band, which insert into the lesser and greater tuberosities, respectively. The ligament is therefore a crucial element of the rotator interval.

The anterior band becomes taut with the arm in external rotation, and the posterior band becomes taut with internal rotation, possibly resulting in resistance to anterior inferior translation during these movements. Rotator interval lesions, which include the coracohumeral ligament, are important, because they increase humeral head translation, and they should be addressed when managing atraumatic types of shoulder instability.

INTRA-ARTICULAR PRESSURE

There is a **negative intra-articular pressure** within the glenohumeral joint, as in most other joints. This can be observed at the time of arthroscopy, when a hiss of air may be heard as the trocar is removed from the arthroscope placed in the glenohumeral joint. This negative pressure is believed to help suck the humeral head on to the glenoid.

SURFACE AREA

The effectiveness of the force transmitted by the humeral head on to the glenoid fossa is dependent upon the surface area of the interface. The relatively small size of the glenoid fossa, which is one-third the size of the humeral head, therefore results in a **small surface area**. This differential in size generates high forces across the joint interface, aiding **glenohumeral stability**.

Dynamic factors

Both static and dynamic stabilizers are important in shoulder stability. This is demonstrated when testing for humeral head translation. The influence of dynamic stabilizers can best be appreciated by examining a shoulder in an anaesthetized patient when the effect of dynamic stabilizers is at a minimum. In this anaesthetized state, there is an increase in translation due to lack of function in the cuff musculature. Active movement of the shoulder results in much less translation, such that the centre of rotation of the humeral head is

related closely to the centre of rotation of the glenoid. This close relationship is possible due to the dynamic constraints of the shoulder, which ensure that glenohumeral rotation is achieved with minimal translation.

Forces acting across the glenohumeral joint cause a **concavity compression force** that maintains stability. Concavity compression is reliant on three factors: the state of the **musculature** compressing the humeral head into the glenoid fossa, the **structural relationship** between the glenoid fossa and humeral head, and, at the limits of motion, the **glenohumeral ligaments**.

Dynamic stabilizers include the following:

ROTATOR CUFF

Contraction of the rotator cuff compresses the humeral head into the glenoid fossa, thereby requiring an increased force to translate the humeral head. The **compressive force** attributed to the rotator cuff contributes to joint stability during the mid-range of shoulder motion as compared with the glenohumeral and coracohumeral ligaments, which contribute at the extremes of motion.

Superior migration of the humeral head may occur in patients with large rotator cuff tears. Isolated tears of the supraspinatus do not, however, usually result in significant superior migration unless there has been extension into the infraspinatus, thereby disrupting the transverse force couple.

BICEPS

The biceps tendon has a Y-shaped origin from the superior labrum. Its role as a secondary head depressor and stabilizer has been debated; however, it is now believed to **reduce translation** in both the **anteroposterior** and **supero-inferior translations**. Its role may become more prominent in the presence of other injuries, such as cuff or labral deficiencies.

SCAPULAR ROTATORS

Scapular position is important, as it influences glenoid version and the amount of superior angulation. Disturbance of normal scapulothoracic dynamics can, therefore, result in increased instability. There is a **rotatory force** couple that enables normal function; the **upper component** consists of levator scapulae, upper trapezius and the upper fibres of serratus anterior, and the **lower component** includes the lower trapezius and the lower fibres of serratus anterior. Any disturbance in these muscle groups, along with the pectoral girdle musculature, which helps coordinate scapulohumeral rhythm, can lead to instability of the shoulder.

DELTOID

The deltoid muscle provides a **superiorly directed shear force** to the humeral head with the arm in adduction. In a cuff-incompetent shoulder, this would result in superior translation of the humeral head and destabilization of the glenohumeral joint. However, in 90 degrees of abduction, its line of action works synergistically with the rotator cuff to increase concavity compression forces.

PROPRIOCEPTION

Proprioception is believed to play a role in shoulder stability. In a normal shoulder, dynamic proprioception is believed to improve hand position sense after movement has been initiated. In individuals who suffer from multidirectional or muscle patterning instability, there appears to be a reduced capacity to recruit proprioceptors and to refine and control motor function of the upper limb, hence compounding the condition and treatment options.

PROSTHETIC REPLACEMENT

In individuals with an intact rotator cuff and deltoid muscle, the positioning of a total shoulder arthroplasty should mimic that of normal glenohumeral anatomy. Failure to do so can result in failure of the implant.

The aim in prosthetic replacement of the humeral head is to choose an implant that replicates the anatomical size of the natural head and to restore the normal centre of rotation. Variables that need to be considered include the angle of stem insertion, the need to replicate both the anteroposterior and medial-lateral humeral offsets, and the need to prevent

any alteration in the natural neck–shaft angle. The alteration of any of these values will change the centre of rotation of the humeral head, resulting in abnormal humeral head translation, decreased range of movement, instability, and abnormal wear patterns between the prosthetic humeral head and the glenoid component.

Thin-stem cemented prostheses give the surgeon the ability to position the stem within the humeral shaft in order to replicate the natural centre of rotation for the humeral head. **Press-fit uncemented stem** designs prevent any adjustment of the humeral head position, as the stem cannot be moved within the shaft. They therefore require the ability to adjust the centre of rotation, and hence anterior posterior and medial lateral offsets, by having an adjustable component between the stem and head, with or without an eccentric Morse taper that is used to 'dial in' the offset. This adjustability of the implant should encourage the replication of normal anatomy, resulting in improved shoulder function.

The complexity of these implants can potentially be avoided with the use of a **surface-replacement arthroplasty**. These implants avoid the potential pitfalls of stem insertion and should replicate normal humeral head anatomy. They do, however, require adequate humeral head bone stock, a requirement that in itself can prevent adequate exposure of the glenoid, thus complicating glenoid component placement in total shoulder arthroplasty.

Glenoid component design and placement is equally important. The glenoid component can be of either a **flat back** or **spherical back** design, with each having different biomechanical properties. Spherical back designs appear to be gaining more favour due to an apparent decrease in lift-off and slip of the component at the bone–cement interface. Malpositioning, in particular retroversion, can also result in instability.

In a cuff-deficient shoulder, an **unconstrained prosthesis** often results in an inadequate result. The lack of the rotator cuff muscles to constrain the prosthetic humeral head results in superior migration of the head on the initiation of abduction. This results in an abnormal centre of humeral head rotation and abnormal articular contact pressures, and subsequent poor function. If used in a total shoulder arthroplasty, the resulting shear forces will cause superior eccentric loading of the glenoid component. This can result in glenoid loosening due to the **rocking-horse phenomenon**.

Fixed-fulcrum devices were introduced in order to accommodate the muscular deficiency. The initial design of these were reverse ball-and-socket-type devices; however, many designs failed due to glenoid component loosening as a result of excessive torque on the glenoid component. Attempts to overcome this resulted in the design of the **Delta reverse prosthesis** (Depuy International Ltd, Leeds, UK), which includes a large glenoid hemisphere with no neck and a humeral cup oriented in an almost horizontal position, resulting in the medialization of the centre of rotation (Figure 22.3).

This results in a more stable head and reduces the torque on the glenoid component compared with earlier designs. The medialization also results in more of the anterior and posterior fibres of deltoid becoming abductors. The humerus is also lowered, resulting in increased tension in the deltoid. The deltoid muscle is, therefore, optimized to act in the presence of a deficient rotator cuff, although rotation, especially external rotation, is rarely restored.

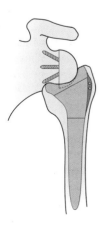

Figure 22.3 *Delta reverse prosthesis.*

Further improvements are needed, as notching of the scapular neck is being reported increasingly. The cause of this is not understood fully, but inferior impingement is the most likely contributing factor, although the degree of bony lysis suggests alternative factors, such as the formation of a polyethylene granuloma.

ELBOW

The main role of the elbow is to provide a functional linkage between the shoulder and the hand, such that the hand can be placed in space. In addition, the elbow must also provide a stable axis for forearm motion and act as a weight-bearing joint. This necessitates complex joint biomechanics in order to maintain stability and function.

ANATOMY

The elbow joint is made up of three separate articulations. The **ulno-humeral articulation**, which acts as a simple hinge, is comprised of the trochlear notch of the ulna and the trochlea of the distal humerus. This is a highly stable and congruent joint, allowing approximately 140 degrees of flexion and extension. In order to maximize the range of movement, the distal humerus is angled anteriorly by 40 degrees and the distal humerus is hollowed out to accommodate the olecranon and coronoid processes.

The trochlear axis, which passes through the trochlea and capitellum, is not perpendicular to the long axis of the humerus but instead forms an angle of approximately six degrees from the perpendicular to the humeral shaft. This results in a valgus angulation of the forearm known as the carrying angle, which varies from 11 degrees in males to 14 degrees in females when measured in extension.

The **radio-humeral joint** is the articulation between the radial head and the capitellum. Unlike the ulno-humeral joint, the radio-humeral joint is much less congruent with the capitellum, having a smaller radius than the radial head. The anatomy of the joint allows for rotational movement at the elbow, regardless of the degree of elbow flexion. The **proximal radio-ulnar joint** is comprised of the articulation of the side of the radial head and the radial notch on the ulna and is stabilized by the annular ligament. The normal range of movement includes 85 degrees of supination and 75 degrees of pronation. The axis of forearm rotation is on an axis through the centre of the radial head and the capitellum.

There are four distinct muscle groups controlling elbow movement. Three muscles control **flexion** – biceps brachii, brachialis and brachioradialis – while triceps and anconeus provide an **antagonistic stabilizing** action. Similarly, pronation and supination each has a group of muscles matched by those acting in the opposite direction. **Pronation** involves pronator teres and pronator quadratus, while **supination** utilizes biceps brachii and supinator.

FREE-BODY DIAGRAM

The forces across the elbow are variable. The forces involved when carrying a mass held in the hand with the elbow flexed to 90 degree can be illustrated in a free-body diagram. Because the forces around the elbow must maintain equilibrium, both the clockwise and anticlockwise moments can be resolved in order to determine the joint reaction force (Figure 22.4).

Clockwise (extension) moment = anticlockwise (flexion) moment

$$(25\,N \times 0.3) + (10\,N \times 0.15) = (B \times 0.05)$$

$$7.5 + 1.5 = 0.05B$$

$$9/0.05 = B$$

$$180\,N = B$$

Joint reaction force + 25 + 10 = 180

Joint reaction force = 180 − 35

Joint reaction force = 145 N

ELBOW INSTABILITY: CLINICAL APPLICATIONS

Like the shoulder, elbow stability is maintained by both static and dynamic structures. **Static**

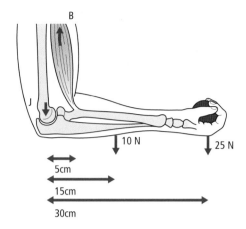

Figure 22.4 *Free-body diagram of the flexed elbow. B, force of biceps; J, resultant force.*

stabilizers include the bony structure of the elbow and soft-tissue stabilizers such as the medial and lateral collateral ligament complexes and the anterior and posterior joint capsule. The **dynamic stabilizers** include the muscles that cross the elbow joint.

Osseous constraints

The olecranon forms the ulno-humeral articulation; however, its role in the stability of the elbow is limited. This is borne out by the fact that in severe injuries to the olecranon, significant bone loss can occur before stability is affected.

The radio-humeral joint is of more importance, particularly as a secondary restraint to valgus stress. If the medial collateral ligament (MCL) is intact, then the radial head has little role in stability. However, the **radial head** is essential for **maintaining stability** if the medial or lateral collateral ligament has been injured or if the distal radio-ulnar joint has been disrupted. If the radial head is excised in the presence of a competent MCL, then care must still be taken, because proximal migration of the radius may cause pain and instability at the distal radio-ulna joint.

The largest joint reaction forces in the elbow are directed in a posterior direction at the distal humerus. This is the result of both the extensor and flexor musculature having a posteriorly directed force. The coronoid is essential to

Table 22.2 Stabilizers of the elbow

Instability	Primary stabilizer	Secondary stabilizer
Valgus stress	Anterior oblique ligament (medial collateral ligament)	Radiocapitellar joint
		Ulno-humeral joint
Varus stress	Ulno-humeral joint	Anterior capsule in extension
		Lateral collateral ligament in flexion
Posterolateral rotatory instability	Lateral ulnar collateral ligament	

resist posterior displacement and provides the major articular contribution to elbow stability. At least 50 per cent of the coronoid process is required in order to maintain ulno-humeral stability, although with this degree of bony deficiency, stability may be lost in full extension. Resistance to posterior displacement with a deficient coronoid is enhanced further by an intact radial head.

Soft-tissue stabilizers

The MCL is made up of three components: the **anterior oblique ligament** (AOL), the **posterior oblique ligament** (POL) and the **transverse ligament** (TL). Although the entire ligament is important in stability, the AOL is the primary restraint and stabilizer of the elbow to valgus strain. It is tight in extension and loose in flexion (Figure 22.5).

In the presence of a radial head fracture, the head can be excised, providing the MCL is intact. However, if the MCL is also attenuated or ruptured, there will be a subsequent valgus

deformity unless a radial head replacement is performed. The POL is tight in flexion and loose in extension. The TL (Cooper's ligament) connects the coronoid to the tip of the olecranon. Its role in the stabilization of the elbow is unclear.

The **lateral collateral ligament** is composed of the **radial collateral ligament** (RCL), **annular ligament** (AL), **lateral ulnar collateral ligament** (LUCL) and **accessory lateral collateral ligament** (ALCL). The LUCL is believed to have a role in posterolateral instability, although other factors, such as increased elbow flexion, also increase the degree of rotatory instability (Table 22.2).

The **anterior capsule** is also likely to play a role in stability on valgus stress as well as during distraction and hyperextension forces. The muscles that cross the elbow joint also play a role in maintaining stability, but their role is dependent on joint position.

PROSTHETIC REPLACEMENT

Total elbow arthroplasty has become increasingly common in the management of elbows affected by rheumatoid arthritis, osteoarthritis and post-traumatic arthritis. There are many different types of elbow replacement, but the majority fall into one of two categories: **linked** and **unlinked**. The choice of implant is dictated by the degree of osseous and ligamentous integrity and the surgeon's personal preference.

The **linked** or **semi-constrained prosthesis** is often referred to as a **sloppy hinge**, as it allows

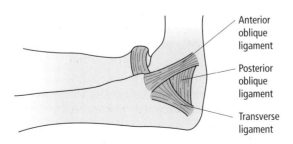

Figure 22.5 Medial collateral ligament.

Anterior oblique ligament

Posterior oblique ligament

Transverse ligament

some varus-valgus laxity, thereby diminishing force transmission at the bone–cement–implant interface. The degree of laxity is variable but ranges from seven to ten degrees, depending on the implant. This may increase further if collateral ligament releases were performed at the time of surgery.

The **unlinked prosthesis** is dependent on the constraint gained from the articulating geometry of the implant and the inherent stability available from surrounding bone, ligaments and muscles. To increase this stability further, some implants include radial head components to act as a further stabilizing factor. The inclusion of this component will reduce varus-valgus laxity, influencing stress distribution at the bone–cement–implant interface. Accurate placement of the implants is, therefore, essential in order to avoid abnormal wear patterns and subsequent implant failure.

Viva questions

1 What anatomical factors are involved in maintaining shoulder stability?

2 How do the muscles of the shoulder girdle control arm elevation and abduction?

3 Discuss the principles in the design of a total shoulder arthroplasty in the cuff-deficient shoulder.

4 Discuss the management of a comminuted fracture of the radial head with respect to maintaining elbow stability.

5 Draw a free-body diagram of an arm held in 90 degrees of elbow flexion and carrying a mass in the hand. Resolve the forces through the elbow and calculate the joint reaction force.

FURTHER READING

Boileau, P, Watkinson, DJ, Hatzidakis, AM, Balg, F. Grammont reverse prosthesis: design, rationale, and biomechanics. *J Shoulder Elbow Surg* 2005;**1S**:147–61S.

Burkart, AC, Debski, RE. Anatomy and function of the glenohumeral ligaments in anterior shoulder stability. *Clin Orthop* 2002;**400**:32–9.

Lippitt, SB, Vanderhooft, JE, Harris, SL, *et al.* Glenohumeral stability from concavity-compression: a quantitative analysis. *J Shoulder Elbow Surg* 1993;**11:2735**.

Morrey, BF, An, KN. Stability of the elbow: osseous constraints. *J Shoulder Elbow Surg* 2005;**1S**:174–8S.

Mura, N, O'Driscoll, SW, Zobitz, ME, *et al.* The effect of infraspinatus disruption on glenohumeral torque and superior migration of the humeral head: a biomechanical study. *J Shoulder Elbow Surg* 2003;**2**:179–84.

23

Biomechanics of the hand and wrist

NICHOLAS SAW AND DAVID EVANS

INTRODUCTION

The biomechanics of the hand and wrist represent a subject of immense complexity, and a thorough understanding is difficult because of:

- the series of joints involved, many of which move together to produce composite movements;
- the muscles that power movement often crossing more than one joint and contracting to produce functional movement in concert;
- the role of ligamentous restraints in the wrist and distal radio-ulnar joint;
- carpal and distal radio-ulnar joint (DRUJ) kinematics not being understood fully.

Nonetheless, some principles can be considered to help us in our appreciation of the hand. This chapter is divided into the hand, the carpus, the DRUJ and the paralysed hand.

THE HAND

JOINTS AND MOVEMENT

For each axis of movement, there should be two motors acting perpendicular to the axis, as seen with flexor digitorum profundus (FDP) and the lateral bands of the extensors at the distal interphalangeal (DIP) joints of the fingers. For three axes of movement – **flexion/extension** (F/E), **abduction/adduction** (A/A) and **rotation**

– six motors are required. This makes for a bulky mass of muscle and increases the complexity of coordination. To simplify matters, no joints rotate in the hand; joints with two axes of movement allow perceived rotation. Rotation is circumduction about joints with non-parallel and offset axes.

PLANES OF MOVEMENT

In the anatomical position, the forearm is supinated, with the palm facing forward. Description of finger and wrist movement is straightforward. The thumb, however, is offset, and so flexion and extension occur parallel to the plane of the palm, abduction and adduction occur perpendicular to the palm, and opposition represents a combined motion to bring the thumb pulp to face the little finger pulp.

INTERPHALANGEAL JOINTS

The interphalangeal (IP) joints are straightforward single-axis hinge joints. They allow **flexion** and **extension** and are powered by two motors. The axis of movement is just anterior to the origin of the collateral ligaments. There is a small trochlea and groove to provide some rotational stability. This is enhanced in most functional positions, as the joint reaction force causes compression of the joint. The **collateral** and **accessory collateral ligaments** and **volar plates** provide further static stability.

METACARPOPHALANGEAL (MCP) JOINTS

These ellipsoid joints have two axes of movement: **F/E** and **A/A**. The F/E axis is transverse about the metacarpal head. The A/A axis, however, is flexed 30 degrees from the metacarpal shaft and is cone-shaped. Therefore, abduction and adduction can occur in the true sense in the anatomical plane relative to the middle finger but can also describe a cone shape with the apex of the cone at the metacarpal head. This is perceived clinically as circumduction.

As an example, try to rotate the extended finger along its own long axis. It is not possible. However, it is possible to describe a circle in the air with the tip of the extended finger with the MCP joint flexed at 30 degrees. The circle is smaller at the DIP joint and smaller still at the proximal interphalangeal (PIP) joint, as in a cone centred at the metacarpal head. As the tip gets closer to this axis, less lateral deviation of the tip is possible. In a precision pinch grip, the pulps of the index and thumb meet along this axis, and no lateral deviation can occur. The remainder of the finger can act as a door on a hinge and pivot about the axis, but the tip does not abduct or adduct.

The compressive joint reaction force and the collaterals and volar plate again provide stability. The ulna collateral ligament of the thumb in particular acts as a passive restrictor of abduction at the MCP joint in pinch.

CARPOMETACARPAL JOINTS

Movement at the carpometacarpal (CMC) joints of the fingers is limited, especially in the index and middle fingers. These two metacarpals are bound rigidly to the distal carpal row and transmit the forces from hand to wrist. The **third metacarpal** acts as a cantilever from which a strong fibrous framework extends, attaching to and holding in place the **flexor sheaths**. This framework, mediated through the collateral ligaments to the deep transverse metacarpal ligament, suspends the flexor mechanisms from the metacarpal heads and transverse arch. In rheumatoid arthritis, the synovitis weakens the radial

collateral ligaments in particular and disrupts the attachments to the arch, with secondary consequences such as extensor tendon subluxation, MCP joint subluxation, ulnar drift and loss of flexion power.

The CMC joint of the thumb is vital to the prehensile hand, and the remainder of this section discusses this joint alone.

The **thumb CMC joint** is a saddle joint and so has two axes of movement: **F/E** and **A/A**. There is no axis of rotation. These two axes are not perpendicular but are skewed relative to each other and to the anatomical plane. The radii of the joint surfaces of the trapezium and metacarpal are also different. The result is an F/E axis across the trapezium that is designed for flexion towards the hypothenar eminence: a functional movement for any grip. The A/A axis is through the metacarpal, but, like the MCP joint described earlier in the shape of a shallow cone, apex volar and ulnar, allows circumduction.

The result is that the thumb metacarpal can **abduct**, **extend** and **pronate** (because of the offset axis and differential radii) to increase the span to grasp an object and oppose the thumb. Flexion and adduction then allow for grip: pulp-to-pulp pinch, key pinch and power grip.

The thumb CMC and MCP joints almost always work in unison, as the motors cross both joints. Therefore, the metacarpal and phalanges usually describe the same movements in different arcs. For example, to flex the metacarpal and extend the phalanges is of little functional use; it is better to extend and then flex both together in order to grasp an object.

Stability of the CMC joint is due to a combination of muscles holding the joint and strong ligaments with thickened capsule. The thumb CMC joint is congruent only at extremes of movement: there is often a degree of translation with focal point loading. In adduction and flexion, the most useful movement for any grip, only the volar surfaces of the CM joint are under load – up to 120 kg in a power grip. The large contact pressures on the volar surface contribute to degenerative change. The **volar oblique** or **beak ligament** between the ulna side of the metacarpal and tubercle of the trapezium is a major restraint to dorsal translation in combination with the **dorso-radial capsule**. The latter should be repaired carefully after trapeziectomy.

MOTORS THAT POWER MOVEMENT

The motors may be divided into **extensors** (supplied by the radial and posterior interosseous nerves), **flexors** (supplied by the median and anterior interosseous nerves) and **intrinsics** (supplied by the median and ulnar nerves). The long flexors and extensors cross many joints and so have the greatest excursions to deal with the range of positions of the hand.

Amplitude of tendon excursion (30–50–70)

Wrist flexors and extensors: 30 mm.

Finger extensors and extensor pollicis longus (EPL)/flexor pollicis longus (FPL): 50 mm.

Finger flexors: 70 mm.

Extensor mechanism

The origins of the extensor muscles are the common extensor origin, radius, ulna and interosseous membrane. **Brachioradialis** (BR) crosses the elbow and acts as an elbow flexor as well as a pronator or supinator, depending on

forearm rotation. **Extensor carpi radialis longus** (ECRL) acts as a wrist extensor and radial deviator as well as a weak elbow flexor. Both BR and ECRL are innervated by the radial nerve and allow the above movements in posterior interosseous nerve (PIN) palsy, whereas **extensor carpi radialis brevis** (ECRB) and the rest of the extensors rely on the PIN for their nerve supply.

The extensor mechanism over the dorsum of the digits represents a complex interplay of extensor and intrinsic function contributing to the accurate positioning of each joint in space (Figure 23.1).

The **long extensors** receive contributions from the **lumbricals** (radial side) and **interossei** to form the **extensor hood** over the **proximal phalanx** with a complex pattern of interweaving fibres that allow for the formation of a differential pulley system. The **intrinsics** and **extrinsics** work in concert to control the tension in the whole system, effecting IP joint extension via the central slip to the middle phalanx and lateral bands to the distal phalanx to allow coordinated positioning. In essence, the long flexors and extensors may be thought to provide the power and the intrinsics the control for hand function.

Flexor mechanism

The **flexor digitorum profundus** (FDP) attaches to the distal phalanx through the chiasma of

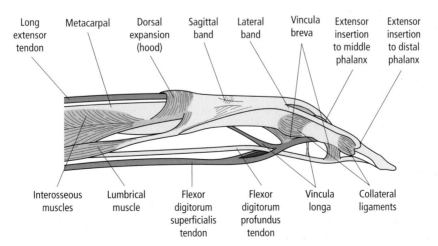

Figure 23.1 *Extensor mechanism of the fingers.*

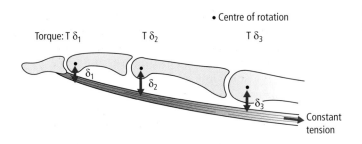

Torque: T δ_1 T δ_2 • Centre of rotation   T δ_3

Constant tension

Figure 23.2 *Increasing torque of the finger flexors proximally.*

the **flexor digitorum superficialis** (FDS) as FDS divides and rotates around FDP to attach to the middle phalanx. FDP is a mass action muscle, although FDP to the index has some independent action. Therefore, if one tendon of FDP is tethered or shortened, the DIP joints of the other fingers will exhibit a degree of flexor lag once the tethered tendon reaches maximum flexion: the **quadriga effect** (analogous to a Roman chariot with four parallel horses controlled by one hand).

The tension generated by the muscle fibres is equal throughout the tendon to its insertion, but the torque generated is dependent on the moment arm. The flexors work with an increasing torque proximally as the moment arm about the axis of rotation increases (Figure 23.2).

When coupled with the addition of successive muscles at each joint, the total torque generated may be large for a relatively small load.

Pulleys

The long flexors tend to bowstring as they contract. This increases their mechanical advantage, but it requires the presence of large webs of skin that make prehension difficult. Moreover, the tendons then effectively take a shortcut and so power is lost, as the muscle cannot then contract fully. Therefore, a system of pulleys is needed to keep the tendons close to the bone.

The pulley system is well known, with thickenings of the flexor sheath creating the annular **A1–A4 pulleys**. The **flexor retinaculum** also functions as a pulley across the wrist. The **cruciate pulleys** (C1–C3) sit between the A pulleys and provide support to the sheath. The **A2** and **A4 pulleys** are most important in that

order and should be preserved or, if damaged, reconstructed.

Intrinsics

Finger intrinsics

The **lumbricals** are unique in their origin from a tendon (FDP) and insertion into the extensor hood (another tendon) on the radial side. They may act as **guy ropes** between the flexors and extensors to allow correct adjustment of tension for finger balance. The **interossei** arise from the metacarpal shafts and are responsible for abduction (mnemonic for dorsal interossei: **DAB**) and adduction (mnemonic for palmar interossei: **PAD**), also contributing to the extensor hood. Both lumbricals and interossei allow for the flexion of the MCP joints and extension of the IP joints on their own (therefore in radial nerve palsy, IP joint extension but not MCP joint extension is possible) and they coordinate the positioning of the fingers for function. The lumbricals are the more effective MCP joint flexors because they have a greater mechanical advantage, being further from the axis of flexion. The contraction of the interossei is also vital to the stability of the MCP joints.

The intrinsics allow finger flexion without curling. The MCP joints flex first, followed by the IP joints. This lets the hand describe a large round shape for grasping. With intrinsic paralysis, attempts to hold an object result in the rolling up of the fingers from distal to proximal (FDP and FDS alone), hyperextension at the MCP joints as a result of unopposed extrinsic extensors, and failure to grasp, i.e. the **intrinsic minus** hand. Intrinsic tightness results in MCP joint flexion and PIP joint extension, i.e. the **intrinsic plus** position (the Bunnell test is used to differentiate intrinsic from extrinsic tightness).

With the lumbricals bridging flexors and extensors, paradoxical extension of the IP joint may occur with attempted flexion. This is seen when the FDP has been divided distal to the lumbricals origin. As the FDP contracts to flex the fingers, the force from the FDP passes through the lumbricals to the extensor mechanism to act as an extensor of the IP joint, i.e. the **lumbrical plus** finger.

The **oblique retinacular ligament** (ORL) **of Landsmeer** is described here. It arises from the proximal phalanx and A2 pulley, passes anterior to the F/E axis of the PIP joint, and attaches on to the lateral slips of the extensor tendon on to the distal phalanx, dorsal to the F/E axis of the DIP joint. As the PIP joint extends, the ORL becomes tighter and tends to passively extend the DIP joint. Therefore, IP joint extension is linked in a controlled way.

Thenar muscles

The **thumb intrinsics** have dual innervation from the ulnar (terminal motor) and median (recurrent motor) nerves. The **adductor pollicis** (AP) is generally under ulnar control, the **abductor pollicis brevis** (APB) median, and the **flexor pollicis brevis** (FPB) and **opponens pollicis** (OP) variable. The latter three arise from the flexor retinaculum and scaphoid or trapezium. OP acts to pronate and flex the metacarpal at the CMC joint. APB and FPB cross both the CMC and MCP joints and therefore act to position the whole thumb in abduction and flexion. APB is unique in being able to abduct the thumb for opposition, and its loss may be cause a significant functional loss (e.g. in severe carpal tunnel syndrome).

The importance of thumb adduction by AP is not so much the action itself but rather the role of resisting abduction, especially working in concert with FPB. In a pinch grip, AP generates the large moment arm required to provide a stable post across the CMC and MCP joints to resist the large forces applied at the tip. It is possible to pinch quite well without a **flexor pollicis longus** (FPL) to flex the IP joint, as the volar plate and collaterals provide a stable extended IP joint to pinch against, at least initially. FPL, however, cannot compensate for the loss of AP. In intrinsic palsy, the AP is denervated. Therefore, in an attempt to hold a sheet of paper between the adducted thumb and index finger, a trick manoeuvre is used. The thumb is pronated sufficiently for FPL to perform a lateral pinch, and there may be some flexion of the index MP joint to facilitate this. This is the basis for **Froment's test**.

As extensor pollicis longus (EPL) crosses the wrist, it acts as a radial deviator. In addition, EPL is also a powerful adductor of the thumb at the CMC and MCP joints and may trick the orthopaedic surgeon in intrinsic palsy. When EPL and FPL contract together, FPL tensions the EPL, which can then provide lateral pinch. The resulting posture of the thumb in this situation is characteristic: there is flexion across the IP and MCP joints (stronger FPL moment arm) and extension at the CMC joint (stronger EPL moment arm). The EPL alone is able to lift the thumb off a flat surface (retropulsion). From its origin, EPL angles around Lister's tubercle in the third dorsal compartment to insert on to the distal phalanx that it extends.

Abductor pollicis longus (APL) and **extensor pollicis** longus and **brevis** (EPB) also aid in positioning the thumb, although supplied by the PIN. APL and EPB are extensors and abductors of the thumb and, acting with AP, stabilize the thumb metacarpal for independent MCP joint flexion. However, they also cross the wrist anterior to the axis of F/E and so abduct and flex the wrist.

Hypothenar muscles

These muscles essentially mirror the thenar muscles, and their significance should not be underestimated. They allow the little finger to oppose the thumb and thereby cup the hand. This allows water to be held, which is a vital act. They also contribute to grip by providing a cushioning mass of muscle and by increasing the breadth of the hand for stability. Try gripping a racket without the little finger to see their contribution.

THE WRIST

The biomechanics of the carpus and DRUJ are horrendously complicated, and their instabilities are beloved of examiners. Fortunately, a complete understanding is unnecessary for examinations and is indeed mostly beyond many surgeons. The instabilities are described here as the section progresses.

Some general observations first:

- The wrist and hand are **suspended off the ulna**, not the other way round.
- The wrist is **inherently unstable**, with the ligaments providing static and the muscles dynamic stability.
- The bones of the proximal carpal row form an **intercalated segment**.

THE CARPUS

The carpus may be divided into the **distal** and **proximal carpal rows. The distal row comprises the trapezium, trapezoid, capitate and hamate. The proximal row comprises the scaphoid, lunate and triquetrum**. The **pisiform** may be considered as the sesamoid of the flexor carpi ulnaris (FCU) tendon and an important stabilizer of the wrist.

The distal row is bound together tightly by interosseous ligaments and functions as a single unit. The proximal row, however, has no tendons attached and functions as an intercalated segment between the radius and ulna and the distal row. Their movement is therefore dependent on the geometry of the bones and the forces applied against the restraining ligaments. These need to be considered.

The radiocarpal joint consists of the articular surface of the radius, with its scaphoid and lunate facets, and the triangular fibrocartilage complex (TFCC). These articulate primarily with the scaphoid and lunate, as the triquetrum is held within the insertions of the TFCC and contact with the ulna disc is limited. The forces generated across the neutral wrist are transmitted primarily through the capitate/scapholunate articulation at the mid-carpal joint, and the radioscaphoid and radiolunate articulations at the radiocarpal joint. The lunate can be considered the key to proximal row movement. It has a wedge shape, being wider volarly and radially, and this shape

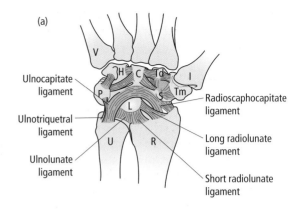

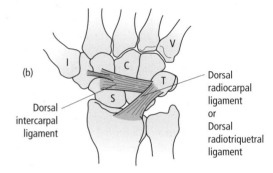

Figure 23.3 *Extrinsic ligaments of the wrist: (a) volar and (b) dorsal. C, capitate; H, hamate; I, first metacarpal; L, lunate; LT, Lister's tubercle; P, pisiform; R, radius; S, scaphoid; Td, trapezioid; Tm, trapezium; U, ulna; V, fifth metacarpal.*

tends to tilt the lunate dorsally when it is under load from the capitate.

The ligaments of the wrist may be classified as extrinsic and intrinsic. The **extrinsic ligaments** are arranged in two V-shapes. The **volar** ligaments arise from the radius and ulna and have the apices on the lunate and capitate, and are the stronger. The **dorsal** ligaments run in a distal/ulnar direction and resist the slide of the carpus down the sloping radius in a volar and ulnar direction (Figure 23.3).

Their names describe the bones to which they attach, such as the radioscaphocapitate (volar) and radiotriquetral (dorsal), these two being the most important. The **intrinsic ligaments** run between the carpal bones, binding tightly to fix the bones (distal row) or somewhat more loosely to allow some intercarpal movement (proximal row). The scapholunate and lunotriquetral ligaments are two such intrinsic interosseous ligaments that allow limited motion.

CARPAL KINETICS

Conceptually, one of the easiest ways to consider carpal kinetics is to remember two points. First, the **scaphoid flexes** in **radial deviation** to get out of the way so the trapezium can approach the radial styloid and **extends** in **ulna deviation** to fill the space vacated by the trapezium. Second, the **lunate** can be thought of as a torque lever suspended between the opposing moments of the **scaphoid (flexion)** and **triquetrum (extension)**. The whole system is under constant and changing tension; therefore, if any part is disrupted, then abnormal and unlinked rotation will occur. The lunate will then tilt with the intact part of the chain. It is the direction of tilt of the lunate that is described in instability.

The F/E axis of the wrist is just distal to the radial and ulnar styloids, and the radio-ulnar axis passes through the capitate. The axis of pronation/supination passes from the radial head to the tip of the ulna styloid and occurs through the radio-ulnar articulation.

A combination of mid-carpal and radiocarpal movement is responsible for flexion (45 degrees mid-carpal, 40 degrees radiocarpal) and extension (25 degrees mid-carpal, 35 degrees radiocarpal). Abduction of 60 degrees and adduction of 20 degrees occurs around the axis of the capitate.

NORMAL WRIST MOVEMENT

In radial deviation, the scaphoid flexes to allow the trapezium to approach the radius. The flexion torque is transmitted to the lunate by the scapholunate ligament (SLL), augmented by the capitate pressing on the volar lip of the lunate. The triquetrum is pulled along with the hamate to a non-articulating position relative to the ulna.

On ulnar deviation, the scaphoid extends to fill the space vacated by the trapezium, passing an extension moment to the lunate via the SLL. The capitate presses on the dorsal lip of

the lunate to tilt it dorsally. The hamate now engages the triquetrum, and the helical shape of the triquetrohamate joint causes triquetral extension, in addition to the torque from the lunotriquetral ligament (LTL).

With axial loading, the greatest force is transmitted across the mid-carpal joint at the capitoscapholunate articulation. The proximal row then changes shape to adapt to the forces. The extensors tend to exert a dorsal force on the capitate, which then tends to tilt the lunate and triquetrum dorsally. The volar facing radial articulation accentuates this. The scaphoid, however, tends to flex with axial loading due to the tension in the volar extrinsic ligaments, so the lunate is under two opposing moments. The stability of the whole construct is dependent on the integrity of the scapholunate and lunotriquetral interosseous ligaments. Disruption allows for independent movement, leading to carpal instability.

The powerful action of radial deviation and extension followed by ulnar deviation and flexion, as in using a mallet, are functionally important and so the muscles that produce these movements are among the most powerful. In this movement, the scaphoid is effectively locked in flexion with the proximal row; thus, this is essentially a mid-carpal movement. In the less common action of moving from ulnar extension to radial flexion, the scaphoid is free to move, and so this is a radiocarpal movement.

ABNORMAL CARPAL MOVEMENT

As described earlier, the carpal bones are held together with ligamentous restraints under constant tension. Disruption may occur by failure of ligamentous restraints or by fractures uncoupling the bony architecture. This may lead to carpal instability. Carpal instability is difficult to describe and understand, but bearing in mind the normal carpal interaction its classification can be explained.

There are many classifications described, including the **Mayo** and that used by the **International Wrist Investigators Workshop**. The mechanics behind the Mayo classification are described, its two main subtypes being **carpal instability dissociative (CID)** and **carpal**

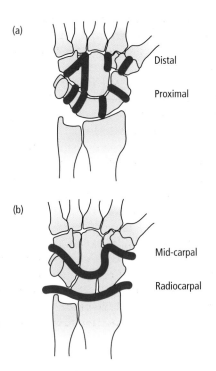

Figure 23.4 *(a) Carpal instability dissociative (CID) and (b) carpal instability non-dissociative (CIND) classifications of abnormal carpal movement.*

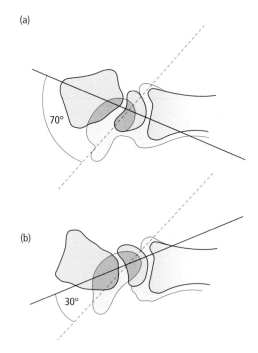

Figure 23.5 *Patterns of instability: (a) dorsal intercalated segmental instability (DISI); (b) volar intercalated segmental instability (VISI).*

instability non-dissociative (CIND) (Figure 23.4).

Carpal instability dissociative

This is instability, **ligamentous** or **osseous**, **within a carpal row**. It may be visible without loading (**static**) or only under load or movement (**dynamic**). CID includes disruptions of the SLL or LTL so the proximal carpal dynamics are affected. Initially, the injury may not be seen on plain radiographs but may be seen only under stress views or under screening (dynamic instability). If untreated, the disruption may become more permanent and visible on plain radiographs (static). The scapholunate gap can be variable, especially in children, so never forget to compare with the contralateral wrist.

Note that the scaphoid tends to flex and the lunate and triquetrum extend. The SLL and LTL hold this proximal row under balanced tension. If the SLL is disrupted, the scaphoid flexes, the lunate extends with the triquetrum via the intact LTL, and a **dorsal intercalated segmental instability** (DISI) pattern occurs.

If the LTL fails, then the triquetrum extends and the lunate tilts volarly, as the flexed scaphoid transmits its torque via the intact SLL to the lunate. This results in a **volar intercalated segmental instability** (VISI) pattern. The pattern of instability is named after the direction in which the lunate tends to abnormally tilt (Figure 23.5).

There may be nothing to see on plain radiographs, or there may be a visible gap between the bones, flexion of the scaphoid (ring sign of seeing the flexed scaphoid end on) and reduction of the carpal index as the capitate slides dorsally or volarly shortening the carpus (Figure 23.6). Abnormal measurements on radiographs indicative of carpal instability are shown in Table 23.1.

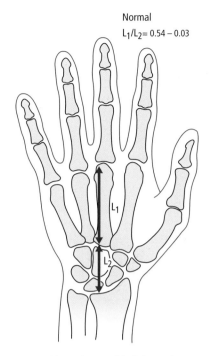

Normal
$L_1/L_2 = 0.54 - 0.03$

Figure 23.6 *Normal carpal height ratio.*

Carpal instability non-dissociative

This describes carpal instability **between** the **distal** and **proximal rows** (mid-carpal instability, MCI), at the radiocarpal joint, or both. The rows themselves are intact. This pattern is less common than CID and results from significant **disruption** of the **extrinsic ligaments** that uncouple the dynamics of the carpus. The patient often describes a 'clunk', as occurs in MCI when the distal row suddenly reduces on

to the proximal row in ulnar deviation. In individuals with ligamentous laxity, such as gymnasts, there may be MCI without significant trauma.

If the very strong radiocarpal ligaments are disrupted, then the carpus may slide down the ulna inclination of the radius, uncoupling the radiocarpal articulation. Ulnar translation is seen on radiographs when more than 50 per cent of the lunate projects beyond the ulnar edge of the radius. The whole carpus may slide (**type 1 ulnar translation**) towards the ulna, increasing the gap between the radial styloid and the scaphoid.

Depending on the direction in which the lunate is tilted, a DISI or VISI deformity may be seen. However, as the proximal row is intact, the scapholunate angle is normal. As the lunate is tilted, the capitolunate angle is abnormal and the carpal height ratio may be reduced.

Carpal instability complex

Carpal instability complex (CIC) results when **instability within** and **between rows** is combined. CIC results from significant disruption of intrinsic and extrinsic soft tissues, or fractures, and the movement of the carpal bones reflects the disruptions.

It is simplest to describe the CIC by the individual components. For example, if the SLL is disrupted, then the end result may be a CID with a DISI deformity. If the radiocarpal ligaments are disrupted, then the result may be a CIND in isolation with translation of the

Table 23.1 Abnormal measurements on radiographs in dorsal intercalated segmental instability (DISI) and volar intercalated segmental instability (VISI)

	DISI	VISI	Normal
Scapholunate angle	<70°	<30°	30–60°
Capitolunate angle	<–30°	<30°	–20° to +10°
Radiolunate angle	<–15°	<20°	–20° to +10°
Carpal height ratio	<0.54	<0.54	0.54 ± 0.03
Scapholunate distance (compare with other wrist)	≥3 mm	<2 mm	<2 mm

whole carpus. However, if both the SLL and the extrinsic ligaments are disrupted, except for the radioscaphoid ligament, then the scaphoid would remain in position while the lunate slides ulnar-wards, and a **type 2 ulnar translation** is seen. The combination of the SLL and extrinsic ligamentous injury creates a CIC.

Combined LTL and SLL injuries may result in CIC. This is seen most commonly in perilunate injuries. As described by **Mayfield**, the stages of perilunar injury progress in a clockwise manner from SLL to capitolunate to LTL to radiolunate disruption. This is as seen from the dorsal aspect of the right wrist. The reverse Mayfield pattern may also be seen, usually in association with TFCC or DRUJ injuries, starting with the LTL. These injuries probably do not happen in a precise sequence, but they show how a CIC can develop with combinations of ligamentous injuries.

Time plays a factor in the evolution of the CIC patterns, as untreated CID increases the strain on the extrinsic ligaments that may have been damaged in the initial injury anyway. These extrinsic ligaments may then become gradually attenuated and dysfunctional, resulting in a CIC.

Adaptive carpus and scaphoid fractures

The alignment of the carpus is dependent on the geometry of the bones and the soft tissues. It follows that if these are altered, then the carpus will adapt in order to compensate for these changes. In situations where there is a malunion of the distal radius, especially following Colles' type fractures, the radial articulation may lose its normal volar tilt. The carpus will adapt to this new alignment, usually with the proximal row translating and tilting dorsally. The distal row exhibits a compensatory flexion, and an adaptive DISI deformity may be seen (**carpal instability adaptive, CIA**).

The scaphoid itself is under two opposite moments. There is a flexion moment exerted on the distal pole (as described earlier) and an extension moment exerted proximally by the triquetrum and lunate via the LTL and SLL. The radioscaphocapitate ligament acts as the fulcrum for scaphoid movement. If the

scaphoid fractures across the waist, these moments are uncoupled and the classic humpback deformity of the flexed distal pole is seen. There may also be a DISI deformity as the lunate and the proximal scaphoid tilt dorsally. The situation is the same in perilunate transcaphoid injury, with the additional ligamentous disruption causing a combined instability, i.e. CIC.

Axial instability

This pattern of instability results from longitudinal or crushing forces disrupting the carpus and the CMC joints. The line of the force disrupts the wrist axially and may affect the radial or ulnar side, or both.

IMPLICATIONS OF CARPAL INSTABILITY

The carpus is designed to function as a whole. Uncoupling of the normal intercarpal and radiocarpal movement affects the axis of movement, causing restriction, and affects joint loading, leading to degenerative change. Both cause pain. The most commonly examined patterns of degenerative change are the **scapholunate advanced collapse** (SLAC) and **scaphoid non-union advanced collapse** (SNAC). Although the pathogenesis is complex, the progression of degenerative change can be simplified and understood from the biomechanics, most of which have already been covered in this chapter.

SLL disruption uncouples the flexing scaphoid from the extending lunate, initially causing a dynamic instability. The capitate is still under the axial loading forces pulling it proximally and may widen the gap on stress radiographs. The carpal height may therefore be shortened. Left untreated, a static DISI deformity may develop. The scaphoid tends to stay flexed and impacts on the rim of the radius, causing abnormal loading of the radiocarpal joint in addition to any chondral damage from the initial injury. Degenerate change occurs between the radial styloid and scaphoid (**SLAC stage 1**). This progresses on to a degenerate scaphoid facet (**SLAC stage 2**). The capitate continues to push down on the widened scapholunate joint, and degenerate change occurs at the lunocapitate articulation (**SLAC stage 3**).

The SNAC wrist is similar, except that the uncoupling of the forces occurs across the fractured scaphoid rather than through the scapholunate joint. The pattern of forces across the wrist is similar, with scaphostyloid arthrosis occurring initially (**SNAC stage 1**). The proximal pole of the scaphoid extends with the lunate, so the capitate impinges on the proximal scaphoid, leading to scaphocapitate arthrosis (**SNAC stage 2**). Unchecked, the lunocapitate articulation becomes affected (**SNAC stage 3**). Ultimately, the carpus is shortened and collapses, and degenerative change progresses to affect the radiocarpal articulation.

THE DISTAL RADIO–ULNAR JOINT COMPLEX

Pronation and **supination** of the wrist involve the proximal and distal radio-ulnar joints and the interosseous membrane. Whilst bearing in mind that proximal disruption will affect wrist movement, only the DRUJ will be considered here.

The **ulna** is the fixed structure around which the radius rotates. The axis of rotation has been described. The extent of the ulnar articular surface (130 degrees) is greater and the radius of the curvature smaller than the shallow sigmoid notch of the radius, so the contact areas vary in rotation. There is about 60 per cent joint contact with the wrist in the neutral position, and this decreases to 10 per cent in full pronation or supination. Relative to the ulna, there are also volar translation and proximal migration of the radius in pronation and dorsal translation and distal migration in supination (the radius slides forwards or back on the ulna). There is also a normal proximal migration of the radius – up to 7 mm – with axial loading resisted by the interosseous membrane and proximal radiocapitellar joint. Like all joints, the stability of the DRUJ is dependent on ligaments and muscles. The TFCC is also discussed here.

The **TFCC** describes a complex structure linking the DRUJ to the ulnar carpus and consists of the articular disc and meniscal homologue, the volar and dorsal radio-ulnar ligaments, the ulnocarpal ligaments and the extensor carpi ulnaris sheath. The TFCC binds the radius, ulna and carpus to form a stable platform for movement. In addition, the extensor carpi ulnaris (ECU) and pronator quadratus (PQ) contribute to dynamic stability.

The volar and dorsal radio-ulnar ligaments arise from the edges of the radial notch and attach to the fovea and base of the ulna styloid. There is debate as to the specific contribution of each ligament to the stability of the DRUJ (which is tight/loose in pronation/supination?), but in essence they bind the radius to the ulna through the whole arc of movement, becoming tight at full pronation and supination. The ulnocarpal ligaments comprise the ulnolunate, ulnocapitate and ulnotriquetral. These ligaments link the carpus to the ulna and so help to stabilize the DRUJ. The axis of pronation and supination can be thought to pass along the ulnotriquetral ligament.

The ECU is bound to the distal ulna by its own sheath, and so its relationship to the ulna is fixed. The sheath itself provides stability, but the ECU also has a major dynamic role dependent on its position relative to the radius. When the wrist is loaded in pronation, e.g. when holding a pen, the ECU acts to compress the DRUJ by squeezing it together. In supination, the carpus tends to sublux dorsally, and the contraction of the ECU exerts a counterforce to prevent this. If the ECU is displaced from its normal position, as in rheumatoid arthritis, then subluxation of the ulna head becomes more pronounced. The contraction of PQ compresses the DRUJ, particularly in supination, to prevent subluxation.

It is worth pointing out that although by convention we normally describe dorsal or volar subluxation of the ulna head, what in fact occurs is subluxation of the radius and carpus relative to the ulna, with supination of the carpus.

WRIST MOTORS

These are all the muscles that cross the wrist, including long flexors and extensors. The dedicated wrist motors, ECU and FCU, and flexor carpi radialis (FCR) and extensor carpi radialis longus/brevis (ECRL/B), often work in controlled antagonism to provide a stable platform for hand movement. For power grip, wrist extension is necessary, and this synergism of movement is of use in transfers.

THE PARALYSED HAND

This section describes the tendon transfers that may be used to restore function following nerve injury or tendon rupture. Before contemplating a transfer, several principles need to be considered:

- The joint must be **passively mobile**.
- The **gain in function** must be greater than the potential loss.
- The **motor** must be of sufficient power (generally 1 grade will be lost) and excursion.
- Ideally there should also be:
  - **one motor per joint** to be moved;
  - a **straight line** of **pull**;
  - **synergistic** transfers;
  - **sensibility**.

The number of motors available also affects what can be achieved. In severe neurological loss, as in brachial plexus injuries, the role of tenodesis and fusion (simplify the machine) cannot be forgotten. Below is a list, though by no means exhaustive, of transfers. When there is a selection, those in italics are suggested.

Radial nerve

Loss: wrist and MCP joint extension.
Transfer:
- pronator teres (PT) to ECRB (less radial deviation than ECRL);
- *palmaris longus to EPL*; or
- FDS IV to EPL;
- FCR (better) or FCU to EDC.

Low ulnar nerve

Loss: intrinsics.
Transfer:
- To prevent clawing:
  - FDS tenodesis;
  - MCP joint capsulodesis;
  - *FDS to lateral band*;
  - ECRL plus graft to lateral band.
- Thumb adduction:
  - ECRB plus graft;
  - *EIP through second metacarpal space*;
  - FDS IV rerouted through fascial pulley.
- First dorsal interosseous (DIO):
  - *often not needed: flex all fingers to form post for pinch*;
  - ECRL or APL to first DIO.

High ulnar nerve

Loss: the above plus FCU and FDP.
Transfer:
- suture FDPs together;
- ?FCR to FCU (remaining radial flexors: PL and APL).

Low median nerve

Loss: thumb opposition.
Transfer:
- PL to APB;
- *EIP to APB*;
- *FDS IV to APB*;
- abductor digiti minimi (AbDM) to APB.

High median nerve

Loss: the above plus PT, finger and thumb flexors (except ulnar FDP).
Transfer:
- AbDM or EIP to APB;
- suture FDPs together;
- re-route biceps or ECU to radius for pronation;
- *ECRL to FPL*;
- BR plus graft to FPL.

Viva questions

1 What is an intrinsic plus/intrinsic minus/lumbrical plus hand?

2 What is Froment's test? What is its anatomical basis?

3 What is carpal instability? What are the common types seen clinically?

4 What are the principles of tendon transfer?

5 What tendon transfers are suitable for a median/ulnar/radial nerve palsy?

FURTHER READING

Brand, PW, Hollister, AM. *Clinical Mechanics of the Hand*. London: Mosby, 1999.

Buchler, U (ed.). *Wrist Instability*. London: Taylor and Francis, 1996.

Cassidy, C, Ruby, LK. Carpal instability. *Instr Course Lect* 2003;**52**:209–20.

Gilula, LA, Mann, F, Dobyns, JH, Yin, Y. Wrist terminology as defined by the International Wrist Investigators' Workshop (IWIW). *J Bone Joint Surg Am* 2002;**84**:1–66.

Goodman, HJ, Choueka, J. Biomechanics of the flexor tendons. *Hand Clin* 2005;**21**:129–49.

24

Biomechanics and joint replacement of the foot and ankle

ROHIT MADHAV, DEBORAH EASTWOOD AND DISHAN SINGH

INTRODUCTION

The foot and ankle have three main functions: to **support** the body during stance, to act as a **lever arm** for propulsion during gait, and for **shock absorption** controlling the acceleration and deceleration forces associated with walking and running. The foot projects forwards from the ankle, providing a lever to control anterior and posterior sway of the human body when the feet are together, i.e. it helps in body balance. The joints transmit half the body weight at rest, up to three times the body weight in walking, and up to 13 times the body weight in sprinting.

In biomechanical terms, this area is immensely complex. The foot structure must be flexible to accommodate uneven ground and allow stability in the stance phase of gait. This flexible structure must, however, convert to a rigid lever arm for heel strike and push-off. In walking and running, the muscles and tendons controlling the position of the foot successively absorb and release energy in a way that assists the body to move in its path so that the centre of gravity is not subjected to rapid acceleration and deceleration forces and the eye level undergoes minimal movement.

NOMENCLATURE

Embryologically, the foot is initially aligned with the leg but then rotates through 90 degrees during development. Therefore, hindfoot movements are described in the axis of the leg, while forefoot movements are described at 90 degrees to this.

There is no general agreement regarding the terms used to describe foot movements, and there is particular disagreement between the definitions used by paediatric orthopaedic surgeons and those preferred by foot and ankle surgeons. The terms described here are based on those of the American Orthopaedic Foot and Ankle Society (AOFAS).

AOFAS definitions of foot and ankle movements

Dorsiflexion/plantarflexion: sagittal plane movements up and down (e.g. ankle).

Varus/valgus: coronal (frontal) plane angulation towards or away from midline (e.g. hindfoot).

Adduction/abduction: transverse plane movements towards and away from midline (e.g. midfoot).

Pronation/supination: describes movement in three planes and three joints, i.e. supination is ankle plantarflexion, hindfoot varus and midfoot adduction.

Inversion/eversion: specific to the subtalar joint, as one axis of rotation produces movement in two planes (hindfoot varus, forefoot supination/hindfoot valgus, forefoot pronation).

Concentric contraction: musculotendinous unit shortening while muscle contracting.

Eccentric contraction: musculotendinous unit lengthening while muscle contracting.

BODY MOTION DURING GAIT

The centre of gravity displaces in vertical, horizontal and lateral directions during the gait cycle. The coordinated actions of the hip, knee, foot and ankle convert individual series of motion arcs into a smooth sinusoidal curve in each of the planes. Vertical and lateral displacements average 4–5 cm and require controlled acceleration and deceleration.

Horizontal movement (propulsion) occurs with each rotatory movement of the pelvis, resulting in torques of approximately 7–8 Nm in the tibia with an average rotation of 19 degrees. During the first third of the stance phase of gait, the lower leg undergoes internal rotation. External rotation occurs during the subsequent two-thirds of stance (Figure 24.1).

BIOMECHANICS OF THE ANKLE

ANATOMY AND KINEMATICS

The **talar dome** is wider anteriorly (mean difference 2.4 ± 1.3 mm) than posteriorly. Its medial side has a narrower radius of curvature and a smaller articular facet compared with its lateral side. Anatomically, the shapes and articular surfaces of the talus and mortise represent a section of a frustum of a cone (Figure 24.2), with its apex medial (mean conical angle 24 ± 6 degrees). The axis of rotation of this diverging cone is the same as that of the ankle joint.

The ankle joint is basically a **uniplanar hinge joint** with motion occurring about a transverse

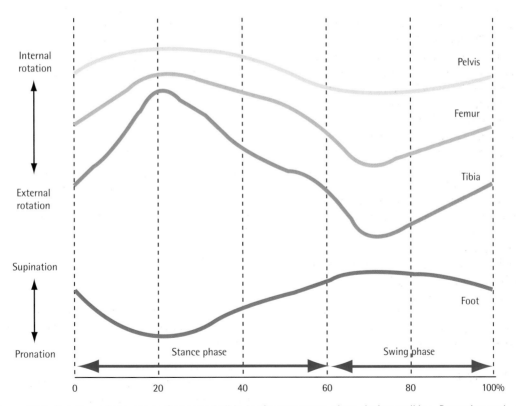

Figure 24.1 *Rotation of the pelvis, femur and tibia in the transverse plane during walking. Pronation and supination of the foot are also shown.*

(a)

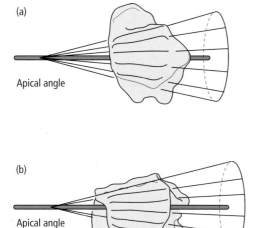

Apical angle

(b)

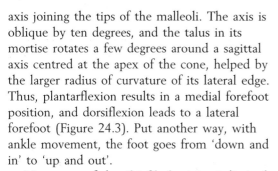

Apical angle

Figure 24.2 *(a) Talus and (b) ankle mortise fit geometrically as a section of a frustum of a cone.*

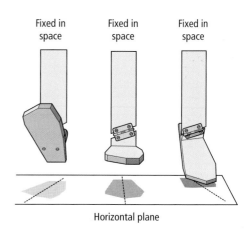

Fixed in space   Fixed in space   Fixed in space

Horizontal plane

Figure 24.3 *Effect of the oblique orientation of the ankle joint on forefoot position with dorsiflexion and plantarflexion.*

axis joining the tips of the malleoli. The axis is oblique by ten degrees, and the talus in its mortise rotates a few degrees around a sagittal axis centred at the apex of the cone, helped by the larger radius of curvature of its lateral edge. Thus, plantarflexion results in a medial forefoot position, and dorsiflexion leads to a lateral forefoot (Figure 24.3). Put another way, with ankle movement, the foot goes from 'down and in' to 'up and out'.

Movement of the **tibiofibular joint** is limited to 2 mm due to the tight syndesmotic ligaments and the interosseous membrane. The contact area of the articular surface is large in all positions of the ankle, resulting in lower contact stresses, which may explain the lower incidence of osteoarthritis in this joint compared with other large joints. Minor deviations of the inclination of the axes of the ankle due to epiphyseal injury, ligamentous injury or malunion of a fracture can result in severe pathological alterations in the joint, although symptomatic degenerative change remains relatively uncommon. The total range of motion of the ankle joint in the sagittal plane is approximately 10–20 degrees of dorsiflexion to 25–30 degrees of plantarflexion. Even with the most oblique axis, a normal ankle provides only 11 degrees of tibial rotation. An average of 19 degrees is required for propulsion, and thus the

subtalar joint needs to be a significant contributor to rotational movement.

The normal pattern of ankle joint motion during gait has been studied extensively. At **initial contact** (heel strike in normal gait), the ankle is in **neutral** to **slight plantarflexion**. The ground reaction causes immediate **plantar flexion** (at 7 per cent of the gait cycle), but the motion rapidly reverses to **dorsiflexion** during mid-stance as the body passes over the supporting foot (at 35 per cent of the cycle). The motion then returns to **plantarflexion** with heel-rise during the late stance phase (from 40 to 62 per cent of the cycle). At **lift-off** at the beginning of the swing phase, the ankle is in **plantarflexion**. The motion reverses towards **dorsiflexion** in the middle of the swing phase (foot clearance) and changes again to slight **plantarflexion** and **pre-positioning** for initial contact (Figure 24.4).

At normal walking speed (about 6 km/h), an individual averages 60 cycles per minute and spends 60 per cent of each cycle in stance phase on each leg. The first 10 per cent of the gait cycle after heel-strike is a period of double stance, i.e. both feet are in contact with the ground. As the individual walks faster, the period of double stance becomes reduced, until eventually, as the individual begins to jog or run, double stance disappears altogether and is

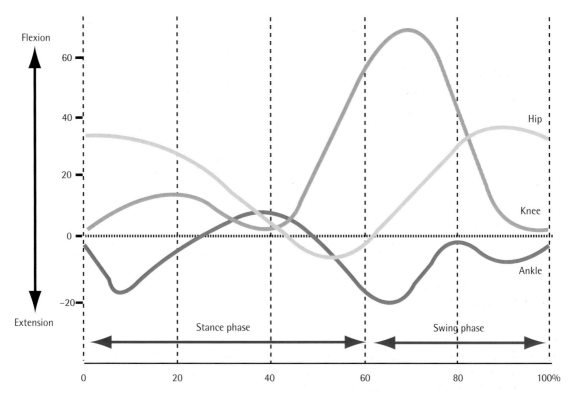

Figure 24.4 *Ankle plantarflexion and dorsiflexion in comparison with hip and knee sagittal plane motion during gait cycle.*

replaced by periods when neither foot is on the ground. In sprinting, heel-strike is replaced by forefoot strike.

KINETICS OF THE ANKLE

Owing to the large load-bearing surface of the ankle (11–13 cm^2), lower stresses are generated across this joint compared with the knee and hip. Changes in the tibiotalar contact area are produced by lateral talar shift, a frequent sequelae of major sprains and fractures of the ankle. If talar shift is not corrected, it can lead to significant biomechanical alterations in the joint. A 1-mm talar shift reduces the ankle joint surface contact area by 42 per cent, leading to a significant rise in joint contact stress and, hence, early degenerative changes.

When an individual stands on both feet, each ankle supports approximately one-half of the body weight. The line of gravity of the body passes a few centimetres anterior to the transverse axis of the ankle joint, and hence the body weight produces a dorsiflexing torque on the joint that varies between 3 Nm and 24 Nm as a result of body oscillations. Therefore, standing with the body weight distributed evenly on both feet requires some activity in the plantar flexor muscles. The main **compressive force** in the ankle during gait is produced by contraction of the **gastrocnemius** and **soleus muscles** and is transmitted through the **Achilles tendon**. When these and other muscles in the lower leg are involved in balancing the body, the joint reaction force at the ankle increases in proportion to the amount of muscle force used for these balancing activities. For an individual standing on tiptoe, the joint reaction force is about 2.1 times the body weight and the Achilles tendon force reaches about 1.0 times the body weight (a total of three times the body weight). This explains why a patient with degenerative arthritis has pain when rising up on tiptoes.

ANATOMY OF THE ACHILLES TENDON

The tendo Achilles has a **spiral arrangement**, with its medial fibres inserting posteriorly and the lateral fibres inserting anteriorly on to the **calcaneal tuberosity**. Thus, when performing a percutaneous lengthening via two incisions, the cuts must be made perpendicular to the fibres, i.e. distal-anterior and medial proximal (**DAMP technique**) in order to cut the correct bundles and achieve a slide. In paediatric practice, a three-cut technique is commonly used, with incisions approximately 3 cm apart in one plane (medial, lateral, medial technique), dividing 50 per cent of the tendon each time.

BIOMECHANICS OF THE SUBTALAR JOINT AND THE FOOT

As discussed earlier, the unique qualities of the foot allow it to be flexible when necessary, as in when walking barefoot, and yet suitably rigid, converting the 26 bones (28 with the sesamoids) and 57 joints into a solid unit, as required for ballet dancing *en pointe*.

ANATOMY AND KINEMATICS OF THE SUBTALAR JOINT

Sometimes the foot functions as a single unit, and at other times it functions as a subtle grasping appendage. The potential of the normal foot to be a prehensile limb has been well demonstrated by patients with complete amelia of the upper extremities and who dress themselves, feed themselves and even write with their feet and toes.

The **talus** is a bone with **no muscle attachments**. It sits atop the calcaneum stabilized only by the ligaments and cradled by all the tendons passing from the leg to the foot. The subtalar joint is commonly referred to as a **torque converter**, and it has been modelled as a **mitred hinge**, transforming tibial rotation into forefoot pronation and supination via inversion and eversion (Figure 24.5).

On average, the subtalar joint can be inverted 20 degrees and everted about 5 degrees. Throughout the stance phase of gait,

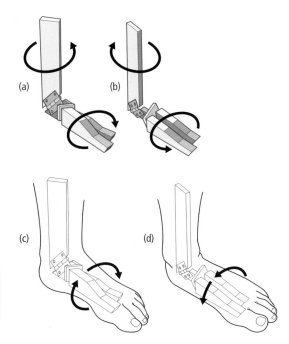

Figure 24.5 *In the mitred hinge model of the subtalar joint, tibial rotation causes subtalar joint inversion (a) and eversion (b) and forefoot supination (c) and pronation (d).*

the average range of motion of the subtalar joint is only 6 degrees in normal feet and 12 degrees in flat feet, a so-called **functional range of motion**. The foot rests in slight supination during the swing phase; at heel-strike, it rotates into slight pronation as the lower limb is internally rotated in the first 15 per cent of the stance phase and the heel strikes the ground slightly lateral to the longitudinal axis of the leg (Figure 24.6).

One degree of tibial rotation would yield 1 degree of foot motion if the axis was at 45 degrees. The flatfooted individual has a more horizontal subtalar axis, and thus the same tibial torsion has greater rotatory effect on the foot; the opposite occurs for the cavus foot. If movements at the subtalar joint are congenitally blocked, as in tarsal coalition, then the ankle joint remodels into a ball-and-socket joint to allow inversion and eversion.

The subtalar joint also demonstrates **linear motion**, i.e. anteroposterior movement. This is likened to the **Archimedes spiral screw** (mean helix angle 12 degrees), where rotational

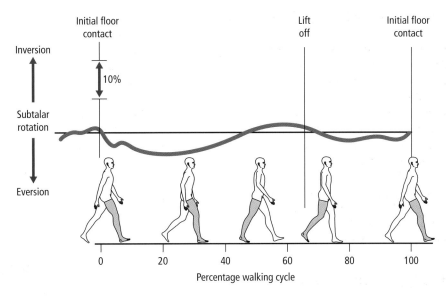

Figure 24.6 *Subtalar inversion and eversion during the gait cycle.*

movements are converted to linear motion. The calcaneum moves forwards in inversion and backwards in eversion.

For practical purposes, foot motion can be considered to be of two distinct types – non-weight-bearing and weight-bearing. Active weight-bearing motion of the foot differs from passive motion because of forces produced by the body weight and by muscle contractions that act to stabilize the joints. When an individual stands on the ball of the foot, the hindfoot inverts slightly and the midfoot is in plantarflexion and the forefoot exhibits some pronation, creating an arch. Standing flatfooted on an externally rotating leg also raises the arch by moving the heel into slight inversion and causing the forefoot to twist into pronation. Rotating the leg internally has the opposite effect: it lowers the arch.

MID-TARSAL/TRANSVERSE TARSAL JOINT MOTION

The transverse tarsal joints (**Chopart's joints**) lie just anterior to the talus and calcaneum and are associated closely with the subtalar joint. They represent motion between the **talus** and **navicular** and between the **calcaneum** and **cuboid**. The **talonavicular joint** is a ball-and-socket type, whereas the **calcaneocuboid joint** is saddle-shaped. The axes of these two joints are positioned in a frontal plane; the superior axis passes through the talar neck and the inferior axis passes through the calcaneal body. When the foot is in **eversion** (i.e. with the arch flat or foot pronated), these two axes fall into parallel alignment in the same plane and the midfoot is able to flex and extend with ease in relation to the hindfoot. However, when the heel is **inverted** (i.e. with the arch elevated or foot supinated), the axes diverge, and flexion and extension movements of the midfoot, with respect to the hindfoot, are significantly restricted. During the mid-stance phase, the pronated 'flat' foot is mobile and can adapt to the uneven ground. In the late stance phase, with heel inversion and forefoot supination, the locked Chopart's joints turn the foot into a stiff lever arm to push off with. This mechanism may be why patients are able to tolerate a pronated foot or flat foot more easily than they tolerate a varus or supinated foot as in club foot.

INTERTARSAL AND TARSOMETATARSAL JOINT MOTION

Motion of the surfaces of the intertarsal and tarsometatarsal joints is restricted by the shapes of the bones, the many restrictive ligaments, and surrounding muscles. **Gliding motion** occurs between the **cuneiform** and **cuboid** and also within the tarsometatarsal joints during gait. Since the total extension of any two bones of the intertarsal joints is small, for practical purposes motion may be considered as translation of power into motion (gliding) of one surface across another. Total midfoot motion ranges from just a few degrees of dorsiflexion to about 15 degrees of plantarflexion and is distributed through all the tarsal bones.

The bony arch is supported by tendons, ligaments and plantar fascia, and its shape is affected by the tarsometatarsal joints (known together as **Lisfranc's joint**). In essence, the **dorsum** of the arch is subjected to **compressive stresses** across the articular surfaces, while the **plantar muscles**, **ligaments** and in particular the **plantar fascia** are under **tensile stress** (like a bow and a bow string). The arch may be raised by passive means through external rotation of the tibia during standing and also through extension of the toes and tightening of the plantar fascia.

METATARSAL BREAK

In the latter part of stance phase, as the weight is transferred to the forefoot, there is an axis through which all the toes extend at the **metatarsophalangeal joints**. This **oblique** axis, which overlies the metatarsophalangeal joints, is called the **metatarsal break**. It varies considerably among individuals in its orientation to the long axis of the foot, from 50 to 70 degrees. It is a generalization of the instant centres of rotation of all five metatarsophalangeal joints. The obliquity of this break conforms to the transverse crease formed in shoes.

FUNCTION OF THE PLANTAR FASCIA

The function of the plantar fascia is complex. From its attachment to the calcaneum, the plantar fascia extends forwards to span all the tarsal and metatarsophalangeal joints and to attach to the plantar aspect of the proximal phalanges. The result is a truss-like structure whose links are the tarsal bones and ligaments of the foot, which is held at its base by a tether,

the plantar fascia. The windlass mechanism is formed at the metatarsophalangeal attachment of the fascia. As the metatarsophalangeal joints are extended passively when one stands on the ball of the foot, the plantar fascia is pulled distally across them, shortening the distance from the calcaneum to the metatarsal heads. This process makes the base of the truss shorter. The tarsal joints are locked into a forced flexed position and the height of the longitudinal arch of the foot is increased. Thus, extension of the toes helps to turn the foot into a rigid lever before push-off.

KINETICS OF THE FOOT

During normal stance, approximately 50 per cent of the load is borne by the heel and 50 per cent is transmitted across the metatarsal heads, predominantly the first and between the second and third heads. A slight change in the foot structure alters the load distribution. At heel-strike, the ground reaction force is slightly medial to the centre of the heel pad. When the foot rolls into slight valgus shortly thereafter during the flatfoot portion of stance, the ground reaction force progresses slightly

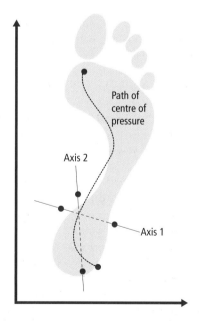

Path of centre of pressure

Axis 2

Axis 1

Figure 24.7 *Path of the centre of pressure during normal gait.*

laterally to lie beneath the cuboid and then forwards towards the base of the first metatarsal. Towards the end of the stance phase, the ground reaction force courses medially to reach beneath the second metatarsal head and then proceeds to the hallux at toe-off. Thus, during the stance phase of gait, the centre of the load progresses forwards rapidly, from the heel to the great toe (Figure 24.7).

The extrinsic muscles provide active control of the foot. The **anterior leg muscles** are active at heel-strike, while **posterior calf muscles** propel the foot forwards to toe-off. The soft tissues of the sole are especially adapted to absorb shock at heel-strike and to protect the bony structures through the stance phase of gait and push-off.

TOTAL ANKLE REPLACEMENT

SUMMARY OF BIOMECHANICAL CONSIDERATIONS

The ankle is not a simple single-axis hinge, and its axis of rotation changes with loading and rotation. The ankle transmits large axial (four to seven times body weight) loads and large shear forces (80 per cent of body weight). These forces are distributed over an articular surface area of approximately 11–13 cm^2. The ligaments contribute significantly to stability in all positions of the joint.

FIRST-GENERATION IMPLANTS

Introduced in the 1970s, the first-generation implants consisted of **two-part constrained** or **unconstrained cemented components**. The constrained-hinge types had high failure rates, predominantly at the implant–bone interface, due to large load transmission. The unconstrained designs relied on malleolar and ligamentocapsular elements for stability. Their positioning was therefore critical, relying heavily on accurate soft-tissue balancing. These failed due to instability in inversion/eversion and internal/external rotation. Cemented implants required considerable bony resection, leaving soft cancellous bone for support, which led to migration and subsidence of components.

SECOND-GENERATION IMPLANTS

The second-generation implants are considered to be **semi-constrained** designs allowing plantar/dorsiflexion and mediolateral or anteroposterior sliding. They usually consist of three components and are uncemented. They provide **full articular congruency** in all joint positions, minimizing wear and deformation of components. The bone–implant interface has reduced non-axial stresses, and soft-tissue balancing is achievable via a range of polyethylene inserts.

Two commonly used types have a **polyethylene meniscus** interposed between the tibial and talar components. These are the low contact stress (LCS) and the Scandinavian total ankle replacement (STAR).

The third type has the **polyethylene secured** into the tibial component, thus essentially becoming a two-part prosthesis (agility ankle system). This prosthesis also incorporates an inferior tibiofibular fusion, thought to provide a larger surface area for implantation and transfer of forces.

The results of the second-generation implants appear more promising but still do not compare favourably with other lower-limb arthroplasties. They can be considered for low-physical-demand patients and patients with subtalar joint degenerative changes. Absolute contraindications include infection, avascular necrosis, neuropathies, poor musculature and malaligned tibiotalar joints.

Surgical technique should involve minimal bone resection and correct orientation. Mediolateral malpositioning can cause soft-tissue impingement and malleolar fractures. Varus valgus angulation can cause higher contact stresses and impingement, leading to accelerated wear. Altered joint-line levels can create muscle and ligament dysfunction.

THIRD-GENERATION IMPLANTS

The third-generation implants have **talar components** shaped like the frustum of a cone and are thus more anatomical. Their long-term results have not been established.

Viva questions

1 What is the ideal position in which to fuse an ankle joint?

2 What is the mechanism by which eccentric contraction of muscle is achieved?

3 Describe the windlass mechanism and its role in gait.

4 Describe changes in the gait cycle with:
 (a) gastrosoleus weakness;
 (b) tibialis anterior weakness.

5 What do you know about ankle joint replacements?

FURTHER READING

Inman, VT, Ralston, HJ, Todd, F. *Human Walking*. Baltimore, MD: Williams & Wilkins, 1981.

Jackson, MP, Singh, D. Total ankle replacement. *Curr Orthop* 2003;**17**:292–8.

Mann, R, Coughlin, M. *Surgery of the Foot and Ankle*, 7th edn. London: Mosby, 1999.

Ramsey, PL, Hamilton, W. Changes in tibiotalar area of contact caused by lateral talar shift. *J Bone Joint Surg Br* 1976;**58**:356–7.

Singh, AK, Starkweather, KD, Hollister, AM, Jatana, S, Lupichuk, AG. Kinematics of the ankle: a hinge axis model. *Foot Ankle* 1992;**13**:439–46.

25

Friction, lubrication, wear and corrosion

GURDEEP BIRING, MARCUS BANKES, JAY MESWANIA AND GORDON BLUNN

INTRODUCTION

Tribology is defined as the science that deals with the interaction between surfaces in motion and consequences of that interaction, i.e. friction, lubrication and wear. Sir William Hunter described the tribological features of synovial joints succinctly in 1743: 'Both are covered with a smooth crust, to prevent natural abrasion; connected with strong ligaments to prevent dislocation; and enclosed in a bag that contains a proper fluid deposited there, for lubricating the two contiguous surfaces.'

Natural synovial joints are subjected to an enormous range of loading conditions; for example, approximately five to ten times the body weight passes through the hip and knee at heel-strike. Articular cartilage has limited ability to repair and, therefore, efficient lubrication is necessary in order to minimize friction and prevent cartilage wear.

This chapter aims to define tribology in normal synovial joints and in joint replacements, with reference to corrosion in the latter.

FRICTION

Friction is defined as the resistance to sliding motion between two bodies in contact. Surface friction comes from the adherence of one surface to another or the viscosity of the sheared lubricant film between the two surfaces. The force required to overcome the fluid's viscosity is much less than the surface adhesion.

For dry friction, three laws of friction have been defined:

- Frictional force (F) = coefficient of friction (μ_f) × applied load (W).
- F is independent of the apparent area of contact or sliding speed (V).
- The kinetic F is independent of V.

In a rotational system, such as a hip replacement, it is important to describe torque rather than force:

$$\text{Frictional torque} = \text{frictional force } (F) \times \text{radius } (r) = \mu_f \times W \times r$$

Even the smoothest polished surfaces appear rough when viewed at high enough magnification. The projections from the surface are called **asperities**. The taller and more numerous the asperities, the rougher the surface and the greater the friction.

Roughness of a surface is expressed as the **mean surface roughness**, or R_a value, which is the average height of the asperities. Comparative R_a values for surfaces in

Table 25.1 Mean surface roughness (Ra) of various orthopaedic surfaces

Material	Ra (µm)
Articular cartilage	1–6
Polyethylene cup	0.25–2.5
Metal femoral head	0.025
Ceramic femoral head	0.02
Charnley stem	1
Matt Exeter stem	0.7–1.3
Polished Exeter stem	0.01–0.03

Table 25.2 Coefficients of friction of various articulations

Articulation	Coefficient of friction (μ_f)
Normal knee	0.005–0.02
Normal hip	0.01–0.04
Metal on polyethylene	0.02
Metal on metal (dry)	0.8
Aluminium on aluminium	2.0

orthopaedics are shown in Table 25.1. The coefficients of friction of various articulations are shown in Table 25.2.

SYNOVIAL FLUID PHYSIOLOGY

Synovial fluid is a **dialysate** of **blood plasma**, without clotting factors, erythrocytes or haemoglobin. Synovial fluid is clear, and sometimes yellowish and viscous, and contains **hyaluronate** (relative molecular mass (RMM) 1–2000 kDa) and **plasma proteins** (20 per cent concentration of plasma; similar to serum). In the synovium, as in all tissues, essential nutrients are delivered and metabolic by-products are cleared by the bloodstream perfusing the local vasculature. Synovial micro-vessels contain fenestrations that facilitate diffusion-based exchange between plasma and the surrounding

interstitium, which equilibrates with synovial fluid and the interstitial fluid of cartilage. Plasma proteins also enter by diffusion, but distribution favours smaller molecules due to a mechanism that limits transfer of these molecules from the plasma. The microvascular endothelium provides the major barrier limiting the escape of plasma proteins into the surrounding synovial interstitium, with larger molecules passing more slowly than smaller molecules. The protein path across the endothelium involves fenestrae, intercellular junctions and cytoplasmic vesicles, but the precise mechanism has yet to be determined.

In contrast, proteins leave synovial fluid through lymphatic vessels, a process that is not size-selective. Protein clearance may vary with joint disease; for example, there is more rapid removal of proteins from joints affected by rheumatoid arthritis (due to increased microvascular permeability) than from those affected by osteoarthritis.

Thus, in all joints there is a continuous passive transport of plasma proteins involving synovial delivery in the microvasculature, diffusion across the endothelium, synthesis and breakdown by the synovium, and ultimate lymphatic return to plasma. The intrasynovial concentration of any protein represents the net contributions of these factors.

SYNOVIAL FLUID MECHANICS

Viscosity is the measure of the internal friction of a fluid. This friction becomes apparent when a layer of fluid is made to move in relation to another layer. The greater the friction, the greater the amount of force required for this movement, known as **shear**. Shearing occurs whenever the fluid is physically moved or distributed, as in pouring, spreading, spraying and mixing. Highly viscous fluids therefore require more force to move than less viscous materials.

Isaac Newton defined viscosity mathematically by the formula:

$$\text{viscosity} = \text{shear stress/shear rate}$$

where **shear stress** is the force per unit area required to produce shearing action (measured in dynes/cm^2), **shear rate** is a measure of the change in speed at which the intermediate layers of fluid move with respect to each other (measured in reciprocal seconds – s^{-1}) and **viscosity** is measured in poise, such that a material requiring a shear stress of 1 dyne/cm^2 to produce a shear rate of 1/s has a viscosity of 1 poise.

Viscosity of synovial fluid from normal knee joints decreases from 500 Pa to 0.5 Pa as the shear rate increases from 0.001/s to 1000/s. This **shear thinning** derives from the alignment of the hyaluronic acid molecules as shear rate increases. Enzymatic degradation of synovial fluid in rheumatoid arthritis leads to loss of non-Newtonian properties, making the fluid a less effective lubricant. In contrast, hyaluronates of synovial fluids from osteoarthritic joints are not degraded and maintain their non-newtonian properties. These properties allow synovial fluid to act as an efficient lubricant as well as allowing nutrition of articular cartilage.

Key facts on synovial fluid

- **Non-Newtonian:** shear stress is not proportional to shear rate.

- **Pseudo-plastic:** undergoes shear thinning.

- **Thixotropic:** undergoes shear thinning with time when sheared at a constant rate.

Important definitions

Rheology: science of deformation and flow of matter.

Shear: rate of deformation of a fluid when subjected to a mechanical shearing stress.

Shear stress: applied force per unit area needed to produce deformation in a fluid.

Viscosity: measure of the resistance of a liquid to flow (internal friction).

Newtonian fluid: fluid or dispersion whose rheological behaviour is described by Newton's law of viscosity. Here, shear stress is proportional to shear rate, with the proportionality constant being the viscosity, e.g. water, thin motor oils, synovial fluid in rheumatoid arthritis (enzymatic degradation makes it a less effective lubricant).

Non-Newtonian fluid: when the shear rate is varied, the shear stress does not vary in the same proportion (or even necessarily in the same direction). The viscosity of such fluids therefore changes as the shear rate is varied (envisioned by thinking of any fluid with a mixture of molecules with different shapes and sizes). The most common types of non-Newtonian fluids one may encounter include pseudo-plastic and dilatant fluids.

Pseudo-plastic: describes a non-Newtonian fluid whose viscosity decreases as the applied shear rate increases, a process that is also termed **shear thinning**, e.g. paints, emulsions, synovial fluid.

Dilatant: non-Newtonian fluid whose viscosity increases as the shear rate increases. The process is termed **shear thickening**. Shear thickening is rarer than shear-thinning but is found in fluids containing high levels of deflocculated solids, e.g. sand/water mixtures, clay slurries.

Plastic: describes a fluid that behaves as a solid under static conditions but once flow is induced with a force known as the **yield value**, the fluid may behave as either Newtonian or non-Newtonian, e.g. tomato ketchup.

Thixotropic: describes pseudo-plastic flow that is time-dependent. When sheared at a constant rate, viscosity gradually decreases (common; seen in materials such as synovial fluid, grease, heavy printing inks and paints).

Rheopexy: essentially the opposite of thixotropic behaviour, in that the fluid's viscosity increases with time as it is sheared at a constant rate (rarer than thixotropy).

JOINT LUBRICATION

Several hypotheses have been proposed to elucidate the mechanisms of lubrication that may explain the minimal friction and wear characteristics of cartilage. They fall into two groups:

- **Fluid-film lubrication:** surfaces are separated by a fluid film, the minimum thickness of which must exceed the surface roughness of the bearing surfaces in order to prevent asperity contact.
- **Boundary lubrication:** contact-bearing surfaces are separated by only a boundary lubricant of molecular thickness, which prevents excessive bearing friction and wear.

The biotribological performance of a joint depends on the **lambda (λ) ratio**. This is the ratio of fluid-film thickness to surface roughness: a ratio of 3 represents fluid-film lubrication, while a ratio of less than 1 represents boundary lubrication.

Studies have shown that fluid-film lubrication dominates in synovial joints. In practical terms, all types of fluid-film lubrication and boundary lubrication occur in synovial joints, depending on the specific joint in question and the particular type of loading applied.

TYPES OF FLUID-FILM LUBRICATION IN SYNOVIAL JOINTS

The various types of lubrication in synovial joints are shown in Figure 25.1.

Hydrodynamic lubrication

The speed of sliding and the viscosity of the lubricating fluid are sufficient to create a thin fluid-film capable of supporting the applied load. There is no contact between surfaces and, hence, no wear. Hydrodynamic (HD) lubrication can occur only under **high speeds** and **low loads**, otherwise the surfaces come into contact. HD lubrication is a poor model for synovial joints; however, it may occur during the **high-speed non-accelerating rotatory motion** of the femur during the swing phase of gait.

Elastohydrodynamic lubrication

HD lubrication assumes that the cartilage is rigid and non-porous when in fact it is elastic and deformable. In elastohydrodynamic (EHD) lubrication, deformation of the bearing surface serves to **trap pressurized fluid** and **increase the surface area**. An increased surface area decreases the shear rate, thereby increasing the viscosity of the synovial fluid. These factors increase the capacity of the fluid-film to carry load and decrease stress within the cartilage. Using this model, the thickness of the fluid film has been calculated to be up to 1 μm, which is less than the roughness of articular cartilage ($R_a = 1$–6 μm).

Micro-elastohydrodynamic lubrication

The micro-elastohydrodynamic (MEHD) lubrication model assumes that the **asperities** of articular cartilage are **deformed under high loads**. This smoothes out the bearing surface and creates a film thickness of 0.5–1 μm, which is sufficient for fluid-film lubrication.

Squeeze film lubrication

This occurs when **bearing surfaces** approach each other **without relative sliding motion**. Because a viscous lubricant cannot instantaneously be squeezed out from the gap between two surfaces that are approaching each other, pressure is built up as a result of the viscous resistance offered by the lubricant as it is being squeezed from the gap. This pressure is temporarily capable of supporting large loads before the fluid is squeezed out and surface contact occurs. The pressure may also deform the articular cartilage surface. Squeeze film lubrication may occur during **heel-strike**.

Weeping lubrication

Mechanisms have also been proposed concerning a localized increase or change in the composition of synovial fluid between the bearing surfaces. In weeping lubrication, **tears of lubricant fluid** are generated from the cartilage by the **compression of bearing surfaces**. This is an unlikely mechanism in diarthrodial joints.

Boosted lubrication

Boosted lubrication assumes that, under squeeze film conditions, the water of synovial fluid is

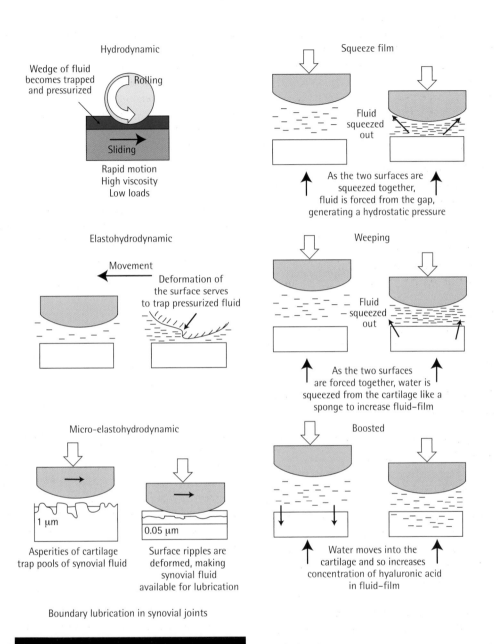

Figure 25.1 *Types of lubrication in synovial joints.*

pressurized into the cartilage, leaving behind a more concentrated pool of **hyaluronic acid–protein complex** to lubricate the surfaces.

BOUNDARY LUBRICATION IN SYNOVIAL JOINTS

Depletion of the fluid-film must inevitably occur after periods of prolonged loading and little movement. A gel-like surface film (thickness 5–20 nm) covers cartilage. This hydrophobic monolayer functions like the pile of a carpet to provide a cushioning layer and protect the articular surface from abrasion. This monolayer is composed mainly of the glycoprotein **lubricin** (RMM 250 kDa), but it also contains **dipalmitoyl-phosphatidyl-choline**, a phospholipid. Enzymatic treatment of cartilage to remove the monolayer leads to increased coefficients of friction.

Lubrication mechanisms are important in the gait, and different mechanisms are thought to act at different stages of the gait cycle (Table 25.3).

Table 25.3 Presumed lubrication in the hip joint during the gait cycle

Phase of gait cycle	Predominant type of lubrication
Heel-strike	Squeeze film
Stance	(M)EHD
Toe-off	Boundary, (M)EHD, weeping
Swing	Hydrodynamic
Prolonged stance	Boundary, boosted

(M)EHD, (micro-)elastohydrodynamic.

LUBRICATION MECHANISMS IN PROSTHETIC JOINTS

The fluid-film is too thin in metal on ultra-high-molecular-weight polyethylene (UHMWPE) articulations, and so **boundary lubrication** predominates. Contact stresses can be up to 20 MPa in total hip replacements (THR) and 30 MPa in some non-conforming total knee replacements (TKR), with the velocity of sliding varying from 0 to 50 mm/s.

Lubrication occurs with a pseudo-synovial fluid, which has a complex and variable biological composition. However, this fluid does not have the rheological properties of healthy synovial fluid. Even though boundary lubrication predominates, mixed conditions do occur, making the role of the lubricant extremely important in determining the coefficient of friction and the wear processes.

Wettability describes the relative affinity of a lubricant for another material. It can be measured by the angle of contact at the edge of a drop of lubricant applied to the surface of the material. Ceramic surfaces show a greater degree of wettability than metals; as ceramics are more hydrophilic, they have improved lubrication and lower friction.

In **metal-on-metal articulations**, true fluid-film lubrication may occur with the latest large-diameter articulations. In metal-on-metal articulations, the **effective radius** is the important determinant of fluid-film thickness. A large effective radius increases contact surface area and decreases interface stress. Radial mismatch or clearance between the femoral head and acetabular cup allows a large effective radius and, therefore, fluid-film thickness. The surface Ra value needs to be small to allow this, so this is only appropriate in metal-on-metal and ceramic-on-ceramic bearings.

Factors determining lubrication

- magnitude and direction of loading;
- geometry of bearing surfaces/surface roughness;
- material properties of surfaces, e.g. wettability;
- velocity at which bearing operates;
- viscosity of lubricant.

WEAR

Wear of bearings is a **progressive loss** of bearing substance from the material as a result of chemical or mechanical action. Chemical wear is usually a result of corrosion. The mechanical conditions under which the prosthesis is functioning when wear occurs have been classified as the four modes of wear:

Mode 1: the generation of wear debris that occurs with motion between the two primary bearing surfaces as intended by the designers.

Mode 2: a primary bearing surface rubbing against a secondary surface in a manner not intended by the designers, e.g. a femoral head articulating with an acetabular shell following wear-through of the polyethylene.

Mode 3: two primary bearing surfaces with interposed third-body particles, e.g. bone, cement or metal.

Mode 4: two non-bearing surfaces rubbing together, e.g. back-sided wear of an acetabular liner, fretting of the Morse taper, stem-cement fretting or neck of femoral component impinging on rim of cup.

Several modes of wear often occur simultaneously, but **mode 1** accounts for the majority of wear in well-functioning hip and knee replacements.

The fundamental mechanisms of wear include **abrasion**, **adhesion** and **fatigue**.

ABRASIVE WEAR (FIGURE 25.2a)

Two-body abrasive wear occurs when a soft material (e.g. UHMWPE) comes into contact with a significantly harder material (e.g. metal). Under these circumstances, the microscopic counter-face asperities of the harder material surface may plough into the softer surface, producing grooves. Some of the softer material may be detached to form wear debris. A femoral head has micro-asperities of height 0.1 μm with an Ra value of 0.025 μm.

Third-body abrasive wear (e.g. sand in one's shoes) occurs when extraneous material such as metallic, ceramic (bearing or coating), bone or cement particles, or even products of corrosion, enter the interfacial region. Such hard material

(a)

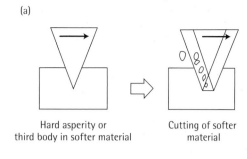

Hard asperity or third body in softer material — Cutting of softer material

(b)

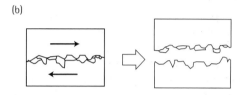

Bond between two materials stronger than the force needed to fracture softer material

Figure 25.2 *(a) Abrasive and (b) adhesive wear.*

may become embedded in the polymer and abrade the femoral head. Raised regions on the originally smooth femoral head then abrade the polymer at a much greater rate than the unblemished surface. A single transverse scratch may increase the wear factor by up to ten times. This is worse with a metal head than with a ceramic head, as the latter does not form heaped-up ridges (i.e. ceramic has a better scratch profile). Abrasive wear can be minimized by manufacturing a hard and smooth femoral head and avoiding extraneous material in the interface.

ADHESIVE WEAR (FIGURE 25.2b)

Adhesive wear occurs when a junction is formed between the two opposing surfaces as they come into contact. The junction is held by intermolecular bonds between solids, and this force is responsible for friction. If this junction is stronger than the cohesive strength of the individual bearing material surface, then fragments of the weaker material may be torn off and adhere to the stronger material. UHMWPE adheres to metal, especially if dry, leading to shearing of UHMWPE.

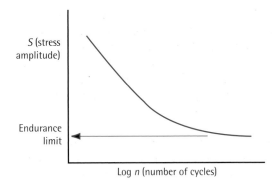

Figure 25.3 *S–n curve.*

FATIGUE WEAR (DELAMINATION)

This is a form of failure that occurs in structures subjected to dynamic and fluctuating stresses. In these circumstances, it is possible for failure to occur at a stress considerably lower than the yield strength for a load. An important parameter that characterizes a material's fatigue behaviour is the fatigue life. This is the number of cycles needed to cause failure at a specified stress level, as taken from the *S–n* plot (Figure 25.3).

Fatigue wear is mainly a problem in TKR, as the joint is less conforming and the UHMWPE is more highly stressed. Repeated loading causes subsurface fatigue failure of the UHMWPE at a depth of a few millimetres, as this is the area of maximum principal stress. Therefore, wear is not related to surface roughness. Cracks appear when the endurance limit is exceeded. This effect can be exacerbated by:

- a subsurface layer of oxidation;
- subsurface faults;
- misaligned or unbalanced implants;
- thin UHMWPE.

A surface layer of UHMWPE therefore breaks off, producing large particles. UHMWPE has macro-asperities two orders of magnitude higher (height 1–10 μm) than the micro-asperities of metal surfaces. These asperities are plastically deformed by loading, producing local contact stress concentrations above the yield stress of the UHMWPE, with subsequent failure by plastic deformation and rupture. This process is known as **micro-delamination**.

VOLUMETRIC AND LINEAR WEAR

Volumetric wear is the volume of material detached from the softer material as a result of wear and is expressed in mm^3/year. **Linear wear** is the loss of height of the bearing surface and is expressed in mm/year.

Measurement in vitro

Volumetric wear can be measured in vitro using simple reciprocating pin-on-plate, rotating pin-on-disc apparatus or more complex joint simulators. Joint simulators aim to mimic the loading conditions in vivo by applying load cycles at 4 Hz, but often with no rest periods. The lubricant and temperature can be adjusted, and wear is measured by loss of weight of softer implant or volume of released particles. However, simulators tend to underestimate wear when compared with wear rates in vivo. It takes 60 days to apply 10 million cycles, with each 1 million cycles being equivalent to approximately 1 year of clinical use.

Measurement in vivo

Cup penetration is commonly measured in vivo by comparison between initial and follow-up radiographs, corrected for magnification, e.g. medial migration of polyethylene hip sockets in millimetres per year. A shadowgraph technique or coordinate machine can be utilized to measure this. Radiographs using the uni-radiographic method or the duo-radiographic method can also measure wear.

Volumetric wear can also be measured by direct examination of explanted cups. Gravimetric methods have been used, whereby the explants are weighed; however, UHMWPE may absorb water, making it heavier, and therefore controls are required.

Laws of wear

Volume of material (*V*) removed by wear increases with load (*L*) and sliding distance (*X*) but decreases as the hardness of the softer material (*H*) increases:

$$V \propto LX/H$$

$$V = k'LX/3H$$

$$V = kLX$$

Where k′ is a dimensionless wear coefficient and k is the wear factor for a given combination of materials that incorporates the hardness of the softer material.

Thus, the wear volume is greater in larger femoral heads because of the increased sliding distance. Wear volume is also dependent on the type of articulation used.

Factors that determine wear

- Patient factors:
  - weight (applied load);
  - age and activity level (applied rate of load).

- Implant factors:
  - coefficient of friction of materials;
  - roughness (surface finish);
  - toughness (abrasive wear)
  - hardness (scratch resistance, adhesive wear);
  - sliding distance for each cycle (depending on the diameter of the head);
  - number of cycles that occur over time;
  - surface damage;
  - presence of third bodies (abrasive wear).

WEAR IN PROSTHETIC HIPS

Penetration of a femoral head into an acetabular cup is a combination of creep and wear. Creep is a visco-elastic property and is defined as time-dependent irreversible plastic deformation in response to a constant load. The amount of creep depends on the applied load and is unaffected by sliding movements between surfaces. Creep usually dominates the initial penetration rate, which hip simulator studies have shown to be of the order of 0.1 mm for the first 1 million loading cycles. This equates to about 1 year of clinical use. The **direction of creep is superomedial**, as this is the direction of the compressive joint contact force in the hip, whereas the **direction of wear is superolateral**, as this is perpendicular to the instantaneous axis of rotation.

Explanted cups reveal the direction of penetration to be superomedial, superior or superolateral. The direction of penetration correlates with the depth of penetration, with low penetration being superomedial due to creep, and high penetration being superolateral due to wear, as roughening of the femoral head, fusion defects in the polyethylene and particulate debris become increasingly important. The magnitude of cup penetration depends on the bearing combination.

CONSEQUENCES OF WEAR AND WEAR PARTICLES

Consequences of wear particles

- synovitis;
- aseptic osteolysis and loosening;
- systemic distribution;
- immune reaction;
- increased friction of the joint;
- misalignment of the joint and catastrophic failure

Osteolysis and aseptic loosening are the most frequently recognized complications of total joint arthroplasty. Both are the direct result of wear debris. Assuming the volume of wear debris is constant, then the number of **wear particles** is inversely proportional to their size. These particles exert their biological activity by being **phagocytosed by macrophages**, stimulating the release of soluble pro-inflammatory mediators, including cytokines and prostaglandins. Particles in the size range 0.1–10 μm are biologically active, with those in the size range 0.1–0.5 μm being the most potent. Mediators released near to bone cause osteolysis, aseptic loosening and ultimate failure of the prosthesis by stimulating bone resorption by osteoclasts, although macrophages may also be able to resorb bone directly by the release of oxide radicals and hydrogen peroxide (Figure 25.4).

Important mediators in this process may **stimulate osteoclasts** [interleukin 1 (IL-1),

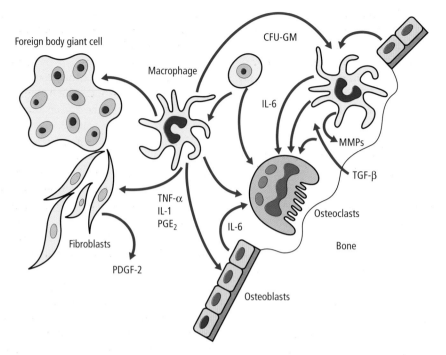

Figure 25.4 *Cascade of cells and mediators involved in osteolysis. CFU-GM, colony-forming units–granulocyte macrophage; IL-1, interleukin 1; IL-6, interleukin 6; MMP, matrix metalloproteinase; PDGF-2, platelet-derived growth factor 2; PGE$_2$, prostaglandin E2; TGF-β, tumour growth factor beta; TNF-α, tumour necrosis factor alpha.*

interleukin 6 (IL-6), tumour necrosis factor alpha (TNF-α), prostaglandin E2 (PGE$_2$), tumour growth factor beta (TGF-β)] or **osteoclast precursors** (monocyte colony-stimulating factors [M-CSF] and granulocyte colony-stimulating factors [G-CSF]), **inhibit osteoblast function** (IL-1) or **directly expose bone** (metalloproteinases such as collagenase).

Several studies have suggested a critical wear volume related to osteolysis; for example, volumetric wear rates above 140 mm^3/year are associated with significant osteolysis around acetabular cups. However, the severity of the osteolytic reaction may also depend on the size of the particles, their shapes and their surface areas.

The major factors that affect the extent of macrophage activation by the wear particles and thus the extent of osteolysis are:

- volume of wear debris;
- total number of wear particles;
- size of particles;
- morphology of particles (irregular shapes are more active than spheres);

- immune response to the particles.

Wear particles are constantly being produced in enormous numbers from prosthetic bearings, and a rough estimate for a 22.225-mm head is that it wears at an average rate of 38 000 submicron particles per step. Osteolysis is self-sustaining and sets up a vicious cycle: as bone resorption and prosthetic loosening progress, abrasion and fretting at the interface may produce increased amounts of particulate debris.

With respect to systemic distribution of wear particles, both metallic and UHMWPE particles are commonly transported to the liver, spleen or abdominal lymph nodes in patients with joint replacements. Wear particles are more prevalent in the liver and spleen in patients with revision implants, implying that these organs are involved only when large amounts of wear debris are generated from mechanical failure. Usually no toxic effects are apparent from these wear particles, although rarely granulomas form in remote organs in response to heavy particulate load.

Increased friction may occur as a result of increased Ra value due to loss of the original polished bearing surface. High wear and penetration rates of UHMWPE in acetabular components lead to impingement, which leads to wear from the site of impingement, loosening, loss of movement and dislocation.

BIOTRIBOLOGICAL CONSIDERATIONS OF DIFFERENT BEARING SURFACES

METAL ON ULTRA-HIGH-MOLECULAR-WEIGHT POLYETHYLENE

The bearing surface of Charnley's original low-friction arthroplasty (LFA) introduced in 1958 was stainless steel on Teflon™. Although this bearing had a very low coefficient of friction, Teflon™ had desperately poor wear characteristics and its use was abandoned in 1961. The following year, UHMWPE was introduced. UHMWPE has a slightly higher coefficient of friction than Teflon™ but much better resistance to wear. This is because its high RMM and its molecular structure produce very high strain energy to failure. Thus, this highly successful bearing combination squeezed out the contemporary metal-on-metal designs, and it has become the gold standard against which other bearing combinations are compared.

The fundamental limitation of UHMWPE is **wear resistance**. UHMWPE has been conventionally **sterilized** using **gamma irradiation** ranging from 2 to 4 Mrads and has been noted to undergo significant oxidative degradation during post-irradiation ageing; this has led to higher wear rates, delamination and gross fracture of the UHMWPE components. In addition to inducing cross-linking of the UHMWPE molecules, radiation causes scission of molecular chains and creates uncombined electrons – **free radicals**. If nothing is done to extinguish these free radicals, with time they may react with oxygen molecules, causing additional chain scission, embrittling the UHMWPE, **increasing its crystallinity** and **decreasing its fatigue strength**, **fracture toughness** and **wear resistance**. Excessive

oxidation occurs in shelf-aged UHMWPE components when free radicals are induced by gamma irradiation and there is time for oxygen to diffuse into the UHMWPE. Maximum oxidation occurs 1–2 mm below the surface, the so-called **subsurface white band**, the thickness of which increases with time.

Cross-linking has been utilized in order to improve the oxidation and wear resistance of polyethylene and can be accomplished with use of **peroxide chemistry**, **variable-dose ionizing radiation** or **electron-beam irradiation**. Cross-linking and oxidation are competing reactions during chain scission in the formation of UHMWPE. Several manufacturers perform gamma sterilization with the UHMWPE component sealed in a suitable **oxygen-free atmosphere**, including **vacuum** or **inert gas** (**argon** or **nitrogen**), where free radicals that are formed recombine and cross-link. Other manufacturers have chosen to sterilize **without irradiation**, using **ethylene oxide** or **gas plasma**, to decrease the production of reactive free radicals. However, these methods do not cross-link the UHMWPE and, therefore, do not improve its wear resistance.

Heating the polymer to above the melting point encourages cross-linking. Although cross-linking dramatically reduces wear rates in vitro and in vivo, re-melting and excessive cross-linking may reduce the fatigue strength and fracture toughness of the UHMWPE, with significant changes in material properties. Interestingly, cross-linked polyethylene releases a relatively high number of **submicrometre**- and **nanometre**-sized polyethylene particles and relatively fewer particles that are several micrometres in dimension; these submicron particles appear to have more functional biological activity in in vitro studies. Therefore, the type of preparation that leads to the least amount of osteolysis is yet to be determined. The response is also dependent on the shape of the particles and on the total volumetric wear. There are many variables, and all of these need to be borne out in clinical studies. Although short-term studies for cross-linked UHMWPE seem encouraging, longer follow-up is required.

FACTORS AFFECTING METAL/ULTRA-HIGH-MOLECULAR-WEIGHT POLYETHYLENE WEAR IN TOTAL HIP REPLACEMENT

- **Surface roughness:**
  - Damaged femoral heads have higher volumetric wear rates, higher total penetration and higher total number of particles produced over the prosthesis lifetime.
  - Damaged heads generate increased numbers of small, more biologically active particles ($< 10\ \mu m$).
- **Thickness of UHMWPE:**
  - Thickness should be at least 8 mm, as contact stress, wear and amount of creep increase dramatically when thickness of polyethylene falls below this level.
  - Adequate UHMWPE thickness can be obtained with a 40-mm cup only by downsizing the femoral head to 22 mm.
- **Type of metal:**
  - Cobalt-chrome has excellent properties, particularly if cold worked, because it is hard, resistant to corrosion and resistant to fatigue.
  - Stainless steel is cheaper but easily scratched.
  - Titanium alloys have poor wear characteristics and a high coefficient of friction compared with cobalt-chrome. They are also sensitive to surface flaws and scratching. Although their use as a bearing surface has been abandoned, they are commonly used for femoral components, particularly uncemented, and almost always for tibial trays of fixed-bearing TKRs.
- **Head size:**
  - The larger the head size, the greater the sliding distance and volumetric wear.
  - From the tunnelling expression, volume of wear debris $= \pi r^2 P$, where P is the penetration and r is the radius of the femoral head. $P \propto 1/r^2$, and therefore the larger the femoral head diameter, the lower the penetration.
- **Modularity:**
  - Modularity is attractive because it allows screw fixation, liner exchange and the use of extended lip liners ('dial-a-prayer').
  - There is increased wear in both cemented and uncemented metal-backed cups due to reduced UHMWPE thickness and increased peak stresses, particularly in the presence of incongruency and gaps between liner and metal backing.
  - Backside wear occurs from relative movement between liner and shell, and is worse if there is a poor locking mechanism or screw holes with sharp unpolished margins. Settling of the cup may lead to increased prominence of screws. UHMWPE may creep through holes, which provide a conduit for wear particles.
- **Third-body wear.**
- **Decreased offset of prosthesis** due to increased joint reaction forces.
- **Production of UHMWPE:** ram extrusion produces linear wear of about 0.11 mm/year and compression moulding of about 0.05 mm/year.
- **Gamma sterilization in air:** oxidation of UHMWPE leads to increased crystallinity and reduction in fatigue strength.

Good design features for uncemented acetabular components

- stable locking mechanism;
- congruency between mating parts;
- avoidance of rough finish or sharp edges around screw holes;
- cluster configuration that can be rotated out of weight-bearing area;
- facility to close off unused holes.

ADDITIONAL FACTORS AFFECTING METAL/ULTRA-HIGH-MOLECULAR-WEIGHT POLYETHYLENE WEAR IN TOTAL KNEE REPLACEMENT

Compared with THR, the tibiofemoral articulation of total condylar knee replacements is non-conforming. The design of fixed-bearing

TKR is a compromise between reproduction of the normal knee kinematics and reduction of contact stresses. **Unconstrained PCL-retaining round-on-flat** tibial inserts produce high contact stresses but allow rotation and femoral rollback without excessive PCL tension. **Conforming PCL-sacrificing round-on-round** designs have lower contact stresses, but at the penalty of reduced rotation. This non-conformity creates areas of high contact stress within the UHMWPE that is design-specific. Concavity in both sagittal and coronal planes ('double-dishing') reduces contact stress. Contact stresses may also be increased by malalignment or ligamentous imbalance due to asymmetrical load transmission.

Contact stresses increase markedly if UHMWPE thickness falls below 8 mm. Maximum stresses on the tibial tray is four times body weight at 15 degrees flexion, which exceeds the uni-axial yield strength of UHMWPE of many knee replacements. High contact stresses produce **delamination**, which is the most important wear mechanism in TKR. Attempts to improve wear characteristics of UHMWPE by heat pressing or reinforcement with carbon fibre rods have instead led to early fatigue failure. **Metal-backed modular** tibial components were developed to provide more secure fixation, improve load transmission and decrease UHMWPE creep, but at the expense of possible undersurface wear.

A **mobile bearing** solves the kinematic conflict by allowing a highly conforming articular surface to exist with free rotation. By eliminating the need for rotation at the femorotibial articulation and allowing rotation of the tibial polyethylene–tibial tray interface, the contact area of the articular surface can be greatly increased, thereby reducing contact stress and wear. Undersurface wear is also reduced by a more conforming implant, particularly with a highly polished cobalt-chrome base plate. There are insurmountable difficulties in the manufacture of polished cobalt-chrome base plates with a suitable locking mechanism for modular fixed-bearing implants. Hence, they are machined from titanium alloy, with inferior wear properties. Despite these theoretical advantages, no study has shown that mobile-bearing TKRs provide improved functional performance, greater activity in younger patients, lower revision rates for mechanical failure or lower wear rates.

CERAMIC ON ULTRA-HIGH-MOLECULAR-WEIGHT POLYETHYLENE

Alumina ceramic has superior wear characteristics over metal. It is one of the hardest materials known (after diamond and carborundum), which therefore makes it resistant to scratching. It can be machined to a **smoother surface** than metal and it is **wettable**, which could explain its excellent friction characteristics under load. Use of ceramic is limited by **expense** and the risk of **head fracture** (0.004 per cent incidence with modern alumina ceramics). Head fractures are associated with small head diameters, large grain size of the alumina and suboptimal fitting of the Morse taper, although modern manufacturing has largely overcome these problems.

Despite these tribological advantages, the ceramic-on-UHMWPE bearing has not consistently shown lower rates of osteolysis. However, the linear wear from the combination of a 22.225-mm alumina ceramic head and cross-linked UHMWPE is only 0.022 mm per annum after bedding in, compared with 0.07 mm per annum with standard metal on UHMWPE. Although lower wear rates have been reported, this reduction is small compared with hard-on-hard bearings and metal on cross-linked UHMWPE. In addition, UHMWPE wear debris and its attendant problems are still produced. These findings emphasize the multiplicity of factors that are involved in wear rates in vivo.

CERAMIC ON CERAMIC

First-generation ceramic-on-ceramic bearings experienced high loosening and fracture rates due to poor-quality ceramic, design faults and cemented all-ceramic acetabular components. Since the 1980s, however, ceramics have gained higher purity, finer grain structure and improved mechanical properties.

Ceramics are very **strong, stiff, bio-compatible** and **bio-inert** and **do not corrode**.

They can be manufactured to a very **smooth surface** finish and are very **hard** (scratch-resistant). They also have **high wettability** compared with metals and polyethylene. Ceramics therefore exhibit very **low friction** and **wear**, with linear wear rates being a fraction of standard metal on polyethylene (linear wear rates 0.025 µm/year). Excellent long-term results have been demonstrated in clinical practice.

However, ceramics are susceptible to **abrasive wear** and **edge-loading**, particularly if the acetabular cup is placed too open. They are also subject to **brittle fracture**, leading to catastrophic failure, although this is a very rare occurrence with modern alumina ceramics. Three types of ceramic are utilized in joint arthroplasty: alumina, zirconia and Oxinium™.

Zirconia is no longer used for the manufacture of femoral heads. Although it has high fracture toughness, it can undergo phase transformation at high temperatures and in wet environments, which substantially weakens the material and roughens the surface, degrading its wear properties. Zirconia is also very costly and is not licensed for use as a bearing surface with zirconia or alumina and therefore must be used with polyethylene. In 2001, zirconia femoral heads were recalled from circulation by the Medical Devices Agency (the regulatory agency in the UK for medicines and healthcare products) because of an observed high rate of fracture.

In contrast with zirconia, **alumina ceramic** is increasing in popularity. Its quality has improved tremendously with reduction of grain size and diminished number and size of inclusions. This has been achieved with the aid of the hot isostatic pressing ('HIPping') process, which has led to a denser, finer grain size in the alumina. In addition, the tapers for both the femoral head and the socket are much better designed in order to accept ceramic bearings. The advantages of a durable ceramic-on-ceramic bearing now outweigh the disadvantage of minimal fracture risk. However, care should be taken when handling this material. Trial reductions with the ceramic liner in situ should be avoided, and there should be no debris or protruding screw heads in the bearing/Morse taper interface. The ceramic bearings should not be struck with a hammer, and careful templating and cup positioning are required due to the reduced liner lip and neck length options.

Oxidized zirconium (OxZr, Oxinium™) was introduced in 2003 as a bearing surface for total hip arthroplasty. This is a metallic alloy with a ceramic surface. Zirconium alloy is heated in air and oxygen diffuses into the alloy and transforms the surface into ceramic, i.e. the surface is not coated. The oxidized surface reaches a depth of 5 µm, with an oxygen-enriched transition layer below. Oxidized zirconium provides superior resistance to abrasion without the risk of brittle fracture, thereby combining the benefits of metals and ceramics. Cross-sectional profiles indicate a uniformly hard ceramic layer on the surface, with a gradual decrease in hardness with increasing distance from the ceramic oxide layer. This minimizes abrasive scratching. Oxidized zirconium can be used in patients with metal sensitivity, as it has undetectable levels of nickel. Knee simulator tests have shown that use of oxidized zirconium can reduce UHMWPE wear substantially.

When revising fractured ceramic femoral heads, total synovectomy, cup exchange and insertion of a cobalt-chromium or new ceramic femoral head minimizes the chance of early loosening of the implants and the need for one or more repeat revisions. The fragments of ceramic are difficult to remove from the tissues and are a major source of third-body wear to subsequent articulations. Total synovectomy is required in order to remove as much debris as possible. Damage to the Morse taper leads to increased fracture risk of an exchanged ceramic head and may be an indication for revision of a well-fixed femoral component. Particulate debris from well-functioning articulations is difficult to quantify, but in vitro studies quantify it to the order of 10 nm. Damaged bearings on the other hand release particles that are in the submicron to micron range, similar to UHMWPE, which can stimulate the inflammatory cascade. However, osteolysis is rare with ceramic-on-ceramic bearings.

METAL ON METAL

Early cemented THRs, such as the McKee-Farrar and Ring devices, featured cobalt-chrome alloy bearings. The first generation of implants had a high failure rate because high frictional torque was transmitted to the cement–bone interface, leading to loosening. In addition, there was high wear because of the thin acetabular shells and a small clearance between the socket and the ball. These early bearings often transmitted load through the equatorial region (**equatorial bearing**) and could even squeak or jam (**clutch coning**). Engineering advances have allowed the manufacture of consistently **polar bearing articulations** with reduction of the frictional torque. Mathematical models have shown that the ideal diametric mismatch (clearance) between the head and the cup to reduce friction and wear should be 90–200 µm. In addition, it is hypothesized that fluid-film lubrication can exist in current surface replacements.

Metals have **good fracture toughness** and so **resist abrasive wear** well, but in order to overcome the adhesive wear the hardness must be increased. This can be achieved by using alloys such as **cobalt-chrome-molybdenum** (CoCrMo) with **high carbide** content. Carbide particles can occupy up to 5 per cent of the surface and have been shown to increase the surface hardness by 10–20 per cent. This reduces the wear rates to approximately 5 µm/year after the first 6 months, when the rate is approximately 10 µm/year.

The metal-on-metal articulation also exhibits the ability to **self-heal**, i.e. to polish out isolated surface scratches caused by third-body particles. However, they seem to exhibit 10–20 times greater wear-in during the initial 1–2 years, but this subsequently reaches a plateau.

The **metal wear particles** are small (50–500 nm) in comparison with those that activate macrophages (0.5–1 µm) and so do not excite such an inflammatory response. Although they are small, more particles (8×10^{12} particles/year) are produced than with UHMWPE (0.4×10^{12} particles/year). Despite this, osteolysis is rarely seen in metal-on-metal articulations. It may be that these particles are transported away from the joint capsule, and therefore this raises concerns about the observed systemic levels of **metal ions** in the body; it has been postulated that these ions may be **toxic** or **carcinogenic**. It is generally agreed that the levels of cobalt and chromium ions are higher in the blood and urine from patients with metal-on-metal implants than from patients without implants. Carcinomas associated with cobalt and chromium implants have been reported in some animal implantation models but, to date, epidemiological studies of patients with joint replacements have not shown a higher incidence of cancer with metal-on-metal prostheses. However, long-term data are awaited, and caution must be exercised in young and/or pregnant individuals. **Metal sensitivity** is another issue, and its association with prosthetic failure is still debated. Current dermatological preoperative screening is not recommended for fear of sensitization of the individual.

Metal-on-metal articulations can be used with conventional THR or as a resurfacing implant. The Metasul™ (Zimmer, Warsaw, IN, USA) bearing system, in which the metal acetabular bearing is embedded in a polyethylene liner, has shown good results. Wear studies have shown that there is a bedding-in period for the first 2 years when the linear wear is 10–20 µm, largely due to third-body abrasion from particles generated as scratches from the original polishing are eradicated and/or from dislodged surface carbides. The main contact zones are eventually worn smoother than the original surfaces, indicating a self-healing or self-polishing effect. This produces a reduction in wear rate, which falls to about 5 µm per year after the third year. This compares with linear wear rates of around 200 µm for metal on UHMWPE and 20–100 µm for ceramic on UHMWPE. Current surface replacements such as the Birmingham Hip Resurfacing (Smith & Nephew, Memphis, TN, USA) have been reported as having 0.02 per cent revision rate at 8.2 years, with little evidence of migration and little effect of bone density.

A comparison of wear rates for alternate bearing articulations is shown in Table 25.4 and

Table 25.4 Wear rates in different articulations with a 28-mm head

	Metal v. UHMWPE	Ceramic v. UHMWPE	Metal v. metal	Ceramic v. ceramic
Linear wear (μm/year)	150–200	75–100	5–10	Negligible
Volumetric wear (mm³/year)	40–80	15–20	0.1–1.0	0.004
Particle numbers	7×10^{11}	–	$4 \times 10^{12} – 2.5 \times 10^{14}$	No reports
Particle size (μm)	0.5–100	0.5–100	0.05–0.5	0.025

UHMWPE, ultra-high-molecular-weight polyethylene.

Table 25.5 Advantages and disadvantages of alternate bearing surfaces

Bearing surface	Advantages	Disadvantages
Ceramic on ceramic	Low wear, biocompatible	Risk of head fracture, abrasive wear, edge loading
Metal on metal	Good long-term clinical results, ability to self-polish	Undetermined effect of elevated ions, undetermined cancer risk, potential metal hypersensitivity
Cross-linked UHMWPE	Reduced wear	Particles more biologically active, excess cross-liking can lead to reduced mechanical properties, short-term clinical results

UHMWPE, ultra-high-molecular-weight polyethylene.

their advantages and disadvantages are summarized in Table 25.5.

The ultimate goal is to eradicate wear from arthroplasties, for which several strategies can be employed (Table 25.6).

CORROSION

Corrosion is defined as the **unwanted dissolution** of a metal in a solution, resulting in its continued degradation. Electrochemical deterioration of a metal happens when positive metal ions are ejected from a reaction site (**anode**) and electrons are allowed to flow to a protected site (**cathode**). The metal has n valence electrons and, by an oxidation reaction at the anode, the electrons are ejected to produce a positively charged metal ion. These ejected electrons must be transferred to another chemical species (cathode) and form the reduction reaction.

Table 25.6 Strategies to reduce wear

Improve bearing surface
   Improved UHMWPEs
   Metal on metal
   Ceramic on UHMWPE
   Ceramic on ceramic

Improved fixation
   Prevention of wear particle migration along the interface
   Seal interface

Prevent osteolysis
   Bisphosphonates
   TIMMPs

TIMMPs, tissue inhibitors of matrix metalloproteinases; UHMWPE, ultra-high-molecular-weight polyethylene.

In situ degradation of metal alloy implants is undesirable for two reasons:

- The degradation process may decrease the structural integrity of the implant.

- The release of degradation products may elicit an adverse biological reaction in the host.

Degradation may result from **electrochemical dissolution phenomena** or **wear,** or a synergistic combination of the two. Electrochemical processes may include **generalized corrosion**, uniformly affecting the entire surface of the implant, and **localized corrosion**, affecting either regions of the device that are shielded from the tissue fluids (**crevice corrosion**) or seemingly random sites on the surface (**pitting corrosion**). Electrochemical and mechanical processes (e.g. stress corrosion cracking, corrosion fatigue, fretting corrosion) may interact, causing premature structural failure and accelerated release of metal particles and ions.

The most commonly used metals for implants are titanium, cobalt-chrome and stainless-steel alloys. These are normally considered to be highly corrosion-resistant due to the formation of a thin passive oxide film that forms spontaneously on their surface. The film acts as a protective barrier to the corrosion processes. This phenomenon is termed **passivity** and is displayed by iron, nickel, chromium, titanium and many other alloys. The mechanism is thought to result from the formation of an adherent and very thin oxide film on the metal surface, which serves as a protective barrier to further corrosion. If damaged, the protective film normally reforms very rapidly. However, a change in the character of the environment may cause a passivated material to revert to an active state and substantial increase in corrosion rates.

GALVANIC CORROSION

This form of corrosion occurs when two **dissimilar metals** are **electrically coupled** together. Metals are considered to be dissimilar in this instance if their surface potential is different. The difference in potential causes electron flow between the two metals. The greater the difference in potential, the more driving force exists for this to occur. The electrochemical series can be used to predict galvanic relationships and determine unsuitable combinations. The more active alloy will become anodic and, thus, the more noble metal will be cathodic. If corrosion occurs in this situation, it will be accelerated on the more active metal, causing greater damage.

CREVICE CORROSION

This is caused by the formation of a **cavity** or **crevice** where **exchange in material** from the bulk solution is limited. This results in a change in the local environment. The solution within the crevice will change, leading to a decrease in the species required for oxygen reduction and a build-up of aggressive species with a decrease in pH. Tighter crevices reduce the amount of electrolyte that must be deoxygenated and acidified and will thus cause more rapid attack.

After oxygen becomes depleted within the crevice, the metal is oxidized and the electrons migrate to areas outside the crevice, where they are consumed in the reduction reaction. High concentrations of H^+ and Cl^- ions have been found in crevices, which can be particularly damaging to the passive films on metal implants. As the corrosion in the crevices increases, the rest of the surface becomes cathodically protected, and corrosion is localized.

FRETTING CORROSION

This is a **synergistic combination** of **wear** and **crevice corrosion** of two materials in contact. It results from micromotion between the two, which disrupts the protective film of a metal. The movement required for disruption of the passive layer can be as little as 3–4 nm and is dependent on the contact load and frequency of movement. This can cause permanent damage to the oxide layer, and particles of metal and oxide can be released into the body from fretting. For example, if the passive oxide film on cobalt-chrome-molybdenum is fractured, exposing the base alloy to an aqueous solution, then the following reactions of chromium (Cr) may occur with similar reactions involving cobalt (Co) and molybdenum (Mo):

$$Cr \rightarrow Cr^{3+} + 3e^- \text{ (dissolution)}$$

$$2Cr + 3/2O_2 \rightarrow Cr_2O_3 \text{ (repassivation)}$$

$$2Cr + 3H_2O \rightarrow Cr_2O_3 + 6e^- \text{ (repassivation)}$$

The Cr in the alloy oxidizes into ionic form (**dissolution**) or reacts with oxygen to reform the oxide film (**repassivation**).

PITTING CORROSION

Pitting is another form of **localized corrosion** attack in which small pits or holes form. The pits ordinarily penetrate from the top of a horizontal surface downwards in a near-vertical direction. This is an extremely insidious type of corrosion, often going undetected and with very little material loss until failure occurs. Pitting results in damage to the implant with a substantial amount of metal ion release. Pits can form at various points that are exposed to a solution containing aggressive species, and these can result from breaks in the protective film, defects in the metal/protective film or voids in the alloy or metal.

Pitting can occur particularly if the solution has a low pH and contains chloride ions. Human body fluids contain approximately 0.9 per cent sodium chloride, and so pitting can occur on metal implants. The early stage of pit formation is sudden and is accompanied by a very high current. Once initiated, the pits are self-sustaining and thus may continue to grow. Dissolution occurs within the pit, and oxygen reduction takes place on the adjacent surfaces. Electrons flowing between the two sites can be seen. The anode of the cell is the small area of active metal, and the cathode is the large passive surface of the remaining metal. There is a large potential difference in this cell, which causes a high flow of current and rapid corrosion.

STRESS CORROSION (FATIGUE)

Metals that are repeatedly deformed and stressed in a corrosive environment show **accelerated corrosion** and **fatigue damage**. A metal implant would be subject to repeated mechanical loads of up to 3×10^6/year, and implants at the lower extremities must support three or four times the body weight. Furthermore, the chemically aggressive environment of the human body makes testing simulating the physiological environment very important.

INTERGRANULAR CORROSION

Metals have a granular structure, with **grain** being the term for areas of continuous structure and the **grain boundary** being the disordered areas between grains. The grain is anodic and susceptible, whereas the grain boundary is cathodic and immune. Alloys are infinitely more susceptible to intergranular corrosion than are pure metals.

INTRAGRANULAR (LEACHING) CORROSION

This occurs due to electrochemical differences within grains.

INCLUSION CORROSION

This occurs due to the inclusion of **impurities**, **cold welding** or **metal transfer**, e.g. metal fragments from a screwdriver.

Practical examples of corrosion in orthopaedics

- stainless-steel wire in contact with cobalt-chromium or titanium alloy stem;
- stainless-steel head in contact with titanium alloy stem;
- titanium alloy screw in contact with stainless-steel plate.

In the absence of relative motion, galvanic coupling of cobalt-chromium with titanium alloy is stable. However, combination of stainless steel with either cobalt-chromium or titanium alloy is unstable, with the steel being susceptible to attack. Couples of similar metals are also stable. In the presence of motion, accelerated corrosion may occur, even when similar metals are used, with its extent depending on the type of fretting motion, the chemistry of the local solution and the microstructure of the metals.

CONCLUSION

This chapter provides the basic concepts and principles of friction, lubrication, wear and corrosion in orthopaedic surgery. The understanding of the basic science of natural and artificial joints is crucial to improving survivorship of implants used in the orthopaedic industry.

Viva questions

1 What do you know about synovial fluid?

2 What are the mechanisms of component wear? How can wear be prevented?

3 What is corrosion? What are the different types?

4 What are the methods of lubrication in synovial and artificial joints?

5 What is the pathological basis for osteolysis?

FURTHER READING

Archibeck, MJ, Jacobs, JJ, Black, J. Alternate bearing surfaces in total joint arthroplasty: biologic considerations. *Clin Orthop* 2000;**379**:12–21.

Campbell, P, Shen, FW, McKellop, H. Biologic and tribologic considerations of alternative bearing surfaces. *Clin Orthop* 2004;**418**:98–111.

Hall, RM, Bankes, MJ, Blunn, G. Biotribology for joint replacement. *Curr Orthop* 2001;**15**:281–90.

Heisel, C, Silva, M, Schmalzried, TP. Bearing surface options for total hip replacement in young patients. *J Bone Joint Surg Am* 2004;**85**:1366–79.

Jacobs, JJ, Gilbert, JL, Urban, RM. Corrosion of metal orthopaedic implants. *J Bone Joint Surg Am* 1998;**80**:268–82.

26
Gait

PRAMOD ACHAN AND FERGAL MONSELL

INTRODUCTION

Descriptive analysis of gait has progressed from the pioneering days of da Vinci, Newton and Galileo. Borelli, a pupil of Galileo, in *De Motu Animalum* in 1682, measured the centre of gravity of the body and described the maintenance of balance. In Germany the Weber brothers described the gait cycle in 1836, and in Paris Marey published a study on human limb movements in 1873. Braune and Fischer in 1895, in their work entitled *Der Gang des Menschen*, determined the velocities and accelerations of various body segments and the contributory forces involved.

Definitions

Gait: particular way or manner of moving on foot, or the translation of the body through space from one point to another.

Analysis: separation of an intellectual or material whole into its constituent parts for individual study.

Bipedalism: process by which one is able to stand upright and ambulate on two limbs.

Gait disorders: slowing of gait speed or a deviation in smoothness, symmetry or synchrony of body movement.

Gage defined gait analysis as 'the systematic measurement, description, and assessment of the quantities that characterize human locomotion'. In orthopaedic practice, the assessment of gait patterns in patients with neuromuscular disease is complex and difficult to analyse in the clinic setting. This has led to the development of motion-analysis laboratories in many specialist centres, which assess gait through several cycles, and in all planes of motion, using split-screen video, three-dimensional computer modelling, force plates and electromyography (EMG). It is useful, therefore, to make the distinction between clinical gait analysis and formal gait laboratory assessment.

The orthopaedic surgeon should be capable of evaluating patterns of movement by observation of the patient in the examination room. In this chapter, a framework is provided for the orthopaedic surgeon to use in order to assess such patterns and determine the features of pathological gait.

NORMAL GAIT

Normal walking has five prerequisites, as defined by Gage (1991):

- stance phase stability;
- adequate step length;
- sufficient foot clearance in swing;

- appropriate swing phase pre-positioning of the foot;
- energy conservation.

In addition, six determinants of gait have been described by Saunders *et al.* (1953). These determinants produce a dampening down of the excessive vertical and lateral movements in gait by interacting to create a smooth pathway for the forward displacement of the centre of gravity:

- pelvic rotation;
- pelvic tilt;
- lateral displacement of the pelvis;
- knee motion;
- knee flexion after heel-strike in stance phase;
- foot and ankle motion.

GAIT CYCLE

The gait cycle is defined as the **time interval** between two successive occurrences of one of the cyclical repeated events of walking. It **begins when the foot strikes the ground and ends when the same foot strikes the ground again**. The cycle represents the rhythmic alternating movements of the lower extremities and results in forward movement.

The gait cycle is divided into two major phases – **stance** and **swing**. The stance phase starts when the foot strikes the ground (initial contact) and ends when the foot leaves the ground, at which point the swing phase commences. In normal walking, initial contact is with the heel and stance ends with toe off. In normal walking, stance makes up 60 per cent of the cycle, with swing making up 40 per cent (Figure 26.1).

Perry (1992) further divided the gait cycle into eight subphases:

- **Stance:**
  - initial contact (IC);
  - loading response (LR);
  - mid-stance (MSt);
  - terminal stance (TSt);
  - pre-swing (PS) (toe-off).
- **Swing phase:**
  - initial swing (ISw);
  - midswing (MSw);
  - terminal swing (TSw).

A formal clinical evaluation of all eight phases is virtually impossible without technological assistance. Therefore, the use of four phases in clinical assessment is advocated:

- **Weight acceptance:** initial contact and loading response.
- **Stance:** mid-stance and terminal stance.
- **Forward progression:** terminal stance and pre-swing.
- **Swing:** initial swing, mid-swing and terminal swing.

Clinical gait analysis involves the following descriptive language, definitions and units:

Step length (metres): horizontal distance travelled along the plane of progression during one step. This is the distance covered from foot contact to the next contralateral foot contact.

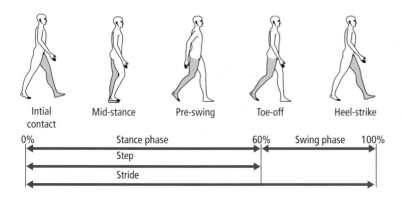

Figure 26.1 *Gait cycle.*

Stride length (metres): horizontal distance travelled along the plane of progression during one stride. This is the distance covered from foot contact to the next ipsilateral foot contact. It is roughly 1.5 m in an adult and $0.9 \times$ height (in metres) for a child.

Cadence (steps/minute): number of steps taken per unit time. Cadence does not change with age and is an individual phenomenon relating to the individual's leg length and body structure. In general, tall people take longer steps at a slower cadence, and shorter people take shorter steps at a faster cadence.

Double-support phase: when both feet are in contact with the ground at the same time.

Float phase: period of time when neither foot is in contact with the ground.

Velocity: stride length/cycle time (metres/second).

Walking base (millimetres): side-to-side distance between the two feet measured from the points of heel contact. It may also be referred to as the stride width or base of support and is normally 50–130 mm.

Foot progression angle (degrees): also referred to as the toe-out angle. This is the angle made between the direction of progression and the midline of the foot (external, negative; internal, positive).

Normal gait also varies with the **age**, **sex** and **body habitus** of the individual.

AGE-RELATED CHANGES

Ninety-seven per cent of children in the developed world are walking independently by the age of 18 months, but their gait is wide-based, non-reciprocating and stiff-kneed. This reflects poor balance and muscle development associated with normal immaturity. Around 3.5 years of age, reciprocating gait develops and resembles that of the adult, albeit with a short stride. By the age of 7 years, the adult pattern of gait is established.

Gait velocity remains relatively constant until the age of 70 years and then declines at approximately 15 per cent per decade for

normal gait and 20 per cent per decade for maximal gait. Step length becomes shorter and accounts for some of the reduction in velocity. The double-support phase increases from 18 per cent of the cycle in young adults to 26 per cent in healthy elderly people. This increased time in double-support improves stability but reduces the momentum of the swing phase, thereby reducing step length further.

SEX-RELATED CHANGES

This area of gait research is controversial, as many authorities believe that there are no differences in gait between the sexes. Leg length and step length may, however, be shorter in females, and, as cadence is identical, females must walk at faster speeds in normal ambulation. During the gait cycle, females have increased hip adduction compared with males, especially in the loading response.

BODY MASS INDEX-RELATED CHANGES

In individuals with a high body mass index (BMI), gait is modified to increase stability at the expense of efficiency, by decreasing stride length, decreasing velocity and spending longer in stance phase. If the BMI is such that the thighs interfere with normal swing of the free limb, then the gait is modified further by circumduction of the swing-phase limb around the stance-phase limb.

VISUAL OR CLINICAL GAIT ANALYSIS

This is the form of gait assessment commonly used in the clinical setting. It requires an **ordered sequence of observation**, starting with a general assessment of the body, including **habitus**, **symmetry**, **limb position, scars, wasting** and **walking aids**, including **prosthetics**. Then, the patient is instructed to walk using an area sufficient for the patient to take at least five strides. Observations are made in the **coronal** and **sagittal** planes, considering one leg at a time, dividing it into stance and swing phases. Personal preference dictates whether the foot or the pelvis is described first.

The normal movements of the major lower limb joints during the gait cycle are given below.

PELVIS

The pelvis rotates **anteriorly** at **heel-strike** and **posteriorly** at **toe-off** in order to increase the effective leg length. It also **lists** (known as **pelvic obliquity**) during the cycle in order to aid leg shortening, thus facilitating swing-through.

HIP

The hip is flexed to 35 degrees at initial contact but commences actively extending until midway through stance. The extensors also provide the tension to prevent collapse of the hip as the **ground reaction force** (GRF) acts in front of the hip joint. As the stance phase continues, the GRF passes posterior to the hip joint and the hip extensors continue to contract, creating a forward momentum for the body. It is only in terminal stance, when the hip is in its maximum extended position, that the hip flexors start to contract again, reaching maximal flexion at terminal swing.

KNEE

Just before initial contact is made, the knee flexors are preparing for absorption of energy by **contracting eccentrically**, with the joint slightly flexed. At loading response, the GRF passes behind the knee, causing a flexion moment that is countered by quadriceps action. As the limb swings over the planted foot, the GRF moves anterior to the knee joint, creating an extensor moment, countered by the posterior capsule, ligaments and knee flexors. At heel-rise, the knee flexes and the GRF passes once again posterior to the knee. Knee flexion continues to increase by toe-off and is maximal at mid-swing in order to allow for ground clearance.

ANKLE

During the loading response phase, the GRF is directed posterior to the ankle joint, generating a decelerating plantarflexion moment. This is controlled by the eccentric contraction of the ankle dorsiflexors so that the foot does not slap down. The anterior compartment muscles thereby act as the first rocker of the ankle joint (Figure 26.2).

As momentum carries the trunk forward on the flat foot, the GRF moves anterior to the ankle, and it is the eccentric contraction of the plantarflexors that allow this to progress in a controlled and smooth fashion as the ankle dorsiflexes. This is the second rocker of the ankle (Figure 26.2).

At terminal stance, the powerful **gastrocsoleal complex** contracts concentrically,

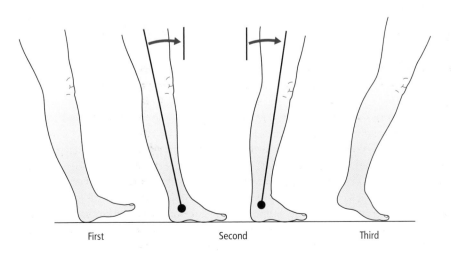

First   Second   Third

Figure 26.2 *Three ankle rockers.*

causing the heel to rise and providing power for toe-off. This action constitutes the third rocker (Figure 26.2).

A graph of ankle kinematics during the gait cycle is shown in Figure 24.4 in Chapter 24.

THREE-DIMENSIONAL GAIT ANALYSIS

Motion-analysis laboratories are used increasingly in the analysis of patients with movement disorders. They are particularly helpful in complex gait patterns, seen in conditions such as cerebral palsy and spina bifida. In combination with a good history and clinical examination, they help the orthopaedic surgeon in planning specific treatment for such disorders.

Most laboratories combine visual analysis with **video-camera** recording of gait to allow repeated slow motion and split-screen playback. In addition, the following are also assessed:

- **Kinematics:** describing the pattern of motion independent of the forces that cause it.
- **Kinetics:** describing forces that produce motion using force plates and computer modelling of the major lower limb joints.
- **Plantar pressure profiles:** demonstrating the weight-acceptance pattern of the foot, and the condition of the medial and longitudinal foot arches.
- **EMG:** assessing the pattern of muscle contraction occurring during the gait cycle in order to direct surgical treatment in the form of muscle or tendon releases or transfers.
- **Ergonomics:** there are a number of techniques to determine the energy consumption and, therefore, efficiency of walking, e.g. physiological cost index and O_2/CO_2 analysis.

Three-dimensional analysis involves the collection of data in the x-, y- and z-axes, which describe the **coronal**, **sagittal** and **transverse** planes, respectively. This information is presented in graphic form, with the graphs showing **one stride length**, **standard deviations** and the **normal values** for age or weight. An example of such a typical graph is shown in Figure 26.3.

ABNORMAL GAIT

In this section, abnormalities of gait are described according to the movements noted on visual analysis of the patient. An idea of the underlying disease process can be gauged from such abnormalities. Abnormal movements may be made either because the patient has no other option, e.g. constraint due to weakness, spasticity or deformity, or as a compensation for another deformity that needs to be identified.

LATERAL TRUNK BENDING/ TRENDELENBURG GAIT

This is an abnormality noted in the coronal plane when the trunk bends towards the side of the stance leg, i.e. an **ipsilateral lean**. This gait pattern is seen most commonly with a painful hip. The causes can be divided into problems due to the following:

- **Motor power:** hip abductor weakness, e.g. pain inhibition, postsurgical, poliomyelitis.
- **Lever arm function:** short femoral neck, e.g. coxa vara.
- **Change in fulcrum:** e.g. hinge abduction in developmental dysplasia of the hip.

ANTERIOR TRUNK BENDING

In this situation, the patient flexes the trunk forwards early in the stance phase, which is best viewed in the sagittal plane. This pattern is seen when compensating for inadequate knee extensors (**weak quadriceps**) by shifting the centre of gravity over the knee. It is seen less frequently with equinus deformity of the foot, hip extensor weakness and hip flexion contracture.

POSTERIOR TRUNK BENDING

This is essentially the reverse of anterior trunk bending and is also evident on the sagittal plane evaluation early in the stance phase. This is a compensation for weak or ineffective hip extensors and again uses the centre of gravity to alter the moment arm across the hip joint.

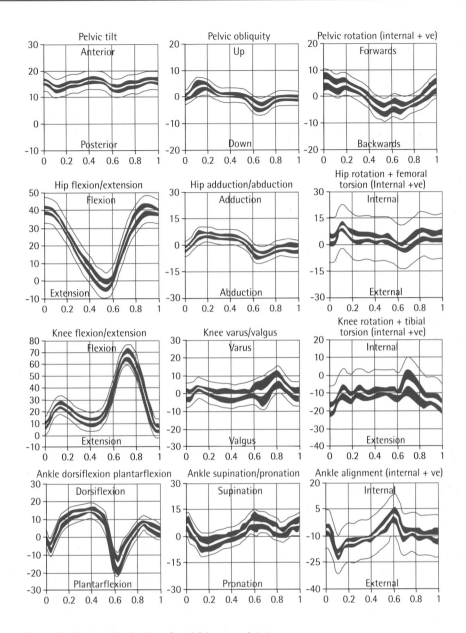

Figure 26.3 *Example of normal gait data for children aged 6–9 years.*

A separate posterior bend may be seen in the swing phase rather than the stance phase, where this movement is used to propel the swing leg forwards in the presence of either **weak hip flexors** or **spastic hip extensors**. This manoeuvre is also evident in patients with **ankylosed** or **arthrodesed hips** and **stiff knees**.

INCREASED LUMBAR LORDOSIS

This is difficult to distinguish from posterior trunk bending, except that the upper trunk remains balanced over the pelvis and the mechanical advantage is gained by increasing the lordosis of the lumbar spine. This pattern is seen in patients with **fixed flexion** at the hip or an **ankylosed hip** joint. It may also be seen following excessive hamstring lengthening in **cerebral palsy**, particularly in the presence of a fixed flexion deformity of the hip, i.e. a tight psoas.

FUNCTIONAL LEG-LENGTH DISCREPANCY

In these patients, due to true or apparent (but functionally real) leg-length discrepancy, the longer leg has difficulty clearing the ground during the swing phase. The patient compensates for this problem by using one of four methods:

- **Circumduction:** rather than swinging the long leg through in the line of progression, the patients swings the long leg around in an abducted position, thus effectively shortening the limb.
- **Hip hitching:** the abdominal-wall and paraspinal muscles are used to hitch the pelvis up on the longer side to gain the same advantage. This is a coronal plane movement, separate from the pelvic obliquity created by abductor function.
- **Steppage:** this is the high stepping gait, where exaggerated hip and knee flexion allow the longer leg to swing through.
- **Vaulting:** here, the shorter leg is plantar flexed in stance on to tiptoes, effectively compensating for the leg-length discrepancy by lengthening the shorter side.

ABNORMAL HIP ROTATION

The whole limb may be affected by rotational abnormalities at the hip, which affect the foot progression angle. This results in an in-toeing gait or an out-toeing gait. Excessive **bony torsion**, e.g. persistent femoral anteversion, is a common cause. Hip malrotation may also be due to **abnormal muscle activity**, as in patients with cerebral palsy, where imbalance between the medial and lateral hamstrings and spasticity in psoas can cause hip rotation. Alternatively, the rotation may be a **compensatory phenomenon** for quadriceps weakness, as seen in polio, where internal rotation of the leg allows the iliotibial band to be used for the swing phase, or external rotation allows the leg

to be moved with less knee flexion. Prolonged abnormal muscle pull on a developing bone alters the shape of the bone and may lead to true bony torsional changes with growth.

EXCESSIVE KNEE EXTENSION

With this gait pattern, the normal knee flexion in the stance phase is lost. Patients often display marked hyperextension in the sagittal plane. Patients with **quadriceps weakness** display this pattern of gait and supplement it with anterior trunk bending. They may use other means of keeping the knee extended, such as placing a hand on the upper thigh. This gait pattern is commonly seen in patients with polio.

EXCESSIVE KNEE FLEXION

Best visualized in the sagittal plane, excessive knee flexion affects subjects during initial contact and heel-rise when the knee is normally in extension. Patients with **fixed knee contractures** or **spastic hamstrings** are unable to extend the knee and adopt this gait pattern.

WEAKNESS OF ANKLE DORSIFLEXION

Weakness of the dorsiflexion results in a **foot-slap** during the first rocker. In addition, **toe-drag** occurs during the swing phase because of the inability to gain foot clearance in swing. This gait pattern can be mimicked by spasticity of the plantar flexors, although in such cases there is rarely a true foot-slap.

INSUFFICIENT PUSH-OFF

This abnormality is best viewed in the sagittal plane when the patient has insufficient ability to push off with the foot during the terminal stance phase. The foot is lifted flat off the ground. It may be seen with **Achilles tendon rupture**, **gastrocsoleus weakness** or **foot pain**.

ABNORMAL WALKING BASE

This may be increased by **neurological causes**, such as cerebellar ataxia, a **fear of falling** or fixed hip abduction. With the first two, a wider walking base allows for a lower, more stable centre of gravity, while fixed hip abduction prevents walking with a narrow base.

Viva questions

1 What are the prerequisites of gait?

2 What are the components of the gait cycle?

3 Describe this patient's gait [based on either a true clinical case or video recording].

4 What are the three rockers of gait?

5 What are the causes of a positive Trendelenburg gait?

FURTHER READING

Chambers, HG, Sutherland, DH. A practical guide to gait analysis. *J Am Acad Ortho Surg* 2002;**10**:222–31.

Gage, JR. Gait analysis in cerebral palsy. *Clin Dev Med* 1991;**121**:101.

Perry, J. *Gait Analysis: Normal and Pathological Function*. New York, NY: McGraw-Hill, 1992.

Saunders, JBM, Inman, VT, Eberhart, HD. The major determinants in normal and pathological gait. *J Bone Joint Surg Am* 1953;**35**:558.

Sutherland, DH, Olsen, R, Cooper, L, Woo, L. The development of mature gait. *J Bone Joint Surg Am* 1980;**62**:336–53.

27
Prosthetics

MANOJ RAMACHANDRAN AND LINDA MARKS

INTRODUCTION

A basic knowledge of the definition, terminology, components and complications of prostheses is essential for the orthopaedic surgeon. This chapter concerns exoprostheses, e.g. artificial arms and legs, but not endoprostheses, e.g. joint replacements.

A **prosthesis is a device or artificial substitute designed to replace, as much as possible, the function or appearance of a missing limb or body part.** Prosthetics is defined as the specialty relating to prostheses and their use.

The aim of **prosthetic rehabilitation** is to enable the patient to achieve maximum functional independence with the prosthesis, taking into account the patient's premorbid abilities, lifestyle and expectations. Note that this aim is not the same as for amputee rehabilitation, which includes wheelchair mobility for patients who are unable to walk. Successful outcome with prosthetic use is dependent on the following:

- **Patient:**
  - premorbid level of activity;
  - ability to learn new skills;
  - pathology in contralateral limb;
  - static and dynamic balance;
  - sufficient trunk control (and upper-limb strength);
  - other comorbidities.

- **Prosthesis:**
  - comfortable to wear;
  - easy to don (put on) and doff (take off);
  - appropriate components;
  - lightweight, durable and reliable;
  - cosmetically pleasing.
- **Teamwork:**
  - Appropriate communication between the surgical and rehabilitation team is essential. For unusual levels of amputation or complex elective cases, a pre-amputation assessment with the rehabilitation team is beneficial. Postoperatively, prompt therapy is critical for maximizing function and independence. The patient's motivation and participation in the programme are pivotal.
  - The surgeon should operate with the prosthesis in mind in order to fashion an organ of locomotion and thus create an optimal stump for limb fitting (see below).

AMPUTATIONS

Upper-extremity amputations are generally more common in the young male population secondary to trauma, while **lower-extremity amputations** are more common in an older population secondary to medical disease (peripheral vascular disease, diabetes,

Table 27.1 Most common indications for amputation by aetiology

Peripheral vascular disease/diabetes	80%
Trauma	10%
Tumour	5%
Congenital malformations/infections	5%

thromboembolism). Table 27.1 lists the most common indications for amputation in developed countries.

For **trans-osseous amputations**, the following should be borne in mind in order to create an ideal stump for limb fitting:

- The **scar** should be **well healed** and **mobile**, away from subcutaneous bony edges and underlying neuromata.
- The **skin** should be as **sensate** as possible.
- The **stump** should have a **cylindrical** or **conical** shape at closure.
- **Excessive soft tissue** distal to the bone section should be **avoided**.
- **Traumatized tissue** must **not** be **retained** in the stump.
- **Myoplastic** techniques (suturing muscles to periosteum) should be attempted, although **myodesis** techniques (direct suture of muscle to bone) may be of use in trans-femoral and trans-humeral amputations.
- **Nerves** should be **sectioned cleanly** under gentle tension and allowed to retract into proximal soft tissue to prevent neuroma formation in an inappropriate location.
- All **bone ends** should be **bevelled** or **contoured**.
- **Non-absorbable sutures** must be **avoided**.

The **optimum level** for amputation to allow limb fitting must be achieved, a common error being that the stump is left too long. For the four main sites of trans-osseous amputation, the levels are as follows:

- **Trans-radial (forearm):**
  - Optimum: junction of proximal two-thirds and distal third of forearm.
  - Shortest: 3 cm below insertion of biceps brachii.

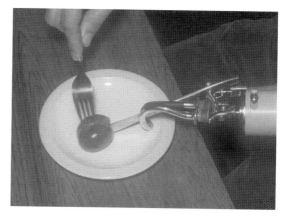

Figure 27.1 *Wrist rotary prosthesis.*

  - Longest: 5 cm above wrist joint, to allow space for wrist rotary prosthesis (Figure 27.1).
- **Trans-humeral (upper arm):**
  - Optimum: middle third of arm.
  - Shortest: 4 cm below anterior axillary fold.
  - Longest: 10 cm above olecranon, to allow space for elbow mechanism (Figure 27.2).

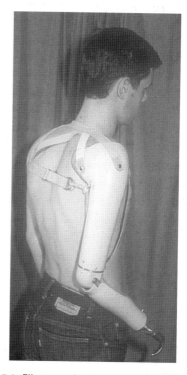

Figure 27.2 *Elbow mechanism.*

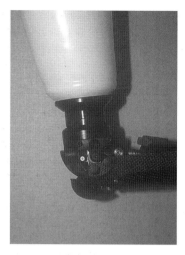

Figure 27.3 *Knee mechanism.*

- **Trans-femoral (thigh):**
  - Optimum: middle third of thigh.
  - Shortest: 8 cm below pubic ramus.
  - Longest: 15 cm above medial knee joint line, irrespective of the patient's height, to allow space for knee mechanism (Figure 27.3).
- **Trans-tibial (leg):**
  - Optimum: 8 cm for every 1 m of height.
  - Shortest: 7.5 cm below medial knee joint line.
  - Longest: level at which a myoplasty can be performed (for final cosmesis of the prosthesis).

For **disarticulation amputations**, the advantages and disadvantages should be considered when fitting prostheses. Advantages include the following:

- The amputation retains the weight-bearing surface.
- The bulbous shape assists suspension of the prosthesis.

Disadvantages include the following:

- The amputation can compromise the choice and/or fitting of prosthetic joints.
- The prosthesis can appear bulky. The exception to this rule is in cases of Symes amputation for congenital absence of the fibula with associated leg shortening. The shortening of the leg allows the bulb of the stump to be masked within the shaping of the external calf prosthesis.

CLASSIFICATION OF PROSTHESES

Prostheses can be classified according to the following:

- **Level of amputation:** e.g. trans-femoral, trans-radial.
- **Structure:** e.g. exoskeletal (where the strength of the prosthesis is in the rigid external structure and all parts are fitted on to or within this structure) or endoskeletal, also known as modular (where the individual components are linked by internal struts and the whole assembly is covered with a soft external cosmesis).
- **Function:** e.g. cosmetic, functional.

Often a combination of these descriptors is used, e.g. 'cosmetic trans-radial prosthesis', 'endoskeletal trans-femoral prosthesis'.

COMMON ELEMENTS OF PROSTHESES

All prostheses have some common elements (Figure 27.4):

- **Socket/interface:** the connection between the residual limb (known as the residium) and the prosthesis. This protects the residium and transmits the forces necessary for standing and ambulation. The socket can either be manufactured using a plaster mould of the residium as a template or it can be manufactured directly from mapping of the residium using computer-assisted technology. The socket may need to be serially adjusted as the volume of the residium stabilizes.
- **Suspension mechanism:** attaches the prosthesis to the residium. This may be in the form of belts, wedges, straps or suction, or a combination of these. Suction suspension can be of two types:
  - **Standard suction:** form-fitting or semi-rigid socket into which the residium is fitted.

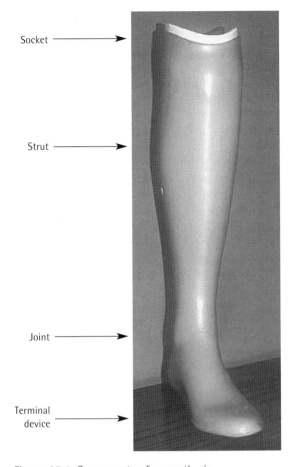

Socket

Strut

Joint

Terminal
device

Figure 27.4 *Components of a prosthesis.*

- **Elastomeric suction:** silicone- or gel-based sleeve that slips on to the residium, which is then inserted into the socket. When combined with a proximal external sleeve and distal valve or vacuum pump, this forms an airtight seal that stabilizes the prosthesis and may assist in controlling stump volume.
- **Struts/tubes (pylons):** intervening structures that restore limb length and attach the socket to the terminal device. These have progressed from simple static tubes to dynamic devices that incorporate components to allow axial rotation, impact absorption and release of energy.
- **Articulating joints (if necessary):** replace missing joint function.
- **Terminal device:** most distal part of the prosthesis.

In the lower limb, the **terminal device** is typically a foot, but it may take other forms for sports and water activities. In the upper limb, the terminal device is a hand, hook, gripper or a more individual functional device, e.g. a billiard-cue support. The terminal device can be either **passive** (less functional but greater cosmesis) or **active** (more functional, controlled by cables attached to a harness – body-power devices – or action potentials from muscle contraction in the residium – myoelectric devices). Active devices are either **voluntary opening**, if they lie closed at rest, or **voluntary closing**, if they lie open at rest.

Note that there are five different types of grip recognized for hand function, making it difficult for prostheses to replicate such complex movements:

- **Precision:** the pads of the thumb and index finger are apposed, e.g. for pinching or picking up a small object (mimicked by a hook or gripper).
- **Tripod:** the pad of the thumb is against the pads of the index and middle fingers (mimicked by most mechanical and electrical hands).
- **Lateral:** the pad of the thumb is apposed to the lateral aspect of the index finger for manipulating small objects, e.g. turning a key in a lock.
- **Hook power:** the small joints of the finger are flexed, and the thumb is extended, e.g. carrying a suitcase (mimicked by preshaped cosmetic hands).
- **Spherical:** the tips of the fingers and thumb are flexed, e.g. turning a doorknob, screwing in a lightbulb.

PROSTHETIC FITTING

In the immediate postoperative period, the key issues are adequate wound healing, pain management, and early therapy for mobility, strength and activities of daily living training. To prepare the residium for the prosthesis, a skin-desensitization programme may be beneficial, consisting of **massage** (to reduce excessive scar formation), **oedema control** (with elastic compression) and **gentle tapping** (on the distal aspect of the residium to mature the site). Pre-prosthetic training may include the use of an early training device, e.g. a pneumatic post-amputation mobility aid (PPAMaid) or an upper-limb gauntlet with a rudimentary terminal device.

In terms of the timing of prosthetic fitting, the following options are available:

- **immediate**;
- **prompt** (around 7–10 days when there is evidence of stump healing);
- **early** (around 3 weeks after the stump has healed);
- **late** (around 3–4 months when the stump is fully mature or if there has been delayed wound healing).

COMMON PROSTHESES

TRANS-TIBIAL PROSTHESES

Socket

The socket of choice used to be the **patella tendon-bearing** (PTB) prosthesis (Figure 27.5). The positive cast is rectified by the prosthetist to take account of pressure-sensitive areas (using **reliefs** – concavities within the prosthesis) and pressure-tolerant areas (using **build-ups** – convexities within the prosthesis). More commonly, sockets are now **total-contact** and, increasingly, **total surface-bearing**, where there is less patella tendon-bearing and weight is distributed more evenly over the entire surface of the residium.

Suspension

There are several options:

- supracondylar cuff;
- supracondylar extension to socket, known as patella tendon supracondylar (PTS);
- sleeve suspension, e.g. neoprene;
- elastic stocking suspension;
- elastomeric sleeve (silicone or gel) suspension with locking pin or lanyard (the latter being a short rope or cord used for fastening), e.g.

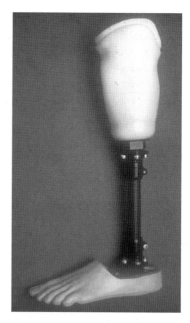

Figure 27.5 *Patella tendon-bearing prosthesis.*

Icelandic roll-on silicone socket (ICEROSS);
- valve/pump suction, using an elastomeric sleeve with a proximal external sleeve and a distal one-way valve or pump.

Articulating joints

In the trans-tibial prosthesis, the articulating joint is the ankle. This can be either:

- non-articulating, e.g. solid-ankle/cushioned heel (SACH);
- articulating: can be uni-axial or multi-axial.

Terminal device

In the trans-tibial prosthesis, this is the foot or a specialized device. Note that the foot and ankle should be considered as one complex. Prosthetic feet/ankles are of three types:

- **Non-energy-storing**, e.g.:
  - SACH: plantarflexion is simulated by compression of the heel and rollover by compression of a plastic or wooden foot;
  - single-axis foot, which adds passive dorsiflexion via compressible wedges, thus increasing stability during the stance phase;

- multi-axial foot, which adds inversion, eversion and rotation, which is useful over uneven ground.
- **Energy-storing:** these feet contain deforming components in the keel (and sometimes also in the heel), which, when compressed at rollover, want to return to their normal configuration and provide some energy return at toe-off (or heel-strike), e.g. the dynamic-response foot.
- **Specialized:** these devices are highly specialized for specific functions and may not look like feet at all. They often contain carbon-fibre composites and are most commonly used for running and sprinting.

TRANS-FEMORAL PROSTHESES

Socket

The socket brim shape is important here, as it conveys how body weight is transferred to the socket:

- **Conventional socket:** shaped to be a plug fit with no defined anatomical features.
- **H socket and Q (quadrilateral) socket:** both are ischial tuberosity-bearing sockets and feature a flat seat at the posteromedial aspect of the brim. The H socket is more pear-shaped and the Q socket more rectangular, but both have reasonably well-defined areas for the anatomical structures at the top of the stump.
- **Ischial-ramal containment (IRC) socket:** also known as a narrow mediolateral (ML) or contour-aligned trochanteric, computer-assisted manufacture (CAT/CAM) socket. Aims to lock on to the pelvis, medially via the inferior pubic ramus and posteriorly by containing the ischial tuberosity, and the transfemoral stump laterally via the greater trochanter. With the pelvis–stump connection controlled, the residium can be coaxed into a more anatomical (adducted) position, maximizing the function of the residual stump musculature.

Suspension

There are several options:

- **Rigid pelvic band:** limits hip to flexion and extension.
- **Double swivel pelvic band:** allows all planes of hip movements.
- **Roehampton soft suspension (RSS):** allows all planes of hip movement.
- **Total elastic suspension (TES) belt:** allows all planes of hip movement.
- **Suction socket (or, more appropriately, muscle-grab socket):** self-suspending socket by means of its intimate sockless fit, aided by active contraction of the muscle mass of the stump.
- **Elastomeric sleeve suspension:** attached with a distal lock or, if less available space, a lanyard.

Terminal device

The terminal devices are ankles and feet, as per trans-tibial prostheses.

Articulating joint

This is a knee joint. Note that the knee joint provides stance and swing control during gait. Stance control can be achieved by:

- alignment alone (hyperextension or geometric);
- lock;
- weight-activated control.

Swing control can be achieved by:

- external front pick-up;
- internal calf spring mechanism;
- pneumatic swing phase control (PSPC) cylinder;
- hydraulic swing phase control (HSPC) cylinder;
- microprocessor control;
- hybrids of microprocessor and pneumatic or hydraulic control.

KNEE AND ANKLE DISARTICULATIONS

For these disarticulations, two different types of socket are available:

- **Differential socket:** the socket is made up of an outer hard cylindrical socket and an inner liner. The liner is made from a plaster cast of the stump and rectified to increase the pressure (grip) over the isthmus of the stump (this is also known as a differential liner). A vertical split allows ingress and egress of the bulb of the stump. The outer aspect of the liner is built up to slide smoothly into the outer cylindrical socket.

- **Windowed socket:** a removable window is cut out of the narrowest area of the socket in order to allow the bulb of the stump to pass through and the socket to be closed, thus maintaining suspension.

HIP DISARTICULATIONS AND TRANS-PELVIC AMPUTATIONS

Prostheses for this level of amputation are bulky. Gait can be grossly abnormal, as the lumbar spine has to be used to swing the prosthesis through for heel-strike. The general components of such prostheses are as follows:

Socket and suspension

- **Hip disarticulations:** the ipsilateral ischial tuberosity is available for weight-bearing and the ipsilateral iliac crest for suspension (although the socket is usually suspended over both iliac crests). Note that the stump can be quite bulky initially.
- **Trans-pelvic amputations:** the extent of the amputation is quite variable and is dictated by the underlying pathology. Usually, the contralateral ischial tuberosity is needed for weight-bearing, and suspension is from the contralateral iliac crest and ipsilateral lower ribs.

Terminal device

The terminal devices are ankles and feet, as per trans-tibial prostheses.

Articulating joint

These are knee joints, as per trans-femoral prostheses, but hip joints can be:

- **Conventional:** joint lies directly under the socket but causes extra bulk under the socket and asymmetry in sitting.

- **Four-bar:** sited anteriorly on the socket and folds away anteriorly for sitting, thus avoiding asymmetry. The connecting tube at the hip and knee joints slants posteriorly to ensure that the prosthetic trochanter–knee–ankle (TKA) line is correct for stance stability.

COMPLICATIONS OF PROSTHESES

Complications can be either **psychosocial** (related to the initial operative procedure, i.e. amputation, and the use of a prosthesis and the perceived associated stigma) or **physical**. The more common physical complications seen are:

- **Dermatological problems:** including blisters and callosities, contact dermatitis, scar problems, excessive sweating and infected epidermoid cysts.
- **Phantom sensation:** sensation that the amputated limb is still present. This may also be accompanied by telescoping, where the patient feels that the amputated limb has shrunk, e.g. the toes are the ankle or the foot is at the knee.
- **Phantom pain:** sensation of pain originating in the amputated part of the limb. The pain can be stinging, burning or cramping in nature and is worse at night (especially if the limb is kept in a dependent position). The pain may or may not be dermatomal and is at its worst immediately after amputation. It is important to acknowledge that this is 'real' and not imaginary pain and to offer reassurance and appropriate treatment, which is usually with anticonvulsants, antidepressants, non-steroidal analgesics or simple analgesics (or combinations of these). For the majority of amputees, phantom pain is temporary.
- **Choke syndrome:** venous outflow obstruction of the residium occurring as a result of narrow proximal part of the socket, in combination with an empty space more distally in the socket. This is the main reason for total-contact/total surface-bearing sockets being preferred. Acutely, choke syndrome presents with red indurated skin with prominent skin pores ('orange-peel'

appearance). Chronically, haemosiderin deposition and venous stasis ulcers may occur.

- **Increase in energy consumption:** may limit ambulation and is not related specifically to use of the prosthesis itself. The level of amputation, the aetiology leading to the amputation, and the aerobic capacity and cardiopulmonary efficiency of the patient affect energy expenditure. In general, the increased levels of energy consumption (percentage above normal) by amputation level are as given in Table 27.2.

Table 27.2 Energy consumption above normal following amputation

Amputation	Increase in energy consumption above normal (%)
Long trans-tibial	10
Average trans-tibial	25
Bilateral average trans-tibial	20–40
Short trans-tibial	40
Average trans-femoral	65
Hip disarticulation	>100
Bilateral transfemoral	>200

Viva questions

1 What is a prosthesis?

2 What are the indications for fitting a prosthesis?

3 Tell me about this prosthesis [prop-based question].

4 As a surgeon, what do you have to consider when fitting a prosthesis?

5 What are the complications of prosthetic use?

FURTHER READING

Colwell, MO, Spires, MC. Lower extremity prostheses and rehabilitation. In M Grabois (ed.). *Physical Medicine and Rehabilitation: The Complete Approach*. London: Blackwell, 2000; pp. 583–607.

Leonard, JA, Jr, Meier, RH, III. Upper and lower extremity prosthetics. In JA DeLisa (ed.). *Rehabilitation Medicine: Principles and Practice*. Philadelphia, PA: Lippincott, Williams & Wilkins, 1998; pp. 669–96.

Luff, R. Amputations. In J Goodwill, M Chamberlain and C Evans (eds). *Rehabilitation of the Physically Disabled Adult*, 2nd edn. Cheltenham: Nelson Thornes, 1997; pp. 172–99.

Smith, DG, Michael, JW, Bowker, JH. *Atlas of Amputations and Limb Deficiencies: Surgical, Prosthetic and Rehabilitation Principles*, 3rd edn. Rosemount, IL: American Academy of Orthopaedic Surgeons, 2004.

28
Orthotics

MANOJ RAMACHANDRAN AND LISA BELLOWS

INTRODUCTION

This chapter reviews the definition, nomenclature and ideal characteristics of orthoses. Furthermore, their functional and biomechanical effects, the materials used in their manufacture, and the complications associated with their use are defined.

> An **orthosis** is a **device** that is **externally applied** or **attached** to a body segment and that **facilitates** or **improves function** by supporting, correcting or compensating for skeletal deformity or weakness.
>
> Department of Health and Social Security (1980)

Orthotics is defined as the **specialty** relating to orthoses and their use.

The word 'orthosis' seems to be derived from a combination of the words 'orthopaedic' and 'prosthesis'. It has now replaced the older terms 'splint', 'brace' and 'calliper'.

NOMENCLATURE

Traditionally, orthoses have been named after a part of the body, a person, a place or an institution, but rarely after function. In the 1960s, the American Academy of Orthopaedic Surgeons (AAOS) set up a task force to suggest standard reproducible terminology for orthoses. According to the AAOS nomenclature, an orthosis is described first by the joint or region of the body that it encompasses and second by a biomechanical analysis of its function. Built into the nomenclature is the ability to indicate functional hinge requirements at each joint. In the USA, prescription charts are in use on which are recorded in diagrammatic form the patient's functional impairment, treatment objectives and orthotic recommendations. In the UK, the use of a combination of AAOS and eponymous nomenclature has persisted.

Regions of the body in AAOS nomenclature

Upper limb	Lower limb	Spine
S = shoulder	H = hip	C = cervical
E = elbow	K = knee	T = thoracic
W = wrist	A = ankle	L = lumbar
H = hand	F = foot	S = sacroiliac

Thus, FO is a foot orthosis, KO is a knee orthosis and KAFO is a knee–ankle–foot orthosis.

Control of designated function

F: free motion allowed.

A: assist, i.e. application of an external force to increase range or velocity of a desired motion.

R: resist movement by external force.

S: stop, i.e. static unit to deter motion in one plane.

H: hold, i.e. elimination of all motion in prescribed plane.

L: lock, i.e. optional lock.

IDEAL CHARACTERISTICS OF ORTHOSES

Orthoses inevitably have to strike a balance between the often-conflicting requirements of function, cosmesis and acceptability. The practical ideal orthosis should aim to have the following characteristics:

- biomechanically effective;
- lightweight;
- durable;
- cosmetically pleasing;
- easy to put on (don) and take off (doff);
- rapid provision and replacement;
- inexpensive;
- washable;
- adjustable;
- comfortable;
- free of pressure areas.

FUNCTIONAL CHARACTERISTICS OF ORTHOSES

The main groups of functions for which orthoses are used are:

- **Provision of support:** to prevent weak muscles or ligaments being stretched, or to support joints by substituting for weakened muscles or ligaments, e.g. thoracolumbar orthosis (TLO) to support a collapsing osteoporotic spine, or KAFO to relieve weight from the lower-leg skeletal mass.

- **Limitation of motion:** e.g. KO to prevent hyperextension.
- **Correction of deformity:** to force the affected joint(s) into near-alignment and redirect growth if possible, e.g. thoracolumbar sacral orthosis (TLSO) to correct an idiopathic scoliosis, or ankle–foot orthosis (AFO) in cerebral palsy. Serial splinting describes the regular readjustment of orthoses to gradually improve the position or range of movement of a joint contracture.
- **Assistance of motion:** e.g. hip–knee–ankle–foot orthosis (HKAFO) to aid walking in myelomeningocele.
- **Miscellaneous:** e.g. warmth, placebo effect.
- **Combination:** many orthoses combine several functions, e.g. KAFO for a leg afflicted by polio gives support, limits movement at the knee (and perhaps the ankle), may help to correct a varus ankle, and may have a spring to assist ankle dorsiflexion.

An alternative functional classification of orthoses comprises two main groups:

- **Static (passive):** has no moving parts and is used to immobilize a part of the body in a particular position.
- **Dynamic (lively):** has moving parts, but movement is controlled by an energy store, e.g. an elastic band. An example is a postoperative outrigger for mobilizing tendon repairs of the hand. Maintaining mobility in joints has advantages in prevention of joint stiffness and muscle wasting, and hastening repair of bone, tendon and ligaments.

For all orthoses, at least three points of pressure are needed for proper control of a joint. For **supportive orthoses** of the resting splint type, the joint must be maintained in optimum anatomical position during rest periods. For **corrective orthoses**, the purpose of the orthosis is to impose or control a set of forces on the body part. Each force has both magnitude and direction, and the resultant must be worked out. The three-point principle (as proposed by Sir John Charnley for fracture immobilization) has long been accepted. Dynamic requirements of an orthosis are less well defined.

BASIC BIOMECHANICAL CONCEPTS

A basic understanding of biomechanics is essential when prescribing orthoses. Newton's third law of reaction, which states that for every **reaction**, there is an **equal** and **opposite reaction**, is vital for comprehension of the principle of **ground reaction force** (GRF) (see Chapter 16). If an orthosis is to be used to modify gait, the prescriber must also be aware of the normal gait cycle in order to diagnose abnormal gait patterns (see Chapter 26). Complex gait problems may require the use of a gait laboratory to determine specific muscle-group inadequacies.

It is important to understand the effects of GRF during the gait cycle (Figure 28.1).

The GRF is the force exerted by the ground on the body. It is equal in magnitude, but opposite in direction, to the force exerted on the ground by the body. If the GRF does not pass through the centre of a joint, then it produces a moment (turning force) on that joint. In mid-stance, the GRF is posterior to the hip, resulting in a hip extension moment that is counterbalanced by the gradual tightening of the anterior hip capsule. The GRF falls anterior to the knee, causing a knee extension moment that is resisted by the tight posterior knee capsule (Figure 28.1a). The GRF falls anterior to the ankle, resulting in an ankle dorsiflexion moment that is resisted by contraction of the gastrocnemius–soleus muscle complex. Thus, in balanced mid-stance, very little muscle activity is needed in order to maintain upright posture. During pre-swing, the force passes behind the knee and acts as a flexor, thus reducing the work requirements for knee flexion (Figure 28.1b).

Forces and moments generated about a particular joint may be calculated using the concept of free-body diagrams (see Chapter 16). Knowledge of such forces and moments is essential when designing an orthosis.

BIOMECHANICS OF ORTHOSES

Orthoses function by application of mechanical forces to the musculoskeletal system. Their success depends on a thorough understanding of biomechanical principles and their correct application.

Regardless of whether the body is stationary or moving, it is always subject to a system of external forces and moments. Normally, the effects of the external moments acting on the body are restricted or controlled by forces generated internally, either in passive tissues such as capsules, ligaments and articular cartilage, or in active tissues such as muscles. Injury or disease of one of these (e.g. ligament rupture, muscle atrophy, spasticity) can lead to an inability to produce the appropriate force to resist the system of external forces. Modifying the system of external forces and moments acting about one or more joints of the body by using an orthosis may restore a more normal function.

There are four ways by which an orthosis may modify the system of external forces and moments across a joint. The first three are **direct** (the orthosis surrounds the joint being influenced) and the last is **indirect** (modification of an external force occurs beyond the physical boundary of the orthosis):

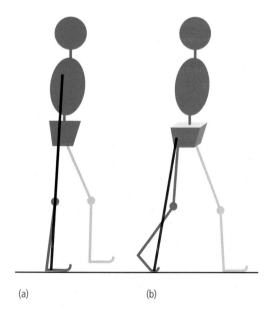

(a)   (b)

Figure 28.1 *Ground reaction force and its line of action during (a) mid-stance and (b) pre-swing.*

- **Control of moments about a joint:** this is the most common reason for prescribing an orthosis. By modifying the moments about a joint, an orthosis may partially or totally restrict the rotational movement at the joint (Figure 28.2). The end result is either a decrease in the range of movement about a particular axis or a limitation of the number of axes about which motion may occur. For an orthosis to be effective in controlling rotation, it must consist of a rigid framework incorporating straps and pads, which apply three forces to the limb. This **three-point fixation** involves one force acting over the joint centre, and the other two forces acting in the opposite direction to the first, placed proximally and distally to the joint. An example is a KO used for medial collateral ligament rupture of the knee, which is designed to eliminate motion in either the coronal or the transverse plane, while allowing motion in the sagittal plane.

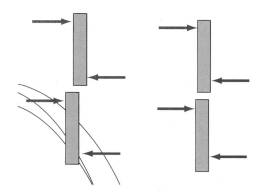

Figure 28.3 *Control of translational forces about a joint.*

anatomical structures and the orthotic exoskeleton and is particularly useful for reducing pain in arthritic joints (Figure 28.4).

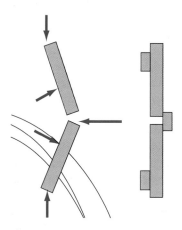

Figure 28.2 *Control of moments about a joint.*

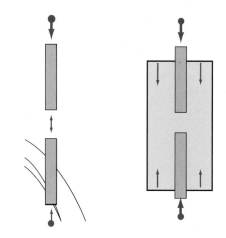

Figure 28.4 *Control of axial forces across a joint.*

- **Control of translation forces across a joint:** translational instability arises only when there are significant shear forces acting across the joint (Figure 28.3). **Four-point fixation** is required to prevent translation. The orthosis can be hinged to allow rotation. An example is a KO used to prevent translation in the transverse plane in posterior cruciate ligament rupture of the knee.
- **Control of axial forces across a joint:** this is achieved by load sharing between the

- **Control of line of action of GRF:** this involves modification of the point of application and line of action of the GRF during either static or dynamic weight-bearing and is relevant only to the lower limb (Figure 28.5). It is particularly useful in modifying abnormally high moments about a joint, but it can also be used to change the alignment of a joint. An example is the use of a lateral heel wedge, which can transfer the GRF from the medial aspect of a varus degenerate knee to the intercondylar eminence or lateral joint line.

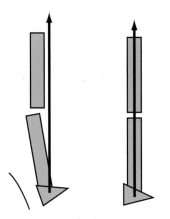

Figure 28.5 *Control of line of action of ground reaction force (GRF).*

MATERIALS USED IN ORTHOTICS

Traditionally, orthoses were made from **leather**, **rubber**, **metal** or **plaster of Paris**. These orthoses tended to be bulky, unsightly and unacceptable to the patient. Leather, such as cattle hide, continues to be used for shoe construction, as it conducts heat and absorbs water well. Rubber has tough resiliency and shock-absorbing qualities and is still used for padding in body jackets and limb orthoses. Metals, such as stainless steel and aluminium alloys, are adjustable and can be used for joint components, metal uprights and bearings. Plaster of Paris continues to be used as the initial mould taken from the patient for the preparation of orthoses.

Gordon Yates in 1968 first described the use of lightweight and more cosmetically pleasing plastic materials in the manufacture of orthoses. The three major materials now in use are:

- **Thermosetting plastics:** e.g. polyester resins, which can be moulded into permanent shape after heating and do not return to their original consistency, even after being reheated. They are formed by pouring liquid plastic resins into moulds, which are then mixed with catalysts that polymerize the resins to set into a rigid form. They are more commonly used in prosthetics than orthotics, where greater rigidity is required.

- **Thermoforming plastics (thermoplastics):** these soften when heated (allowing reshaping by application of pressure) and harden when cooled. They can be reshaped many times and are subdivided according to their moulding temperatures:
  - **High-temperature thermoplastics:** require moulding temperatures between 120 and 190°C. Great skill is required in their manufacture. They are ideal for high-stress activities. These orthoses are made by heating a sheet of polyethylene (e.g. Vitrathene™, Subortholen™, Ortholen™) or polypropylene (e.g. Vitralene™) in a hot oven. The final product is then either vacuum-formed or moulded over a positive plaster-of-Paris cast. Plastics differ in molecular weight, tensile strength, fatigue resistance and mouldability. They are commonly used for making more rigid orthoses such as AFOs and TLSOs.
  - **Moderate-temperature thermoplastics:** require moulding temperatures of 100–120°C. An example is Plastozote™ foam made from polyethylene of closed-cell construction. It is very lightweight and, after heating in a hot-air oven, it can be moulded directly on the patient, as it has low heat conductivity and its surfaces cool rapidly. It is commonly used for making custom-made cervical collars and pressure-distribution pads.
  - **Low-temperature thermoplastics:** require moulding temperatures below 80°C and so can be moulded in a water bath or hot-air oven. Ideal for use in acute splinting by occupational therapists. They can be moulded directly on to the patient, with minor modifications made using a heat gun or hair dryer. As a group, these thermoplastics are less rigid and less durable than other plastics; however, they are cheaper, because less time, skill and equipment are required for fabrication. Note that they may also soften in direct sunlight or near a fire. The common types of polymers in use are transpolyisoprene (Orthoplast™) and polycaprolactone (Polyform™, Aquaplast™), to which synthetic rubber may be added (many

types of Sansplint™). The plastics differ in setting times, rigidity, impact strength and transparency.

- **Self-generating polyurethane foam:** used in Neofract™ corsets and braces, this freshly prepared foam is poured into a cotton pattern and distributed evenly with a roller. The filled pattern is allowed to harden directly over the patient. The custom-made cast is prepared in minutes and is donned and doffed by using a zip fastener. Polyurethane foam is also used to make moulded cushions for wheelchairs and can be used as filler in KAFOs and shoes.

COMMON ORTHOSES

FOOT ORTHOSES

Insoles are commonly prescribed for a variety of foot pathologies. Insoles can be classified into three groups:

- **Simple insoles:** either off-the-shelf or fabricated without casting. Provide poor surface area contact and little if any biomechanical control.
- **Total contact insoles:** made initially by taking an imprint of the patient's foot and then casting this imprint with plaster of Paris. A thermoplastic is then moulded from the positive plaster-of-Paris cast. These are the most commonly used foot orthoses.
- **Functional/biomechanical orthoses:** corrective insoles introduced by Mervon Root, a podiatrist, in the 1960s. The foot is held in its corrected position when the cast is taken. The insole obtained therefore acts to correct the underlying foot deformity when the deformity is flexible. For fixed deformities, an accommodative insole is used.

When the limits for the use of insoles are reached, **custom-made shoes** are considered. Again, these can be corrective or accommodative, with respect to the deformity. A custom-made shoe often requires many fittings before it is satisfactory. Shoes can be modified either externally or internally in order to reduce pressure on sensitive areas by

redistributing weight towards pain-free areas. For **external** shoe modifications, **heels** can be of the following types:

- **Cushioned:** wedge of compressible rubber used to absorb impact at heel-strike or, with a rigid ankle, to allow more rapid ankle plantarflexion by reducing the knee flexion moment.
- **Flared:** medial to resist eversion and lateral to resist inversion.
- **Wedged:** medial to promote inversion and lateral to promote eversion.
- **Extended:** e.g. a Thomas heel projects anteriorly on the medial side to provide support to the medial longitudinal arch.
- **Elevated:** shoe lift to compensate for fixed equinus deformity or leg-length discrepancy of more than about 0.65 cm.

For **external** shoe modifications, **soles** can have the following:

- **Rocker bars:** convex structure placed posterior to metatarsal head, shifting rollover point from head to shaft. Used for ulcers over metatarsal heads in diabetes mellitus.
- **Metatarsal bars:** bar with flat surface placed posterior to metatarsal head to relieve pressure on heads.
- **Wedges:** medial to promote supination and lateral to promote pronation.
- **Flares:** medial to resist eversion and lateral to resist inversion.

For **internal** shoe modifications, the **heels** can have the following:

- **Cushion relief:** soft pad with excavation placed under painful point of heel.
- **Cups:** rigid plastic insert covering the plantar surface of heel and extending posteriorly, medially and laterally to prevent lateral calcaneal shift in the flexible flat foot.
- **University of California at Berkeley Laboratory (UCBL) insert:** rigid plastic insert fabricated over a cast of the foot held in maximum manual correction and encompassing the heel and midfoot, with rigid posterior, medial and lateral walls. Used to control hindfoot valgus and midfoot pronation.

For **internal** shoe modifications, the **soles** can have the following:

- **Metatarsal pads:** domed pads designed to reduce stress from metatarsal heads by transferring load to metatarsal shafts in metatarsalgia.
- **Inner sole excavations:** soft pad filled with compressible material placed under metatarsal heads.
- **Arch supports:** e.g. medial arch support extending from half inch posterior to first metatarsal head to anterior tubercle of the os calcis.

ANKLE–FOOT ORTHOSES

AFOs are used to prevent or correct deformities and reduce weight-bearing. The position of the ankle indirectly affects the stability of the knee, with ankle plantarflexion providing a knee extension force and ankle dorsiflexion providing a knee flexion force. AFOs have been shown to reduce the energy cost of ambulation in a wide variety of conditions, such as the spastic diplegic form of cerebral palsy, the lower motor neuron weakness of poliomyelitis, and the spastic hemiplegia of stroke.

Plastic AFOs include consist of a shoe insert, a calf shell, a heel-retaining strap and a calf strap attached more proximally. Examples include the following:

- **Posterior leaf spring:** narrow calf shell and narrow ankle trim line behind the malleoli to allow some flexibility. Used for compensating for weak ankle dorsiflexors – dorsiflexion assist – by preventing excessive equinus at heel-strike or drop-foot in swing. Allows the tibia to progress forwards during the second rocker of stance phase. Has no mediolateral control.
- **Solid AFO:** wider calf shell with trim line anterior to the malleoli. Prevents ankle dorsiflexion and plantarflexion, as well as varus and valgus deviation.
- **Hinged AFO:** adjustable ankle hinges can be set to the desired range of ankle dorsiflexion or plantarflexion. Commonly, a hinged AFO prevents plantarflexion but allows relatively full dorsiflexion during the stance phase of gait.
- **Ground reaction AFO (GRAFO):** made with a solid ankle at neutral. The upper portion wraps around the anterior part of the tibia proximally to provide strong ground reaction support for patients with weak triceps surae. Prevents knee hyperextension by creating a flexion moment at the knee (Figure 28.6).
- **Dynamic AFO (DAFO) or tone-reducing AFO (TRAFO):** broad footplate used to provide support around most of the foot, extending distally under the toes and up over the medial and lateral aspect of the foot in order to maintain the subtalar joint in

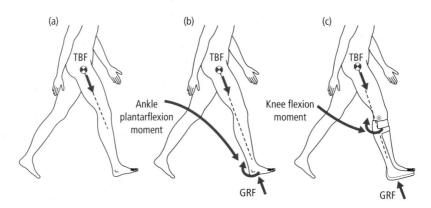

Figure 28.6 *Ground reaction force (GRF) control in the sagittal plane. Before heel contact, no GRF acts on the lower extremity (a). At heel contact with no orthosis, the GRF control acts to plantarflex the ankle (b). At heel contact with an ankle–foot orthosis (AFO), the GRF control acts to flex the knee. TBF, total body force.*

normal alignment. There is some evidence that in cerebral palsy, these are capable of reducing tone in muscle groups above the area braced and, therefore, by reducing tone, improving function – this is the principle of **inhibitive casting**.

Metal and metal–plastic AFOs consist of a shoe or foot attachment, ankle joint and two metal uprights (medial and lateral), with a calf band connected proximally. The mechanical ankle joints can control or assist ankle dorsiflexion or plantarflexion by means of stops (pins) or assists (springs). The mechanical ankle joint also controls mediolateral stability.

KNEE–ANKLE–FOOT ORTHOSES

KAFOs consist of an AFO with metal uprights, a mechanical knee joint and two thigh bands. They can be used in **quadriceps paralysis** or **weakness** to maintain knee stability and control flexible genu valgum or varum. They can be manufactured from metal, e.g. double upright metal KAFO (most common) and Scott–Craig metal KAFO (used for spinal cord injury patients with paraplegia), or from plastic, e.g. ischial weight-bearing KAFO.

TRUNK–HIP–KNEE–ANKLE–FOOT ORTHOSES

A trunk–hip–knee–ankle–foot orthosis (THKAFO) consists of a spinal orthosis in addition to an HKAFO (a hip joint and pelvic band in addition to a KAFO) for control of trunk motion and spinal alignment. A THKAFO is indicated in patients with paraplegia and is very difficult to don and doff. An example is the reciprocating gait orthosis (RGO).

MISCELLANEOUS EXAMPLES

Weight-bearing orthoses

Designed to eliminate weight-bearing through the lower extremities, e.g. PTBO for use in the treatment of diabetic ulcers, neuropathic joints and insensate feet.

Charcot restraint orthotic walker (CROW)

Used in the end-stage foot disease of diabetes, syphilis and leprosy.

Fracture orthoses

Stabilizes the fracture site and promotes callus formation, while allowing weight-bearing and joint movement. Motion at the fracture site is prevented through circumferential compression of the soft tissues (**Sarmiento's hydrostatic compression principle**).

Angular and deformity orthoses

An example is the Denis Brown splint for congenital talipes equinovarus.

Hip orthoses for paediatric disorders

Used to maintain the hip in a flexed and abducted position in order to hold the femoral head within the acetabulum, e.g. Pavlik harness, von Rosen splint. Other types are used to maintain the hip in abduction and keep the femoral head in the acetabulum, e.g. the Scottish Rite, Toronto and non-skeletal-bearing trilateral orthoses.

COMPLICATIONS OF ORTHOSES

Complications can be **psychosocial** (related to the use of an orthosis, particularly any perceived associated stigma) or **physical**. The following are the more common physical complications seen:

- **Compression phenomena:** tight orthoses can encircle limbs, resulting in compression of nerves, arteries and veins, and resulting in pain, paraesthesia, impaired distal circulation and oedema.
- **Heat and water retention:** leading to maceration of skin, impaired wound healing and skin infection, particularly in close-fitting orthoses such as spinal braces.
- **Patient–orthosis interfacial effects:** this interface is defined as the junction between

the body tissues and the orthosis and/or the support surface through which forces are transmitted. Forces may arise at this interface, either because of equal and opposite forces imposed on the body by the support surface (Newton's third law), or because an orthosis has been designed specifically to hold one or more joints in a particular position. These forces may lead to tissue necrosis and skin breakdown, especially if the compressive and shear forces generated are distributed in a non-uniform manner, e.g. over bony prominences with thin overlying subcutaneous tissues (**extrinsic factors**), or if there are contributory patient factors, e.g. decreased skin sensation, decreased level of consciousness, paralysis, dehydration, peripheral vascular disease, malnutrition or systemic disease (**intrinsic factors**). To decrease the pressure effects of an orthosis, the following can be attempted:

- Proper contouring to decrease the tendency of the orthosis to move downwards under gravity.
- Good mechanical design, e.g. leverage to reduce the amount of force exerted on the skin.
- Adequate padding and large contact areas over which the forces can act. Note that a maximal conforming support area will provide a uniform distribution of pressure. This can be applied in two ways. First, the support surface, made of a relatively high modulus material, can be matched in shape to the area of the body it interfaces with, e.g. a spinal brace. Second, the support surface can be flat but made of relatively soft material, which can deform under load, e.g. in seating applications.

Viva questions

1 What is an orthosis?

2 How do orthoses work?

3 Describe this orthosis to me [prop-based question]. How does it work?

4 From what materials are orthoses manufactured?

5 Explain how a GRAFO works.

FURTHER READING

Department of Health and Social Security. *Classification of Orthoses*. London: HMSO, 1980.

Engen, TJ, Lehmkuhl, LD. Lower extremity orthotics. *Curr Orthop* 1989;**3**:194–200.

Jain, AS. Upper limb orthotics. *Curr Orthop* 1990;**4**:259–62.

Morrish, G, Whittle, MW. Spinal orthoses. *Curr Orthop* 1989;**3**:122–7.

Yates, G. A method for the provision of lightweight aesthetic orthopaedic appliances. *Orthopaedics* 1968;**1**:153–62.

29

Inside the operating theatre

MANOJ RAMACHANDRAN AND ALAN WHITE

INTRODUCTION

Joseph Lister wrote in 1867:

> When it had been shown by researchers of Pasteur that the septic property of the atmosphere depended on minute organisms suspended in it, it occurred to me that decomposition in the injured part might be avoided by applying some material capable of destroying the life of the floating particles.

Lister went on to develop his practice of antisepsis, including carbolic acid (phenol) spraying of the air around the operation site, instrument sterilization, and washing of the surgeon's hands. Since Lister's time, much effort has been spent in trying to provide an environment in which orthopaedic surgery, especially joint arthroplasty, can be performed with minimum risk of subsequent infection. This chapter summarizes these efforts and provides a framework for the orthopaedic surgeon when considering the operating theatre environment.

OPERATING THEATRE BASICS

The operating theatre should be located **close to other related facilities**, e.g. the intensive therapy unit (ITU), the accident and emergency (A&E) department, the radiology department, the pathology department and the wards. Areas

of **public circulation** and **non-essential departments** should be **avoided**. Independent orthopaedic theatres are desirable for maintenance of an aseptic environment, efficacy and speed of surgical procedures, and organization of theatre lists.

THEATRE DESIGN

Operating theatres should be of sufficient size to accommodate theatre personnel, the patient and the necessary theatre equipment. Most operating theatres are designed in theatre suites linked by a double or single corridor. It is conventional to think of theatres in four zones:

- The **outer zone** includes the rest of the hospital and theatre reception.
- The **clean zone** comprises the area from the theatre reception up to the theatre doors.
- The **aseptic zone** (Figure 29.1).
- The **disposal zone**.

Theatre design is based around the operating table. Areas that require access to and from the operating table include the anaesthetic room, scrub area, disposal zone and recovery area. To provide optimal conditions for patients and staff, **temperature**, **humidity**, **light** and **ventilation** must all be controlled carefully.

TEMPERATURE AND HUMIDITY

Patients are at risk of **hypothermia** from **paralysis**, **cool intravenous fluids** and large

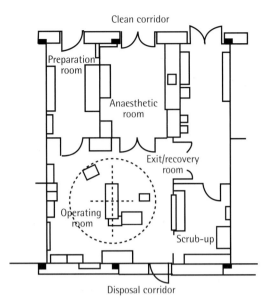

Figure 29.1 *Aseptic zone in the operating theatre.*

exposed wounds. To prevent hypothermia, theatre temperatures of 24–26°C are recommended. However, ideal working temperatures for surgeons are between 19 and 20°C. Therefore, a compromise is achieved by creating a **warm microclimate** for the patient using **warming blankets** or **airflow mattresses**. There is, however, a potential effect on airflow systems in theatre with such devices. Temperature control is particularly important during cementation of arthroplasties, as the temperature affects the polymerization of polymethylmethacrylate cement. Maintaining a constant temperature is also important when operating on young children.

Relative **humidity** in the theatre should be capable of adjustment in the range 40–60 per cent. Both humidity and temperature are controlled most readily by alterations made in the ventilation of the theatre.

ILLUMINATION

High-quality artificial illumination **without shadows** is required in the operating room. The light source should be capable of producing a minimum of 40 000 lux at the incision site. Its direction should be **easily adjustable** by the surgical team. Satellite lights are usually

employed; however, these create heat and subsequent convection currents and may, therefore, alter local airflow patterns.

VENTILATION

A surgical wound can become contaminated from a variety of sources in the operating theatre (Figure 29.2). In general, there are four main sources of infection in the operating room:

- direct contact from the surgical team;
- instruments;
- airborne contamination;
- the patient.

Airborne contamination originates almost exclusively from personnel within the theatre. Ninety-five per cent of wound contamination can be accounted for by the airborne route. An individual may shed 3000–50 000 microorganisms per minute, depending on activity and clothing. Bacteria from the upper respiratory tract (e.g. *Streptococcus*, *Staphylococcus*) are dispersed by, for example, talking and coughing. The skin is regularly contaminated with *Staphylococcus*, which is shed into clothing and the surrounding environment. The axillae and groins are colonized particularly heavily. Ninety per cent of all bacteria emissions come from below the neck level.

It is the role of the ventilatory system in theatres to reduce airborne bacteria to a minimum. The result is judged by the **air cleanliness**, expressed as **bacteria-carrying particles per cubic metre** (BCP/m^3) or **colony-forming units per cubic metre** (CFU/m^3). This is measured most accurately with a **microbiological volumetric slit sampler**, e.g. Casella slit sampler (Casella London Ltd, London, UK), or with settle plates. Slit samplers draw in a set volume of air per minute (30–70 L/min) past culture plates; the plates are incubated for 48 h at 37°C and the colonies formed are counted. According to British Standards, air sampling is recommended in plenum ventilated operating theatres at commissioning or after refurbishing. In ultra-clean operating theatres, air sampling is recommended on a regular basis several times a year (the standard is every 3 months) and should be done inside and outside the enclosed area.

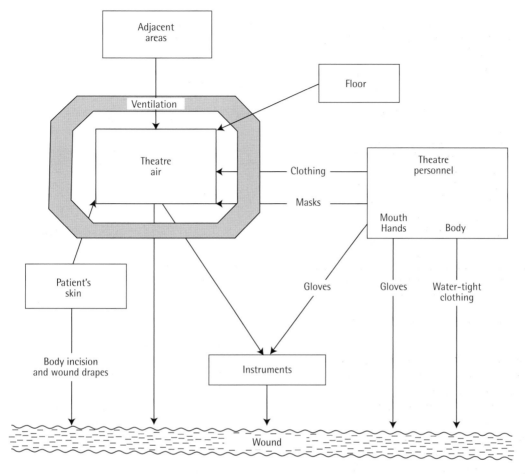

Figure 29.2 *Routes and sources of infection in the operating theatre.*

In terms of definitions of cleanliness, in a standard plenum ventilated operating theatre lying empty, there should be less than 35 CFU of bacteria/m³ of air and less than 1 CFU/m³ of *Clostridium perfringens* and *Staphylococcus aureus*. During operative procedures, there should be less than 180 CFU of bacteria/m³. In ultra-clean laminar flow theatres, there should be less than 20 CFU/m³ at the periphery of the enclosure and less than 10 CFU/m³ at the centre.

VENTILATORY SYSTEMS

To reduce airborne contamination, ventilatory systems must ideally provide a bacteria-free source of air and produce positive pressure to displace contaminated air away from the operational site and to prevent entry of bacteria from contaminated areas.

SOURCE OF AIR FOR VENTILATION

Air is usually taken in at the **roof level** of the theatre suite. It is drawn by a series of **fans** through filters capable of removing bacteria-carrying particles. It is also humidified and warmed or cooled. High-efficiency particulate air (**HEPA**) filters are commonly employed. These are capable of filtering particles of 0.5 microns in size with 99.97 per cent efficiency.

TYPES OF VENTILATORY SYSTEM

Plenum

In this system, pressure inside the theatre is greater than that outside. Clean air is fed via wall or ceiling diffusers and let out of vents paced just above floor level. Air also passes out around doors and other openings. In theory, air from contaminated areas should not enter the aseptic zone. However, the opening of doors and the movement of personnel within theatres makes the system less efficient. For example, opening a standard theatre door transfers 2 m³ of air across the opening, and turbulence is created by such activity. Standard positive-pressure ventilated operating theatres deliver around 15–25 air changes per hour.

Laminar flow

A laminar airflow room is a room in which laminar airflow characteristics predominate throughout the entire air space with a minimum of eddies. **Laminar airflow characteristics involve the entire body of air within a designated space moving with uniform velocity in a single direction along parallel flow lines.** True laminar airflow is not achieved unless there is close to 100 per cent HEPA filter coverage in the ceiling grid system.

There are three main types of theatre air flow:

- horizontal laminar flow;
- vertical laminar flow;
- ex-flow or exponential flow (Howorth enclosures).

However, theatres are usually designed with a vertical downward airflow concept. Only specific processes require horizontal airflow.

It is common for laminar flow to be restricted to an area in the centre of the operating theatre – the **room-within-a-room principle**. The flow of air is around 0.3 m/s and is not perceptible to the individual in the airflow path. The flow is broken around obstructions such as operating lights but quickly reforms.

Horizontal laminar flow

Here, HEPA filters form a wall or part of a wall. The positioning of the scrub team is important, and the use of equipment such as image intensifiers may be restricted (Figure 29.3). Horizontal laminar flow is easier to install than vertical laminar flow in a pre-existing theatre. Of interest, Salvati *et al.* (1982) found that although horizontal laminar

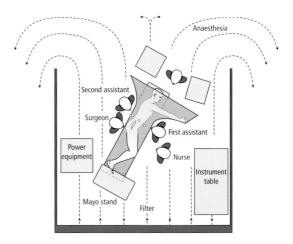

Figure 29.3 *Horizontal laminar flow.*

flow reduced the incidence of deep joint sepsis following total hip arthroplasty, sepsis rates following total knee arthroplasty increased, probably due to difficulties with intra-operative personnel placement.

Vertical laminar flow

An enclosure is formed with panels extending from the ceiling to within 2 m (although this is variable) of the floor. Air is passed through HEPA filters in the ceiling and directed towards the operative field in a vertical direction. Entrainment of the flow, however, can occur from personnel moving within the periphery of the laminar flow area (Figure 29.4). Such entrainment can deflect contamination inwards towards the wound. Full enclosures, however, are free of this problem.

Ex-flow system (Howorth enclosure)

Howorth (1980) described a flow of clean air from the operating theatre in the shape of an inverted trumpet (**exponential flow** or **ex-flow**). The air moves downwards and outwards. Peripheral entrainment therefore cannot occur as with vertical laminar flow systems. This system is theoretically more efficient than laminar flow and, as such, requires fewer changes of air per hour.

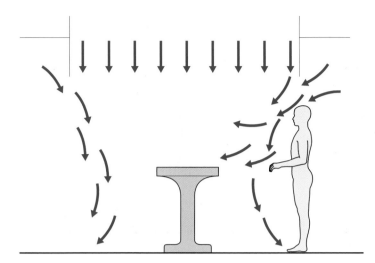

Figure 29.4 *Effect of entrainment on vertical laminar flow.*

CLINICAL EFFECTS OF LAMINAR FLOW

Following the introduction of vertical laminar flow, Charnley (1972) reported a reduction in the incidence of deep infection from 7 per cent to 0.5 per cent in the period 1960–70, during which time 5800 total hip arthroplasties were performed. Charnley attributed the decreased incidence to air factors in combination with better surgical wound closure and surgical apparel. A Medical Research Council (MRC) prospective randomized trial reported by Lidwell *et al.* (1982) confirmed a significant reduction in wound contamination and deep joint sepsis in ultra-clean air theatres and found that vertical laminar flow was more effective than horizontal laminar flow. Certain prophylactic measures (Table 29.1) were also effective in reducing deep joint sepsis.

CLOTHING

The ideal surgical clothing would prevent airborne bacteria dispersion, act as an effective barrier even when wet, and allow air and water vapour circulation. To date, this ideal clothing has not been found. Dispersion of bacteria from clothing may occur at apertures, e.g. at the neck and arm openings; this is significant particularly when combined with local convection currents set up by the radiation of

Table 29.1 Prophylactic measures identified by the Medical Research Council (MRC) trial (1982)

Prophylactic measure	Factor by which deep joint sepsis was reduced
Antibiotic-loaded cement	*11*
Systemic antibiotics	*4.8*
Ultra-clean air	*2.6*
Plastic isolators	*2.2*
Body exhaust suit	*2.2*

body heat. Direct migration of bacteria may occur through clothing, especially when wet; this is known as **moist bacterial strike-through**.

CLOTHING TYPES

Standard (balloon–) cotton clothing

This is **comfortable**, as it is made of an **open weave**, which allows for easy air circulation. However, the pore size is 80 microns and it is therefore inefficient at preventing migration of bacteria-carrying particles. **Moist bacterial strike-through** is a particular problem.

Ventile™

This is cotton product with a **close weave**, giving a pore size of 20 microns. It is effective in reducing bacterial dispersion but is **uncomfortable** to wear as it inhibits air circulation. It has also been employed as a **front pad** to prevent moist bacterial strike-through from the abdominal and lower thoracic areas of the surgeon.

Gore-Tex™

This is woven polyester laminated to a film of polytetrafluoroethylene (PTFE). The **open structure** allows for air exchange, but the pore size of 0.2 microns acts as an **effective barrier**. Dispersion via neck and arm apertures still occurs, and therefore Gore-Tex suits with seals at the neck and arms must be worn. However, such garments tend to be uncomfortable during prolonged procedures.

Disposable non-woven clothing

This is the most common type of surgical gown used in joint arthroplasty. These fabrics, e.g. spun laced fibres, are **unwoven** and appear microscopically as a random mat. Bacteria tend to get entrapped within the fibres. Because of its open structure, air circulation is not impeded. Unfortunately, these gowns are single-use only and therefore are expensive, although the overall cost may be beneficial when compared with reusable cotton gowns.

Body exhaust systems

These work by maintaining a **negative pressure** within the gown, which prevents the admission of bacteria-carrying particles by the wearer. In Charnley's all-enveloping gown and mask, air is drawn off at the helmet by a body exhaust unit. As the gown–helmet system is impermeable, air is drawn in around the operator's legs and passes over the body, cooling the operator. Operators communicate via a special audio system. Disadvantages include feelings of claustrophobia and inability to use microscopes. A variation in the Charnley body exhaust system is the **neck lace and mandarin gown**, which exclude the head of the operator. This system works on the basis that 90 per cent of bacteria-carrying particles are admitted below neck level.

CLINICAL EFFECTS OF CLOTHING

The MRC trial showed a 50 per cent reduction in deep joint sepsis in operations performed in ultra-clean-air theatres. A further 25 per cent reduction was achieved by combining ultra-clean operating theatres with body exhaust systems. The lowest incidence of all (0.06 per cent) was achieved using ultra-clean air, body exhaust systems and antibiotics. The effects of these variables were found to be independent and cumulative.

SURGICAL DRAPES

Skin preparation with antiseptics is augmented by the use of isolation drapes, of which there are three types:

- **Body drapes:** disposable non-woven drapes are preferred in theory to traditional cotton fabrics, for the reasons given in the previous section.
- **Incisional drapes:** these have been adopted widely, chiefly in order to hold down the surgical drapes. There is no evidence that their use reduces the rate of wound infection. If incisional drapes are employed, then it is important that they remain adherent to the wound edge throughout the operation.
- **Wound-edge drapes:** these cover the incised wound. Bacteria persisting in the wound edge may lead to subsequent wound contamination. These drapes are not currently used in orthopaedics.

MASKS AND GLOVES

MASKS

Theatre air may be contaminated by micro-organisms liberated from the upper respiratory tract of theatre personnel. The level of air contamination caused, however, is low compared with that produced from the skin of the same individual. Even so, **all members of the surgical team** must wear masks when operating on trauma and orthopaedic cases. The main purpose is to protect the wound from direct contamination and, in particular, the projectile effects of talking and breathing. Masks should be **changed after each operation**, as they are easily contaminated. There is no evidence to suggest that there is any need for non-scrubbed personnel to wear masks if they are not in the operating area, but the British Orthopaedic Association (BOA) guidelines recommend that all theatre personnel wear masks during orthopaedic operations.

GLOVES

Gloves are worn to **protect the surgical wound** from contamination by any residual bacteria remaining after the surgical scrub. They also function to **protect the surgeon** from haematogenous spread of viral disease. **Glove perforation** during orthopaedic procedures has been recorded to be as high as 40 per cent. **Surface colonization** of gloves during joint arthroplasty has also been noted. For these reasons, **double gloving** together with the changing of top gloves before implant handling is advocated. In addition, there is a significant incidence of contamination of glove tips at the end of skin preparation. Gloves should, therefore, be changed before making the skin incision, or the incision site must be prepared separately, before draping the patient.

Viva questions

1 What is the layout of an operating theatre department?

2 What are the main sources of infection in an operating theatre environment?

3 What different types of ventilatory system are used in theatres?

4 What factors can be altered in operating theatres in order to help reduce the incidence of deep joint sepsis following joint arthroplasty?

5 What is moist bacterial strike-through? How can it be prevented?

FURTHER READING

British Orthopaedic Association. *British Orthopaedic Association Recommendation on Sterile Procedures in Operating Theatres.* London: British Orthopaedic Association, 1995. www.boa.ac.uk/PDF%20files/Sterile%20Procedures%20in%20Operating%20Theatres.pdf.

Charnley, J. Postoperative infection after total hip replacement with special reference to air contamination in the operating room. *Clin Orthop Relat Res* 1972;**87**:167–87.

Howorth, FH. Air flow patterns in the operating theatre. *Eng Med* 1980;**9**:87–92.

Lidwell, OM, Lowbury, EJ, Whyte, W, *et al.* Effect of ultraclean air in operating rooms on deep sepsis in the joint after total hip or knee replacement: a randomised study. *Br Med J (Clin Res Ed)* 1982;**285**:10–14.

Salvati, EA, Robinson, RP, Zeno, SM, *et al.* Infection rates after 3175 total hip and total knee replacements performed with and without a horizontal unidirectional filtered air-flow system. *J Bone Joint Surg Am* 1982;**64**:525–35.

Appendix

Common bone disorders

PETER BATES AND MANOJ RAMACHANDRAN

A detailed understanding of the breadth of disorders affecting bone is vital for the orthopaedic surgeon. In this appendix, some of these disorders (excluding fractures) are covered in detail in systematic note form, allowing the reader to review rapidly the pertinent facts. The following definitions are worth committing to memory:

> **Metabolic bone disease:** generalized disorder of skeletal homeostasis.
> **Osteopenia:** radiological appearance of decreased bone density. The term is neither a disease nor a diagnosis, and implies no aetiology.
> **Osteoporosis:** state of decreased mass per unit volume (density) of normally mineralized bone matrix. When this decrease produces an increased risk of skeletal fracture, pathological osteoporosis exists.
> **Osteomalacia:** increased, normal or decreased mass of insufficiently mineralized bone.

DISORDERS OF BONE MINERALIZATION

HYPERCALCAEMIA

Symptoms and signs

- May be **asymptomatic**.
- **Bones:** excessive bone resorption.
- **Stones (renal):** polyuria, polydipsia, dehydration, kidney stones.
- **Groans (gastrointestinal):** constipation, anorexia, nausea, vomiting.
- **Psychic moans (central nervous system, CNS):** confusion, stupor.

- **Other effects:** stiff joints, myopathy, hypertension.

Causes

1. Primary hyperparathyroidism

AETIOLOGY

- Solitary parathyroid adenoma (80 per cent).
- Parathyroid hyperplasia (15 per cent).
- Multiple parathyroid adenomas (4 per cent).
- Parathyroid carcinoma (1 per cent).

EFFECTS

- **Plasma calcium** is **high** from all three sources (gut, kidney, bone).
- **Plasma phosphate** is **low** due to increased renal excretion.
- Result is **bone resorption** and **inadequate repair** (due to lack of phosphate).

SYMPTOMS AND SIGNS

- Of hypercalcaemia.

ELECTROCARDIOGRAM (ECG)

- Decreased Q-T interval

BLOODS

- High calcium.
- High parathyroid hormone (PTH).
- Low phosphate.

URINE

- High phosphate.

X-RAYS

- Predilection for **cortical bone** (cancellous-sparing).

- **Osteopenia**.
- Osteitis fibrosa et cystica, or **brown tumours** (fibrous marrow changes).
- **Subperiosteal resorption** (especially radial borders of proximal phalanges and tufts of distal phalanges; also seen at the medial end of clavicle, femoral neck and upper tibia).
- **Pepper-pot skull** (diffuse multiple areas of resorption).
- **Chondrocalcinosis** and **metastatic calcification** of soft tissues.
- **Loss of lamina dura around the teeth** is specific.

HISTOLOGY

- Within brown tumours, increased giant cells and fibrous tissue with haemosiderin staining is seen.
- Osteoblasts and osteoclasts active on both sides of trabeculae (as in Paget's disease), with widened osteoid seams.

2. Malignancy

- Humoral hypercalcaemia of malignancy:
  - secretion of PTH-related protein;
  - especially squamous lung carcinoma.
- Solid tumours with bone metastases, e.g. breast, kidney, thyroid, prostate:
  - cytokine-related effects [e.g. interleukin 1 (IL-1), interleukin 6 (IL-6), tumour necrosis factor alpha (TNF-α)] via activation of osteoclasts.
- Haematological malignancy:
  - clonal plasma cells resorb bone in multiple myeloma via cytokine-related effects;
  - lymphomas can synthesize 1,25(OH)$_2$ D3.

3. Less common causes of hypercalcaemia

- **Familial:**
  - pituitary adenomas in multiple endocrine neoplasia (MEN) I and II:
    - MEN I: pancreatic and pituitary tumours;
    - MEN II: thyroid medullary carcinoma of the thyroid and bilateral phaeochromocytomas;
  - familial hypocalciuric hypercalcaemia (defect in calcium-sensing receptor, leading to poor renal clearance of calcium).

- **Endocrinopathies:**
  - hyperthyroidism;
  - Addison's disease.
- **Exogenous:**
  - vitamin D excess;
  - steroid administration.
- **Metabolic:** milk-alkali syndrome.
- **Granulomas (synthesize 1,25(OH)$_2$ D3):** sarcoidosis.
- **Tertiary hyperparathyroidism:** occurs after prolonged primary hyperparathyroidism, where the glands act autonomously, secreting excess PTH, which results in hypercalcaemia. Treatment is the same as for primary hyperparathyroidism.

Note that in **secondary hyperparathyroidism**, there is excess PTH as an appropriate response for low calcium – this is seen in dietary vitamin D deficiency and renal osteodystrophy in chronic renal failure (see below).

Treatment

- Treat underlying cause.
- Rehydration with normal saline (saline diuresis).
- Loop diuretics with or without dialysis (severe cases).
- Specific pharmacotherapy.
- Bisphosphonates (to inhibit osteoclastic activity).
- Chemotherapy in malignancy, e.g. mithramycin.

HYPOCALCAEMIA

Low PTH and low vitamin D can both lead to hypocalcaemia.

Symptoms and signs

Acute

- **Neuromuscular irritability:**
  - tetany;
  - seizures;
  - Chvostek's sign (tapping over parotid gland in region of facial nerve causes muscle twitches);
  - Trousseau's sign (carpopedal spasm if brachial artery occluded with blood-pressure cuff).

- Depression.
- ECG shows prolonged Q-T interval.

Chronic

- Cataracts.
- Fungal nail infections.

Causes

1. Hypoparathyroidism

AETIOLOGY

- Usually iatrogenic following thyroidectomy.

EFFECTS

- Decreased PTH leads to low plasma calcium and high plasma phosphate.
- Alkaline phosphatase normal.

SYMPTOMS AND SIGNS

- Of hypocalcaemia.
- Vitiligo, hair loss.

TREATMENT

- Vitamin D analogues, e.g. alfacalcidol.

2. Pseudo–hypoparathyroidism (PHP)

AETIOLOGY

- Rare hereditary disorder due to failure of target cell response to PTH.
- Pathology can be:
  - PTH receptor abnormality;
  - signalling abnormality, e.g. cyclic adenosine monophosphate (cAMP) defect, G-protein abnormality;
  - lack of necessary cofactors, e.g. magnesium.
- One form of PHP, Albright hereditary osteodystrophy, presents with (use the mnemonic BORESS):
  - brachydactyly: short first, fourth and fifth metacarpals and metatarsals;
  - obesity;
  - reduced intelligence;
  - exostoses;
  - skull X-rays show basal ganglia calcification;
  - subcutaneous ossification.

EFFECTS

- Increased PTH but low calcium.
- Increased phosphate.
- Normal or increased alkaline phosphatase.

Note that in pseudo-pseudo-hypoparathyroidism, the same clinical features as in PHP are present but biochemistry is normal and there is a normal response to PTH.

3. Renal osteodystrophy

DEFINITION

A group of disorders of bone mineral metabolism seen in chronic renal failure.

AETIOLOGY

HIGH-TURNOVER RENAL BONE DISEASE

- **Uraemia** and **phosphate retention** from glomerular dysfunction.
- **High plasma phosphate** leads to hypocalcaemia by:
  - impairing synthesis of $1,25\ (OH)_2$ vitamin D_3 by inhibiting renal 1-α hydroxylase (note that synthesis of the renal vitamin D metabolite is also directly impaired by tubular damage in renal failure);
  - direct lowering of calcium, which stimulates PTH secretion;
  - direct stimulation of PTH secretion.
- Low serum calcium produces **secondary hyperparathyroidism** (and ultimately hyperplasia of the chief cells of the parathyroid gland and **tertiary hyperparathyroidism**).
- As renal function deteriorates, acidosis exacerbates the negative calcium balance.

LOW-TURNOVER RENAL BONE DISEASE

- Slowed bone formation and turnover (**adynamic** lesion of bone).
- Slowed mineralization (osteomalacia).
- **Aluminium deposition** (impaired renal excretion) produces osteomalacia:
  - inhibition of proliferation and differentiation of osteoblasts;
  - inhibition of PTH release from parathyroid gland.
- **No secondary hyperparathyroidism.**

EFFECTS

- Hypocalcaemia:
  - rickets or osteomalacia;
  - osteoporosis.
- Slipped upper femoral epiphysis in children.
- Secondary hyperparathyroidism:
  - osteitis fibrosa et cystica (bone-marrow replacement by fibrous tissue);
  - osteosclerosis (20 per cent of cases):
    - from secondary hyperparathyroidism and increased osteoblast activity;
    - lucent and dense bands in the spine ('rugger-jersey spine');
  - metastatic calcification: calcium and phosphate solubility may be affected, producing ectopic calcification in the conjunctivae, blood vessels, skin and periarticular tissues.
- Amyloidosis:
  - as a result of beta-2 microglobulin from chronic dialysis;
  - clinical effects include pathological fractures (from amyloid deposits – amyloidomas), arthropathy, carpal tunnel syndrome;
  - diagnosis made on histology by staining amyloid pink with Congo red stain.

LABORATORY CHANGES

- Raised serum urea and creatinine.
- Normal to low serum calcium and high phosphate.
- Raised alkaline phosphatase (osteoblasts) and high PTH levels.

DIAGNOSIS

Tetracycline-labelled bone biopsy.

MANAGEMENT (PREDOMINANTLY MEDICAL)

- Adjust serum phosphate to normal:
  - reduce dietary phosphate (less milk, cheese and eggs);
  - phosphate binders, e.g. calcium carbonate.
- Adjust serum calcium to normal:
  - increase calcium absorption with $1,25(OH)_2$ D3;
  - calcium supplementation.
- Suppress secondary hyperparathyroidism with $1,25(OH)_2$ D3 (or may require parathyroidectomy).

- Chelate bone aluminium in cases of aluminium retention (with desferrioxamine).
- Manage chronic renal failure with dialysis or renal transplant.

4. Osteomalacia/rickets

DEFINITION AND SUMMARY

Osteomalacia is **deficient** or **impaired mineralization** of bone matrix (osteoid). **Rickets** is the **juvenile form**, with **impaired mineralization** of cartilage matrix (chondroid), affecting the physis in the zone of provisional calcification.

The common causative factor in all aetiologies is inadequate serum calcium and phosphorus level to allow mineralization of newly formed osteoid/chondroid. Treatments are aimed at restoring calcium and phosphate levels to normal so that mineralization can occur.

AETIOLOGY

DIETARY DEFICIENCY

- Calcium or vitamin D deficiency.
- Dietary chelators (phytates in chapattis, oxalates in spinach).
- Phosphorus deficiency (aluminium-containing antacid abuse).

GASTROINTESTINAL MALABSORPTION

- Post-gastrectomy.
- Biliary disease.
- Intestinal defects.
- Short bowel syndrome, coeliac disease, Crohn's disease.

RENAL TUBULAR DEFECTS (LOSS OF PHOSPHATE)

- **Hypophosphataemic vitamin D-resistant rickets/osteomalacia:**
  - most common form of rickets;
  - X-linked dominant (mutation in P-EX gene);
  - impaired renal tubular reabsorption of phosphate;
  - characteristic deformity of bilateral symmetrical anterolateral femoral and tibial bowing;
  - normal glomerular filtration rate but reduced vitamin D response;
  - radiographs resemble ankylosing spondylitis, with ligamentous calcification and ossification (enthesiopathy);

- phosphate replacement and high-dose vitamin D3 necessary.
- **Multiple renal tubular defects leading to aminoaciduria (Fanconi's syndrome):**
  - inherited, e.g. cystinosis;
  - acquired, e.g. multiple myeloma.
- **Renal tubular acidosis:**
  - inherited:
    - proximal (bicarbonate wastage);
    - distal (H^+ gradient defect);
  - acquired: ureterosigmoid anastomosis.

RENAL OSTEODYSTROPHY
See above.

HEREDITARY VITAMIN D-DEPENDENT RICKETS (TYPES I AND II)
Very rare.

- Clinically severe rickets with alopecia totalis, epidermal cysts and oligodontia.
- Inherited defect of $25(OH)_2$ vitamin D_3 hydroxylation:
  - Type I:
    - renal 1α-hydroxylase deficiency;
    - autosomal recessive (chromosome 12q14).
  - Type II:
    - end-organ insensitivity to $1,25 (OH)_2$ vitamin D3;
    - abnormality in nuclear receptor.

HYPOPHOSPHATASIA
- Autosomal recessive disorder of phosphate synthesis.
- Due to low levels of alkaline phosphatase.
- Increased urine phosphoethanolamine is diagnostic.
- Trend towards distinguishing hypophosphatasia as a clinical entity separate from osteomalacia.

MISCELLANEOUS
- Oncogenic osteomalacia (haemangiopericytomas, non-ossifying fibroma, fibrous dysplasia, neurofibromatosis).
- Anticonvulsant medication (phenytoin, phenobarbital).
- High-dose bisphosphonates.
- Heavy-metal overdose.
- Chronic alcoholism.

RICKETS

CLINICAL
GENERAL
- Retarded bone growth and short stature.
- Pathological fractures (Looser's zones on compression side).
- Symptoms of hypocalcaemia (see above).
- Proximal myopathy (vitamin D receptors present in skeletal muscle).

FROM SKULL TO TOE
- Delayed fontanelle closure and frontal and parietal bossing.
- Dental disease.
- Enlargement of costochondral junction (rachitic rosary).
- Harrison's sulcus (indentation of lower ribs at diaphragm insertion).
- Centrally depressed 'codfish vertebrae', dorsal kyphosis ('cat back').
- Bowing of the knees, 'sabre shin'.
- Waddling gait

BLOODS
- Increased PTH; therefore, low normal calcium and low phosphate.
- Low vitamin D levels.

X-RAYS
- Physeal increase in height and width (continues to grow but cannot mineralize).
- Metaphyseal cupping, flaring and jagged appearance.
- Small ossific nuclei.
- Coxa vara.
- Flattening of the skull.

OSTEOMALACIA

PLAIN X-RAYS
- Looser's zones (microscopic stress fractures on concave border of long bones).
- Milkman pseudo-fracture on compression side of long bones (fractures that have healed but not mineralized).
- Biconcave vertebral bodies – can lead to severe kyphosis.
- Thin cortices; indistinct, fuzzy trabeculae.
- Triradiate pelvis.
- Signs of hyperparathyroidism.

BONE BIOPSY (TRANSILIAC)
- Widened osteoid seams.
- Tetracycline labels abnormal.

DISORDERS OF BONE MINERAL DENSITY

OSTEOPOROSIS

World Health Organization (WHO) definition, 1994

A skeletal disease characterized by **low bone mass per unit volume** and **deterioration** of the **micro-architecture** of bone tissue, with a consequent increase in **bone fragility** and susceptibility to **low-trauma fractures** (vertebral most common).

Diagnosis

Estimation of bone mineral density is measured against the population mean in young adults:

Normal bone mineral density is within 1 standard deviation (SD) of that mean.
Osteopenia is considered 1–2.5 SD below the mean.

Osteoporosis is considered >2.5 SD below the mean.

The **T-score** is the number of standard deviations below the mean for a sex- and race-matched healthy young adult population (aged 25–35 years).

The **Z-score** is the number of standard deviations below the mean for an age-, sex- and race-matched young adult population.

These values are guidelines rather than diagnostic standards. It is important to differentiate between osteomalacia and osteoporosis (Table A.1).

Risk factors

Age
- The normal ageing process, in which men and women are almost equivalent.
- With each decade, there is a 1.4–1.8-fold increased risk.

Oestrogen deficiency
- Oestrogen appears to block the action of PTH on osteoclasts and marrow stromal cells, thereby preventing bone loss.

Table A.1 Osteoporosis versus osteomalacia

	Osteoporosis	Osteomalacia
Definition	*Bone mass decreased, mineralization normal*	*Bone mass variable, mineralization deficient*
Age of onset	*Elderly, postmenopausal*	*Any age*
Aetiology (examples)	*Idiopathic, age-related, endocrine abnormality, disuse, alcoholism, calcium deficient*	*Vitamin D deficiency, abnormality of vitamin D pathway, hypophosphatasia, renal failure*
Symptoms	*Pain when fractures occur*	*Generalized bone pain*
Laboratory tests	*Serum Ca normal*	*Serum Ca low or normal (high in hypophosphatasia)*
	Serum PO_4 normal	*Serum PO_4 low or normal*
	ALP normal	*ALP elevated (unless hypophosphatasia)*
	Urinary Ca high or normal	*Urinary Ca normal or low (high in hypophosphatasia)*
Bone biopsy	*Tetracycline labels normal*	*Tetracycline labels abnormal*

ALP, alkaline phosphatase.

- Oestrogen levels in women may fall below those in age-matched men following menopause.
- Early menopause confers greater risk.

Genetic factors

- Ethnicity: people of northern European and Far Eastern descent are at greater risk than black people and people of Polynesian descent.
- Family history.
- Low body mass index (BMI) (<19 kg/m^2).

Environmental/lifestyle factors

- Nutrition:
  - Low calcium intake and absorption are associated strongly with fracture risk.
  - Anorexia and excessive exercise leading to amenorrhoea at a relatively young age reduce peak bone mass.
- Breastfeeding.
- Sedentary lifestyle or immobilization: mechanical loading inhibits resorption.
- Smoking.
- Excess alcohol.

Drugs

- Chronic corticosteroid therapy.
- Excessive thyroxine.
- Anticoagulants, e.g. heparin.
- Anticonvulsants, e.g. phenytoin.
- Chemotherapy.

Chronic disease

- Chronic kidney, lung or gastrointestinal disease.
- Liver cirrhosis.
- Hyperthyroidism.
- Hyperparathyroidism.
- Cushing's disease.
- Rheumatoid arthritis.
- Malignancy, e.g. multiple myeloma.

Clinical factors

- Previous history of fragility fracture (wrist, hip, vertebra).
- Loss of height, kyphosis.
- Osteopenia or loss of vertebral morphology on plain X-ray.
- Strong family history of osteoporosis or fragility fractures.

Pathophysiology

The two major determinants in the development of osteoporosis are:

- peak bone mass (usually achieved in the third decade of life);
- rate of bone loss thereafter.

Histology

Bone resorption is greater than bone formation:

- **Cancellous bone:** trabeculae are thinned and decreased in number. Some are lost completely. This loss of bony struts leaves adjacent areas unsupported and therefore significantly weakened.
- **Cortical bone:** decreased size of osteons and enlargement of marrow space. The cortices of long bones become thinner with age, while the overall bone diameter expands.

Management

History

- Risk factors.
- Symptoms of fractures.

Examination

- Kyphosis (dowager's hump).
- Hip and distal radius fractures.

Plain X-ray

- More than 30 per cent bone loss is required to be seen on X-ray, making subjective osteopenia an insensitive test.
- Old wedge fractures may be seen in the thoracolumbar spine:
  - anterior wedging;
  - centrally depressed 'codfish' vertebrae.

Blood tests

- Full blood count (FBC), erythrocyte sedimentation rate (ESR), biochemistry, bone profile, thyroid function.
- Prostate-specific antigen (PSA), testosterone and gonadotrophin levels in men.
- Serum PTH (hyperparathyroidism).
- 25(OH)-D$_3$ levels (vitamin D body stores).

- Plasma electrophoresis (multiple myeloma).
- Urinary free cortisol (Cushing's disease).

Bone biomarkers

- Serum bone-specific alkaline phosphatase (osteoblast activity).
- Serum osteocalcin (bone matrix protein).
- Collagen degradation products in urine (bone resorption):
  - telopeptides, i.e. amino-terminal cross-linked telopeptides of collagen I (NTx), carboxy-terminal cross-linked telopeptides of collagen I (CTx);
  - pyridinolines.

Transiliac bone biopsy

- Tetracycline-labelled biopsy to exclude osteomalacia, e.g. in young osteopenic patients and in chronic renal failure.

Bone mineral density (g/cm²)

This is measured in the vertebra, hip and wrist. It is the gold-standard clinical test for osteoporosis and its response to treatment.
- **Dual-energy X-ray absorptiometry (DEXA):**
  - Twin X-ray beams of different energies are passed through the chosen bone and their emerging strength is measured.
  - Low radiation, accurate, quick, simple to perform.
  - Can be performed on the hip or vertebra (most predictive of fracture) or wrist.
  - According to current treatment guidelines from the British Orthopaedic Association:
    - if over age 75 years and one insufficiency fracture, start treatment;
    - if under age 75 years and one insufficiency fracture, order DEXA scan;
    - scanning also recommended for patients on corticosteroids.
- **Quantitative computed tomography (CT):**
  - The vertebra is scanned alongside an artificial phantom, and the two are compared.
  - Measurements are taken from the centres of T12 to L4, and a mean is calculated.
  - Precision and accuracy are good, but cost and radiation dose are much higher than with DEXA.

- **Quantitative ultrasound:**
  - Non-invasive, inexpensive, portable, no radiation dose.
  - Still relatively experimental, and not used to diagnose osteoporosis.

Prevention

- Avoid risk factors: avoid smoking, avoid excess alcohol, avoid drug abuse, adequate diet, prevention of falls.
- Encourage load-bearing exercise in young women.
- Monitor patients on corticosteroid treatment and with strong family history.

Treatment

PREVENT BONE LOSS

- **Calcium and vitamin D with physical activity:**
  - Decreases bone resorption but does not increase bone mass or density.
  - Minimum recommended daily amount (RDA) should be achieved:
    - RDA calcium = 1400 mg;
    - RDA vitamin D = 600–800 IU.
  - Adding 500 mg Ca and 700 IU vitamin D reduces fractures by 50 per cent over 3 years in people over age 65 years (Dawson-Hughes, B, Harris, SS, Krall, EA, Dallal, GE. Effect of calcium and vitamin D supplementation on bone density in men and women 65 years of age or older. *New Engl J Med* 1997;**337**:670–6).
- **Oestrogen therapy (hormone-replacement therapy, HRT):**
  - Helps to decrease bone resorption and slow progression of osteoporosis, but does not increase bone mass.
  - Should be initiated within 6 years of menopause.
  - Risks of cardiovascular side effects and breast malignancy.
- **Bisphosphonates:**
  - See Chapter 4.
  - Shown to dramatically reduce fragility fractures when given weekly.
  - Newer bisphosphonates may be given less frequently, e.g. ibandronate (every 3 months) and zoledronic acid (once a year).

- **Calcitonin:**
  - See Chapter 4.
  - Inhibits osteoclastic resorption in the short term, but bone mass stabilizes in the long term.
  - Significant side effects are a problem, e.g. nausea, flushing, vomiting, anti-salmon antibodies.
- **Selective oestrogen receptor modulators, e.g. raloxifene:**
  - Work like oestrogen to prevent bone loss but may enhance menopausal symptoms, so not indicated within 5 years of menopause.
  - Good evidence for vertebral but not hip fractures.
- Various combination therapies.

STIMULATE BONE FORMATION

- **Physical activity.**
- **Sodium fluoride:**
  - Stimulates osteoblastic activity but not shown to reduce fracture rate (although slow-release fluoride may be better).
  - Significant side effects are a problem, e.g. gastrointestinal symptoms, distal tibial stress fractures as bone formed may be abnormal.
- **Teriparatide (recombinant PTH):**
  - See Chapter 4.
  - Licensed in subcutaneous form for women with postmenopausal osteoporosis.
  - Reduces likelihood of both vertebral (by 65 per cent) and non-vertebral (by 53 per cent) fractures.
- **Strontium:**
  - See Chapter 4.
  - Increases bone formation and decreases bone resorption.
  - Excellent for reducing risk of both vertebral and non-vertebral fractures.

OSTEOPETROSIS (MARBLE BONE DISEASE)

Group of disorders characterized by increased bony sclerosis loss of medullary canal caused by impaired osteoclast function.

Histology

- Osteoclasts lack the ruffled border required for effective resorption.
- Marrow spaces filled with necrotic calcified cartilage.

Types

- Autosomal recessive infantile or 'malignant' form is most severe.
- Autosomal dominant benign form (Albers-Schönberg disease).

PAGET'S DISEASE OF BONE

Epidemiology

- Age >40 years: 3 per cent prevalence.
- Age >80 years: 10 per cent prevalence.
- Strong geographical prevalence (high in UK and USA; rare in Scandinavia and Asia), especially mining communities, e.g. Lancashire, UK.
- Familial history (15–30 per cent of cases).
- Increased incidence in HLA-DQw1.
- No racial differences in incidence.
- Slight male preponderance.
- Monostotic 17 per cent, polyostotic 83 per cent.

Aetiology

- Probably **viral** (paramyxovirus, e.g. measles, respiratory syncitial virus): osteoclasts contain viral-like inclusion bodies.
- **Genetic** predisposition: chromosome focus for familial expansile osteolysis, an analogous disease, has been found.

Pathophysiology

- **Increased osteoclast size** and **number,** leading to **increased bone resorption.**
- This is followed by a **compensatory increase** (up to 40 times) in **disorganized osteoblastic bone formation,** i.e. accelerated and chaotic process of bone turnover and remodelling.

Phases

Use the mnemonic 'LAB'.

- **Lytic phase:** a 'front' of osteoclastic resorption is seen, usually near the metaphyseal region of a long bone or osteoporosis circumscripta in the skull.
- **Active phase:** both osteoclastic resorption and osteoblastic bone formation occur in the same area of bone. Bone is laid down in chaotic fashion, leading to areas of sclerosis and areas of relative osteopenia.
- **Burnt-out phase:** a dense mosaic pattern of bone is seen, with little cellular activity.

Histology

- Multiple resorbing and forming surfaces are characteristic with mosaic appearance.
- The chaotic process produces disorganization of collagen fibrils, making the matrix brittle and susceptible to pathological fracture and deformity.
- The marrow becomes fibrous, with scanty marrow cells.
- Fracture healing in pagetic bone is slower than normal.

Diagnosis

Clinical

- Usually **asymptomatic** (95 per cent).
- **Bone pain** unrelated to activity, and often worse at night.
- **Secondary osteoarthritis** in joints affected by Paget's disease in supporting bone.
- **Pathological fracture**, e.g. femoral neck.
- **Deformity**, e.g. bowing of long bones, enlargement of the skull ('tam-o'-shanter' or large soft beret).
- **Nerve compression:**
  - conductive hearing loss due to temporal bone enlargement;
  - basilar invagination;
  - spinal stenosis or cauda equina syndrome (exacerbated by steal syndrome).
- Vascular shunting leading to **high-output cardiac failure**.
- **Gout** (increased nucleic acid turnover).

- **Osteosarcoma** – suspect this when a previously asymptomatic lesion becomes painful.

Plain X-rays

EARLY

- Lytic areas in any bone.
- Metaphyses of long bones – candle-flame areas of porosis (flame or arrow sign).
- Osteoporosis circumscripta in the skull.

LATER

- **Cortices** become **thickened**, sclerotic and irregular.
- **Loss** of **corticomedullary differentiation.**
- **Loss** of **normal bony architecture, coarse trabeculae.**
- **Widened bones** and bowing.
- Disease progression from one end of a bone (usually proximal).
- **Fissure fracture** (on the convex side of long bones).

Laboratory tests

- Raised serum alkaline phosphatase (marker of osteoblast activity).
- Raised serum acid phosphatase (marker of osteoclast activity).
- Raised urine hydroxyproline and collagen-derived cross-linked peptides (marker of collagen turnover).

Bone scintigraphy

- Hot spots seen in areas of active Paget's disease (occasionally with cold areas centrally due to necrosis).
- Only 65 per cent of lesions seen on bone scan will be seen on X-ray.

Indications for medical treatment of Paget's disease

- Bone pain and deformity.
- Before orthopaedic surgery (e.g. arthroplasty) in order to reduce bleeding.
- Pagetic spinal stenosis or nerve entrapment.
- Prevention of fracture or deformity in severe osteolytic cases and in young patients.
- Secondary high-output cardiac failure.

Treatment

- Open reduction and internal fixation for fractures.
- Due to slow bone healing.
- Osteotomy or arthroplasty for secondary degenerative joint disease.
- Calcitonin: not used frequently.
- Bisphosphonates (alendronate/etidronate/pamidronate): taken for 2–3 months before elective surgery.

Malignant sarcomatous change

- Up to 30 times increased risk of osteogenic sarcoma (1–6 per cent of all patients with Paget's disease).
- Usually in diffuse, long-standing, polyostotic disease.
- 50 per cent are osteogenic.
- Less commonly, fibrosarcoma, chondrosarcoma and giant-cell tumour.
- Prognosis very poor.

OSTEONECROSIS (ON)

Definition

Death of the cell population within a segment of bone following loss of blood circulation. Organic and inorganic components of the matrix are unaffected, but the cells die.

Clinical features

- **Age:** 20–50 years (average 38 years).
- **Site (descending order of frequency):**
  - femoral head
  - medial femoral condyle;
  - humeral head;
  - talus;
  - lunate (Keinbock's disease);
  - capitellum (Panner's disease);
  - metatarsal heads (Freiberg's infraction);
  - tarsal navicular (Kohler's disease).
- **Symptoms:**
  - Slow insidious onset of pain, starting initially on exercise and later at rest/at night.
  - Pain may subside after 6–8 weeks.
  - Pain may precede X-ray changes by many weeks.
  - Early sign in the hip is loss of internal rotation.

Pathogenesis

- **Idiopathic (40 per cent):** half of these are bilateral.
- **Arterial disruption:** fracture (acute or stress fracture), dislocation or infection.
- **Arteriolar occlusion:** thrombosis, embolism, sickle cell crisis, Caisson disease (nitrogen bubbles from acute decompression).
- **Vessel-wall damage:** vasculitis (systemic lupus erythematosus, SLE), irradiation.
- **Capillary occlusion from fatty infiltration:**
  - steroid treatment: >30 mg prednisolone for >30 days carries 37 per cent risk, 80 per cent bilateral;
  - high alcohol intake: 20 per cent;
  - Gaucher's disease: marrow cavity packed with Gaucher's macrophages filled with cerebroside;
  - pancreatitis;
  - hyperlipidaemia;
  - other: renal transplant, haematological malignancies, diabetes, sepsis, inflammatory bowel disease.

Aetiology

The actual mechanism of ischaemia leading to osteonecrosis is not understood fully in most cases. Proposed mechanisms include:

- **Intraosseous hypertension:** 'compartment syndrome of bone' – increased pressure found within bones with early ON, but it is not clear whether this is a cause or effect.
- **Abnormal extra-osseous blood flow:** loss of transcortical blood flow has been demonstrated in pre-radiographically defined ON.
- **Fat embolism:** resulting from a fatty liver, disruption of depot or marrow fat, or coalescence of plasma lipoproteins. This mechanical blockage leads to a release of prostaglandins and subsequent intravascular thrombosis.

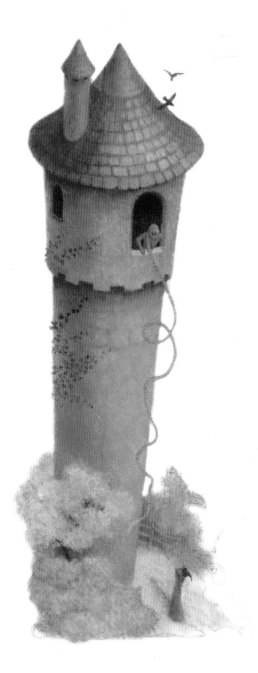

Contents

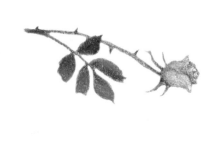

Sleeping Beauty

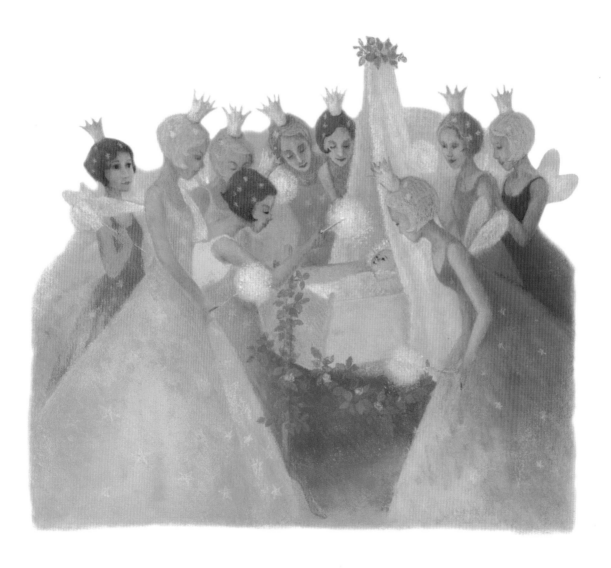

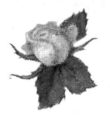

As sharp as a needle, the sun broke through and shone on the royal palace. How could the sun not shine, on such a happy day? All the dukes and duchesses were there, all the barons and baronets and countesses. Musicians were playing, chefs cooking, and chroniclers scribbling in their history books:

'Today the Princess Beauty is christened, first and beloved child of the king and queen, heiress to the throne. Never has this kingdom of ours seen such celebrations! Here have come wizards and wise men, and fairies of every colour, all with magical gifts for our baby princess . . .'

But no. Look again. One name is not on the list. The Grey Fairy was not invited. 'She has a tongue as sharp as a needle,' the queen had said, when the guest lists were drawn up. 'Must we invite her?'

So now all colours of fairies but grey stood before the cradle and touched the baby with their glittering wands:

'I give her Love.'

'And I give her Laughter.'

'I give her Beauty.'

'And I give her Health.'

Suddenly, a log in the great fireplace spat, and an ember flew out on to the carpet. Up from the ember sprang the Grey Fairy. 'And I say that before she is full grown, she shall prick her finger at a spinning wheel and DIE!' The fairy hurled her curse into the cradle like a handful of rusty nails, and the baby began to cry.

'No, no!' cried the queen.

'Take that back!' roared the king.

'Please!' begged the assembled guests. But the Grey Fairy only turned to grey smoke and curled away up the chimney.

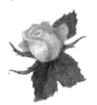 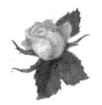 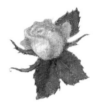

Only one fairy remained who had not yet given her christening gift. Now, this Lilac Fairy raised her wand in blessing over the screaming baby. 'The Grey curse cannot be lifted—but it can be blunted. My gift to you, Princess Beauty, is this: you shall not die but only sleep until a greater magic than mine can wake you!'

The christening broke up in confusion and panic. Soldiers were sent out through the whole city, through the whole kingdom. 'Destroy all the spinning wheels! Burn them on bonfires!' commanded the king. 'If there are no spinning wheels, she can never prick herself. Hurry! Burn every one! And find the Grey Fairy! Perhaps she can be made to eat her words!'

No trace was found of the Grey Fairy, but spinning wheels by the hundred were smashed and burned, their sharp spindles pulled out like the stings out of wasps. The sheep in the fields went unsheared for want of wheels to spin their wool. But Princess Beauty grew, unharmed, into a toddler, a girl, a young woman.

Naturally, no one spoke to her about the dreadful matter of the Curse, and thanks to the fairy blessings (and her own good nature) she was the sweetest, most beautiful, most loved princess in the history of the nation.

On her sixteenth birthday, Beauty was playing hide-and-seek with her cousins. When it was her turn to hide, she opened a cupboard door and slipped inside. At the back of the cupboard, she noticed a small door. Beyond the door, a staircase, steep and spiral,

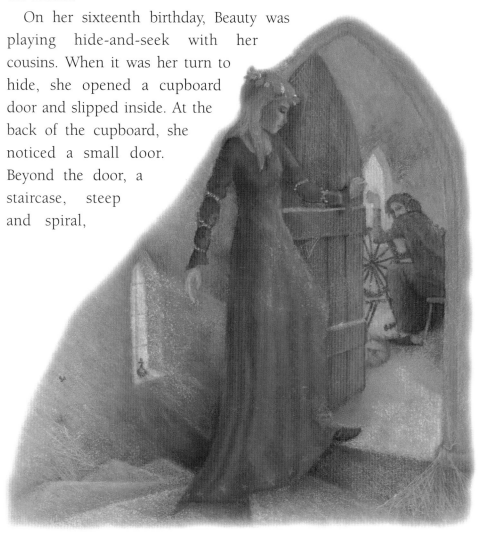

wound up past arrow slits and alcoves draped with cobwebs. And there at the top was a turret room she had never known existed before. The door stood open and from inside came the whirra-whirra-whirr of a wheel, spinning.

'Come in, dearie. Have you never seen a spinning wheel? No? It's for twining wool into thread. Come closer and see how it's done.' The spinner was a woman all in grey. Even her hair and face were grey—like something that has lived out of the sunlight too long. But her grey smile was inviting enough. 'Would you like to try, dearie? Just take hold of the spindle . . .'

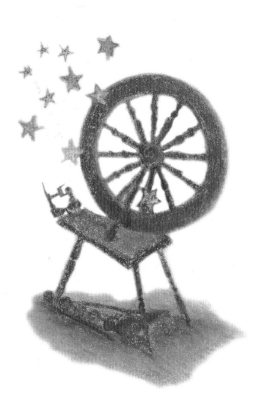

'Oh! My finger!' Beauty showed the prick to the grey lady, but the spinner only laughed at the drop of blood on her fingertip. Laughed and laughed and laughed.

Beauty ran back to the door, back down the stairs. But her head was swimming, so that the spiral stair seemed to be unwinding under her feet. She stumbled through the cupboard and out into the hall, holding up her finger: 'Mother! Mother, look!' And then the black and white flagstones heaved like the sea, and Beauty felt herself falling, falling, falling . . .

Asleep.

The queen grieved as though her daughter were dead already. She kissed her—over and over—but for all she loved Beauty, hers was not Love's Kiss. Beauty did not wake. 'She may as well be dead,' said the queen bitterly, as Beauty was carried to her bed in the west tower. 'Shall I ever live to see her eyes open again?'

The king did his best to comfort her, but his kiss did not wake Beauty either, and he did not know how long his daughter might sleep.

In Fairyland, all the candles guttered and went out. That was how the fairies knew that the Curse had been fulfilled. Beauty had fallen into her terrible sleep. 'Let us take pity on the king and queen and everyone who loves Beauty,' they said. 'Let all sleep, and not her alone. Let sleep shroud the palace, and magic protect them from harm until Love's Kiss arrives.'

So, one by one, the members of the royal household fell asleep. The guards by the doors, the cooks making supper, the dogs by the fire, the king blowing his nose. Just as sheets are hung over the furniture of an empty house, sleep was thrown over the entire court. The horses in the stables, the doves in the cote fell into a magical sleep, keeping Beauty company on her long dream-journey.

Around the castle, the hedges grew, as unsheared

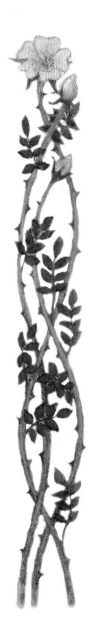

as the sheep. The flowers in the garden beds ran wild. Briars and brambles rolled in from the forest. Trees grew up from acorn to oak, from conker to horse-chestnut, from stone to plum tree. And the royal rose garden tumbled among the trees, weaving a magical web of thorny suckers no outsider could break through.

Now no one could reach the royal palace. Many tried but turned back. The people of the kingdom were sorry to lose their king and queen and princess, but time eased their sorrow, and they had lives to live. They told their children about the Fairy Curse, but it sounded more like a story than history. And in time the trees grew so tall, the rose thorns so dense, that nothing of the palace could be seen from the highway. Nothing.

*   *   *

One hundred years later, a bee with a sting as sharp as a needle stung the horse of Prince Charmant as he rode along the highway of a foreign kingdom. The horse bolted, and carried the prince off the highway and into a wood. He thought he saw, among the treetops, the gleam of sun shining on a distant window, and tried to ride

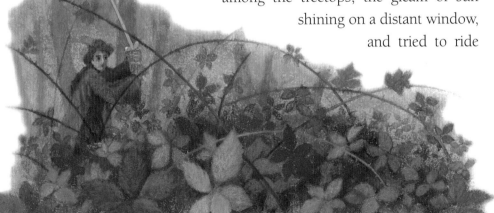

towards the building. But he found no pathway through the briars and brambles.

A woman sat on a log, stringing lilac flowers into a daisy chain. 'What building is that?' he asked her.

'A castle. There's no road to it. You must cut your way through the briars if you want to reach it. They say there's a princess asleep inside. A very beautiful princess . . .'

Prince Charmant was intrigued. His heart raced a little, at the thought of the beautiful princess. He drew his sword and struck at a thorny bramble. But either his sword was sharper than he knew, or the bramble died at that very moment, for it dropped to the ground at his feet, withered and brown. 'Did you see that?' he said, turning back to the woman. But she had gone. There was no sign of her anywhere.

On and on, hacking and slicing at the dense undergrowth, Prince Charmant forged a path towards the castle. He could see it more clearly now: a turret, a dome . . . It was hard work, but not so hard as he had expected, for the wood seemed to be dying, withering, dropping its autumn leaves on his head like coloured blessings. At last, scratched and panting, he stood on the palace steps listening to a soft purring sound—like a thousand contented cats—coming from inside. He put his ear to the lock. It could not be . . . Yes, it was! It was snoring. The guards in the inner courtyard stood about, back-to-back, snoring and sound asleep!

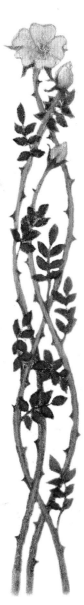

Charmant leaned his shoulder against the door, and it swung open. There were flowers and flags festooning every wall—as though time had stopped in the middle of a grand celebration. A cake with sixteen candles stood, unnibbled—even the mice in this castle were asleep!—the sixteen candles not yet lit. And everywhere, there were people—strewn untidily about, hats awry, sleeping in heaps on the floors and sofas and stairs.

Charmant climbed over them. A curious sensation of excitement gripped him—as though he was about to make the most important discovery of his life. Something like a strain of music was throbbing inside his head, telling him to go on, to hunt and search, to look for the princess.

'She could be any one of these,' he told himself, as he stepped over a ring of sleeping schoolgirls in party dresses. 'But she is not,' said the music in his head.

He searched the east tower and the chapel. He found the king and queen, she with her face all salty with dried tears, he in the act of blowing his nose. Then Charmant climbed the west tower and came to a bedchamber especially full of flowers. The bed had white damask curtains and the cover was embroidered with intertwining roses.

And there on the pillow he saw a face which stabbed his heart like a needle—the most beautiful face he had ever seen. So deathly white was the princess that he took hold of the hand on the cover, thinking it would

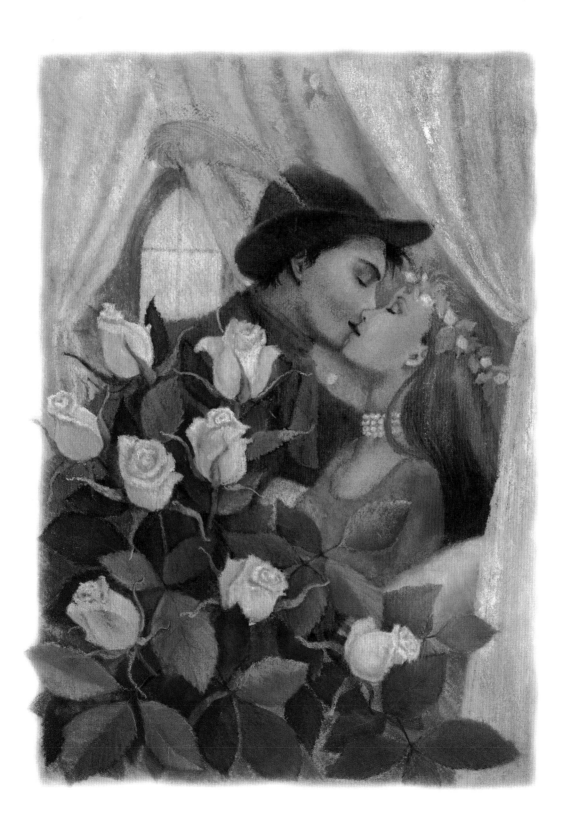

be cold. A drop of blood on the princess's finger smeared his hand, warm and wet.

Then Prince Charmant did something most improper for a prince of the royal blood. He should have waited. He should have asked permission of the king, of the queen, of the girl herself. But he could not help it. Her beauty had worked a kind of magic on his heart. He bent and kissed the sleeping princess on her lips.

Something brushed his face. It was the princess's lashes, a-flicker. 'Look, mother. I pricked my finger,' she murmured, and sat up.

Throughout the palace, dogs scratched, horses stamped, cats stretched. Guards overbalanced, viscounts sneezed, the king blew his nose. The guests picked themselves up off the ballroom floor, and little girls asked if it was time to eat the birthday cake. Noise filled up each room and staircase and hall like a goblet filling with wine.

But up in the white chamber in the west tower, neither Prince Charmant nor Princess Beauty spoke. They just looked at one another in wonder, she a hundred years older than he, yet not a day's difference in the age of their hearts.

'Will you marry me?' he said.

'I suppose I should, now that you've kissed me,' said Beauty. 'But first we'd better finish the game, hadn't we? Whose turn is it to count to fifty?'

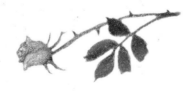

Rumpelstiltskin

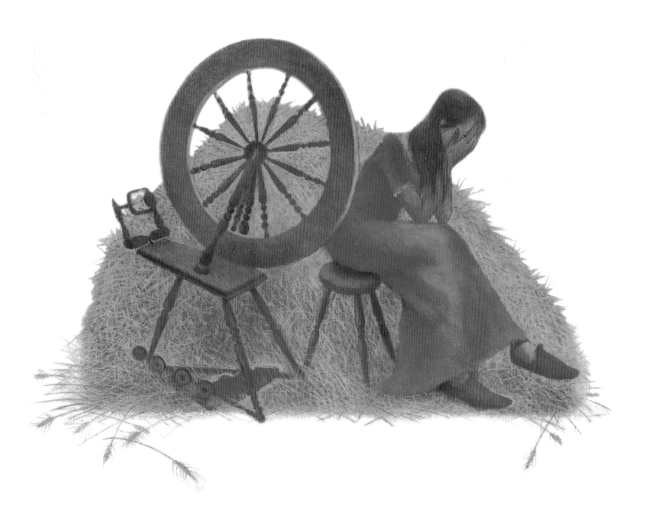

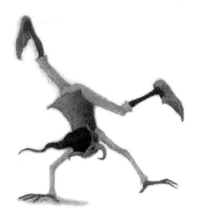

Fathers like nothing better than to talk about their children—to show them off, to sing their praises. Miller Thumb talked about his daughter all the time. In fact he boasted and bragged and began to embroider the truth.

'My Polly sweeps up the mill every night!' (True.)

'My Poll spins at her wheel every morning!' (True.)

'In fact, my Poll can spin straw on that wheel of hers!' (Unlikely.)

'Yes, yes; in fact, no word of a lie: my Poll can spin straw into gold!' (Oh dear.)

'No!' His friends at the inn were so astonished that one ran and told the lord of the manor; the lord told the king.

'Send your daughter to the palace,' said the letter delivered next day to the mill. 'By order of the King.' Miller Thumb was thrilled. 'He must have heard how pretty you are and wants to marry you!' he said to Polly.

'Don't be foolish, father,' said Polly. 'Kings don't marry country girls.' But she brushed her hair and went to the palace, and the king's eyes flashed with pleasure at the sight of her.

'Come with me,' he said, and with a grip disagreeably tight on her wrist, he led Polly to a small tack-room behind the stables.

Strange place for a spinning wheel, thought Polly.

'I can't abide braggarts,' said the king. 'Spin this bale of straw into gold by morning, or I shall cut off your father's head and put a stop to his boasting.'

The door banged. The bolt shot shut. The horses in the stable next door stamped their hard-shod feet. And Polly wept. 'Oh, father, father, what have you done, and what can I do to put it right? Spin straw into gold? It's never been done in the history of the world, and I'm not the one to do it first!'

'But I am!'

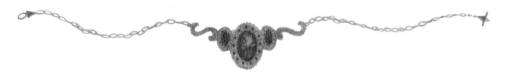

From a bin of bent, discarded horseshoes, a strange old man poked out a poker-long nose. It was as bent as a horseshoe and red as rust. 'I'll do your spinning for you. At a price.'

'What can I give you, except my thanks?' gasped Polly.

'That necklace of yours would do.'

And so the bargain was struck. Polly gave up her necklace, and the little man gave up his night, spinning the wheel till it whistled. Straws twined together, then fell from the spindle like golden woodshavings, curling and coiling on the dirty floor. Long before morning, the straw was all gone, and gold strewings covered the floor. The little spinner climbed back into his barrel, and Polly fell asleep.

When the king opened the door, he stared. 'It was true! The miller was telling the truth!' He was sorry now that he had given Polly only one bale of straw to spin. 'Come with me.' And with a grip disagreeably tight on her arm, he led her to the royal sewing room.

Strange place for a haystack, thought Polly, as men with pitchforks piled twenty bales of straw in the centre of the room.

'Spin all this into gold before morning,' said the king, 'or I'll cut off your father's head—and yours too!' You see, the king was as fond of gold as the miller was of boasting.

The door slammed, the bolt shot shut. The courtiers in the room next door sniggered and shuddered and went away. And Polly wept. 'Oh, father, father, what have you brought me to, and how am I to get myself out of it? Spin straw into gold? I'd need the luck in a barrel of horseshoes to do that!'

'But I wouldn't,' said a voice. Out of the coal scuttle wriggled the

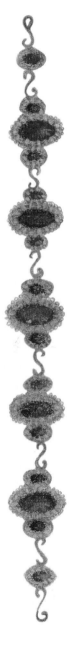

same little man, spilling coals across the turkey rug. 'I'll
do your spinning for you. At a price.'

'But what can I give you, except my thanks?'

'That bracelet of yours would do.'

So the bargain was struck. Polly gave up her bracelet,
and the little man gave up a day and a night to spinning.
The wheel spun so fast that its three feet danced on the
floor. The spinner was gone when Polly awoke, and the
whole big room was carpeted in shavings of gold.

When the king opened the door, he danced a little
caper and beamed. 'No fluke! No trick of the eye! You
really can spin straw into gold! Come with me.' And
holding her prisoner-tight, for fear she escape him, he led
her to the ballroom of the palace. Behind them trotted the
prime minister carrying the spinning wheel. Men were
pitching bale after bale of straw in through the windows,
filling the vast hall from floor to ceiling. 'Spin this into
gold by morning, and I shall marry you to my son!'
declared the king.

'No, I can't—' Polly began to say.

But the double doors slammed, their bolts shot shut.
The king's voice echoed back down the long corridor:
'Then you shall die, girl!'

Polly sat down and wept. 'Oh, father, father, what did
I ever do to deserve this? Spin all this straw into gold? It
would take all the magic in the land to do it, and I haven't
one speck.'

'But I have,' said a voice. Out from amid the stacked

straw, like a hamster emerging from its nest, burrowed the ugly little man, cracking his skilful finger joints. 'I'll spin all this and make you the prince's bride. At a price.'

Polly looked down at her bare arms, touched her bare throat. 'I've nothing but my pinafore and petticoat to give you,' she said.

'Don't want them.'

'A kiss, then.'

'Save it for the prince.'

'My thanks, then. What else?'

'A promise. Promise to give me whatever you hold in your arms on the happiest day of your life, and I'll spin the straw into gold.'

Polly thought of her wedding. Isn't that the happiest day of any girl's life? She thought of the wedding bouquet she would be holding that day, and imagined tossing it to the little goblin.

So the bargain was struck; Polly gave her promise, and the little man gave his all to spin the straw. Gold fell like shavings from a lathe, and the spinning wheel turned so fast that its three little feet wore pits in the polished floor. Its spokes whistled and its hub threw out sparks. But unspun straw still towered over them both in sweet-smelling cliffs.

Just as morning light crept in at the windows—just as the king's steps echoed down the corridor—the last thread of gold trickled from the spindle, and the goblin disappeared in a flash of golden chaff.

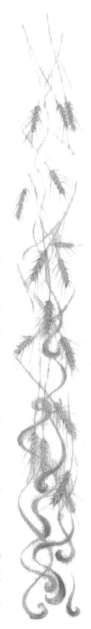

When the king opened the double doors, he had never seen so much gold in all his life. He skipped and jumped and clapped his hands. 'Excellent! You shall marry my son and spin gold for him every day of your life!'

Fortunately, the prince had other ideas of married life. 'My bride will never sully her hands with spinning!' he said, caressing Polly's fingers in a most agreeable way. In fact he was a wonderful husband in every respect, and their wedding was the happiest day of Polly's young life. But although she peered around from the church steps, cradling her bouquet, looking for the little spinner, she saw no sign of him—no poker nose, no squint, no long, crackling fingers.

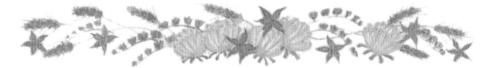

The old king died and the prince became king, Polly his queen.

Polly forgot all about her bargain. She was very happy. In fact her happiness grew every day until, three years later, her baby son was born. Then, cradling him in her arms and gazing at his curling lashes and tiny, perfect hands, Polly realized that wedding days were nothing compared with joy like this.

'I'll take him now,' said a voice. And out from the brand new cradle clambered the spinner, cracking his long, skilful finger joints. 'You swore to give me whatever you were holding in your arms on the happiest day of your life. Here it is, and here am I. Give me the child!'

'No, no!' cried Polly. 'Take anything! Take all I have, but don't take my baby!'

'I want nothing else. I, who can spin straw into gold? What else could I possibly want? All I ever wanted was the child. Now waiting and work have brought round the hour. Hand him over to me! That's the rules of the game.'

'But it's not a game!' cried Polly. 'Or if it is, why did I never have a chance to win? Oh, spinner, spinner, give me a fair chance in an unfair world!'

The spinner gave a hideous cackle and flexed his crackling fingers. 'Very well. I've waited three years. I can wait three days longer. Here's a riddle for you—to make the game fairer:

> *What's my name?*
> *That's the game.*
> *Search about.*
> *Find it out.*
> *If you can,*
> *Keep your wee man.*
> *If you can't,*
> *Then you shan't.*
> *Three times I'll come,*
> *Then playing's done:*
> *I keep your son!'*

Turning a single cartwheel, he disappeared, leaving a smell in the air like rotting straw.

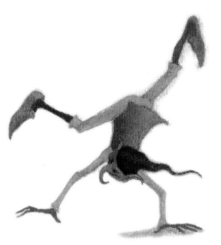

Polly called out the army and had them search the town. They emptied every barrel of horseshoes, every coal scuttle, and pulled apart every hayrick in the realm. The young king offered rewards, and gathered in every church register of christenings. The goblin came back for the first time, and they asked him: 'Is your name Aaron or Bernard, Yves or Zachariah? Is your name Africa or India, Russia or Franz?'

But he only laughed and disappeared in a puff of flour shrieking, 'Guess again! You'll never guess!'

The king posted suggestion boxes on every street corner, and the people (who loved their new king and queen dearly) thought of all the

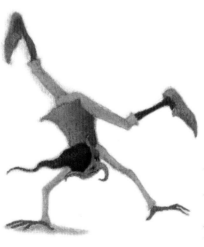

names they had ever heard. The goblin came back for the second time, and Polly asked him: 'Is your name Horse or Monkey or Lion? Is your name Pixie or Elf or Goblin?'

But the spinner only laughed and disappeared in a sprinkling of crumbs squealing, 'Guess again! You'll never guess!'

In desperation Polly rode the kingdom from end to end, from top to bottom, from the mountains to the sea. She eavesdropped from roof-tops, listened at locks, and jotted down names on her cuffs and the palm of her hand. But in her heart of hearts she knew that no one knew the spinner's name except the spinner himself.

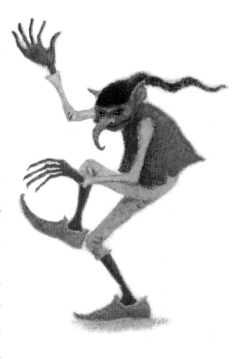

She was riding back to the palace, her baby asleep on her back, when the road passed through a forest dark with more than shadow. Far off she saw the glimmer of a fire, and heard a crackling like twigs. Creeping closer, she saw the spinner himself, dancing in a frenzy of joy round the campfire. He was wriggling his long, noisy fingers in the air and singing:

> *Move every stone, drain every bog;*
> *Ask all the cats and every dog;*
> *Dig up the sea with a single oar:*
> *You won't find what you're looking for!*
> *Search the night with candleshine:*
> *Soon your baby will be mine.*
> *Guess again and lose the game,*
> *For Rumpelstiltskin is my name!'*

Polly turned her face to the moon and smiled, then tugged on her reins and quietly rode on through the wood.

Next day, the spinner came for the third and last time, carrying a willow basket under his arm to put the baby in.

'Is your name Avril or Maggie or Sandra?' said Polly. 'Is your name Mars or Venus or Saturn?'

The spinner reached into the royal cradle to tickle the royal baby. 'No, no! Ha ha! I win! I win!'

'Or is it Rumpelstiltskin?' said Polly, and the name crackled on her tongue.

The spinner gave a shriek and his nose uncurled with rage. 'Who told you?! Spies and traitors! Who told you?! I'll cut out their tongues!' Such a temper seized him that he stamped and stamped, feet dancing just where the spinning wheel had danced as it spun straw into gold.

All of a sudden, the floor gave way, and a gaping hole swallowed Rumpelstiltskin like a well swallowing a bent penny. Purple smoke filled the air, and when it cleared there was no trace of the spinner but for that gaping hole and a scream of rage echoing through the palace: 'RUMPELSTILTSKIN!!'

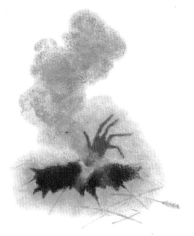

Rapunzel

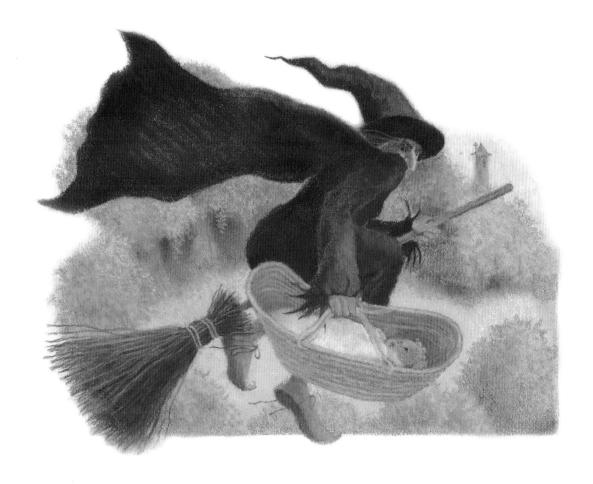

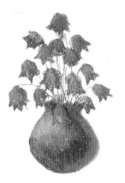

Once, in the salad days of the world, there was a plant called a bell-flower, or sometimes rapunzel. It was not grown for its pretty bell-shaped flowers but for the root beneath the ground, which made a healthy salad. You probably would not eat it: I'd rather not. But Greta wanted more than anything in the world to eat a plate of rapunzel. She was ill: thin and frail and sickly, and her beauty was withering fast like the flowers of an unrooted plant.

'Gil! Gil!' she whispered to her husband. 'Fetch me bell-flowers, or I shall die before the week is out!'

Unfortunately, the only bell-flowers in the whole county grew in their neighbour Grizzel's garden. And Grizzel was a witch.

Gil loved his wife dearly. He was terribly afraid of the witch, but more afraid of losing his darling Greta. So that night he climbed over the garden wall, picked the bell-flowers and put them in a vase by his wife's bed.

'Where are the roots?' groaned Greta. 'Can I eat flowers, you fool? Bring me the roots!'

So Gil went back next night with a trowel, and treading softly, creeping silently past the belladonna and snapdragons, dug up the roots of the sweet rapunzel.

'Thief! Villain! Vandal!' The witch stood over him, a broom held high, its burning twigs lighting up the garden and his guilty deed. 'You'll pay for this!'

'Anything! I'll pay you anything! My dearest possession! But please let me have some rapunzel, or I'm sure my wife will die!'

'Your dearest possession?' mused Grizzel.

'Name it.'

'Pay when I ask you for payment,' said the witch, suddenly calm and smiling. 'Here are some I picked earlier.' And from under her cloak she took a small basket of roots, clean and ready to eat.

The salad was the best medicine in the world for Greta. At the very sight of it, her face brightened; at the very taste, she felt better. Within a week she was strong and well. Within the year, she was expecting a baby.

It was the prettiest baby, too—fit and beautiful, with lots of golden hair. Greta and her husband would stand for hours in silent wonder, looking down at their first child, their baby daughter.

'We'll call her Bell-flower,' said he.

'Rapunzel, yes,' said she. And Rapunzel was their dearest possession.

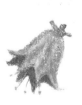

'Pay me now as you promised me then!' Suddenly Grizzel stood on the other side of the crib, a moses-basket under her arm and a grin on her wizened face.

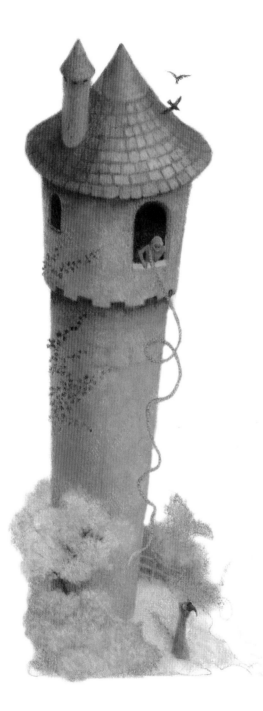

'What does she mean, Gil? What does she want?'

'No! You can't take our daughter! Not Rapunzel! No!'

'I've thought of nothing else since I first planted the seed in my garden. Give her over! A promise is a promise, and promises must be kept!'

Neither tears nor pleading would change Grizzel's mind: she had planned this terrible bargain all along. Putting the baby girl in her basket, she flew away, far and farther than far.

Grizzel had always wanted a child. She had always dreamed of having a little daughter all to herself—someone to love her despite her ugly face and nastier nature. So she flew on her broomstick into the deepest forest in the world—to a tower already prepared for her precious prize. Taller than the trees, and without any stairs, the tower stood like a lighthouse in a sea of green, one room at the very top.

And no door.

As the years passed, twining plants climbed the brickwork, almost as high as the single window at the top.

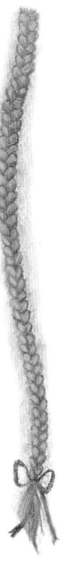

Inside, Rapunzel also grew—from a pretty baby to a beautiful young woman, though there was no mirror for her to look in and realize this. She saw no other human being. Only Grizzel who came and went by the window.

Rapunzel's hair grew as long as the twining plants outside—a glossy hank of shining golden hair. It was Grizzel's pride and joy. It was also very useful.

When her broomstick wore down to a flightless stump, the old witch could still visit her precious prisoner. She would stand at the base of the tower and call:

'Rapunzel! Rapunzel! Let down your golden hair!'

And Rapunzel would let fall her plait, like a rope, for the witch to climb. She loved the witch (who else was there to love?) though she felt an emptiness inside her which she could not understand.

'Is there truly no one else in the world but you and I?' she would ask.

'No one you would want to meet, dearie. No one you need ever meet.'

All day long, Rapunzel was alone—alone and lonely. So she sang, and her voice thrilled the birds for miles around. One day, a young man lost in the wood heard her singing and walked towards the sweet sound. The singing brought him to a clearing, and in the clearing he saw a tower. At the foot of the tower, an old crone was calling: 'Rapunzel! Rapunzel! Let

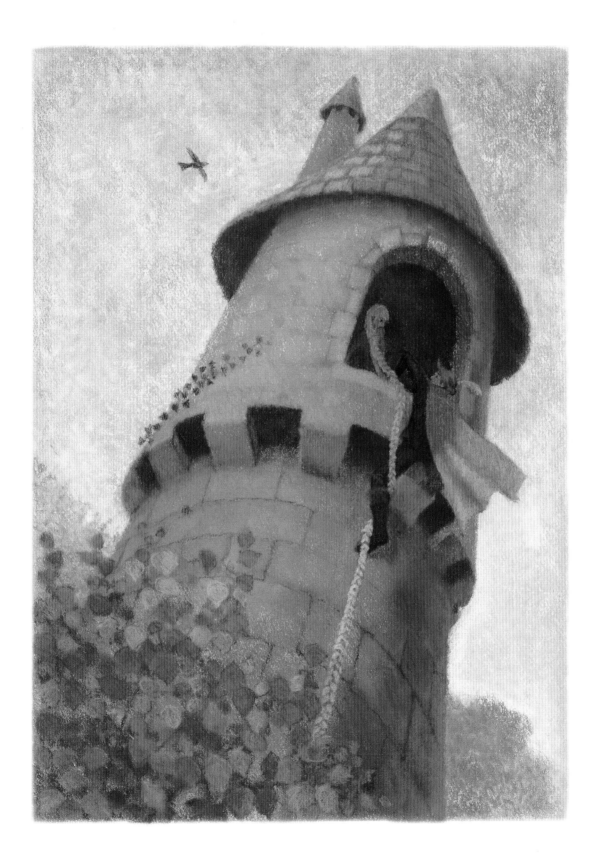

down your golden hair!' And lo and behold! a beautiful girl came to the window and uncoiled her shining golden plait. The young man hid and watched until he saw Grizzel finish her visit and leave, climbing down the rope of hair. He waited a while, then came out of hiding.

'Rapunzel! Rapunzel! Let down your golden hair!'

Rapunzel was startled. 'Come day, go day,' she said to herself. 'It seems only a moment since Grizzel was here yesterday.' But being a good obedient girl (and very afraid of Grizzel's temper) she let down her plait at once.

Goodness! How heavy the old woman seemed today! How big a breakfast she must have eaten!

Then—one, two—over the windowsill came the hands which should have been old and veined, the hair which should have been grey and thin, the face which should have been ugly and toothless. And they were none of those things! The most beautiful creature Rapunzel had ever seen climbed in through her window.

'Oh!' she said. 'I've seen deer and boar. I've seen weasels and foxes. But what are you?'

'I'm Prince Florian,' said the young man, staring almost as much.

Then they talked and talked. Rapunzel found out the truth about the world, and the prince found out the truth about himself—that he was in love with Rapunzel and wanted to marry her.

'Tomorrow I shall come back for you! Tomorrow, when I've found my way out of this forest. I'll bring a rope for you to climb down and we shall ride away together—to the cities and fields and places you've never seen!'

The emptiness inside Rapunzel was gone. She knew now that Grizzel had lied to her, deceived her, imprisoned

her, but she was too full of happiness to be angry. Her lover climbed
down her hair, and the forest swallowed him up from sight, but she
stayed by the window till the darkness was as thick as tar, watching the
way he had gone. Then she fell asleep with her forehead on the sill.

'Rapunzel! Rapunzel! Let down your golden hair!'

Rapunzel started awake. 'So soon? Have you come back so soon, my
love?' she said, hurrying to tumble her hair down the tower. 'Quickly! Quick!
We must get away from here before Grizzel comes on her daily visit!'

Over the sill—one, two—came veiny hands, grey hair, toothless ugly
face. 'So! Have I found you out, little Miss Liar? Have I come too early

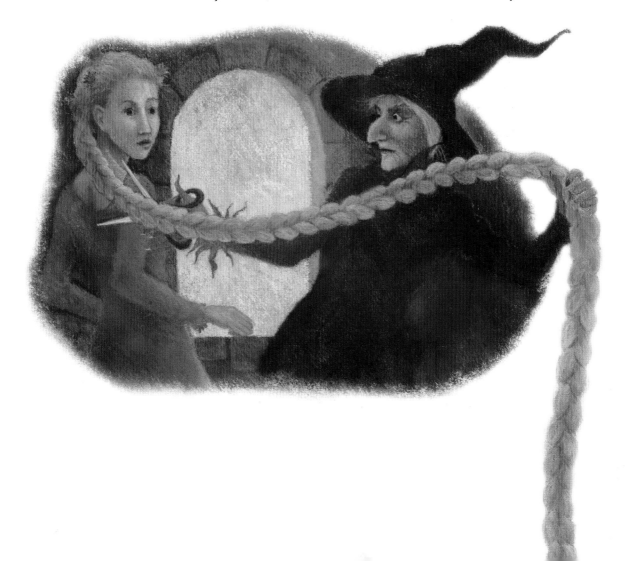

for your liking?' The jealousy in Grizzel's face blazed like a furnace. Her treasure, locked up in its treasure chest of stone, had been grasped by other hands, kissed by other lips. A pair of scissors flashed in the sunlight and—SNICK SNACK!–she cut through Rapunzel's lovely hair, cut through the love between them.

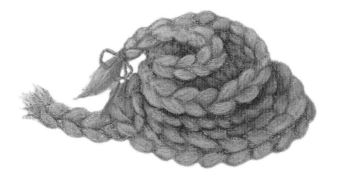

Lowering Rapunzel to the ground with her own severed plait, Grizzel screeched after her: 'Go! Get away! See how you fare in the wilderness without me to wait on you hand and foot! Go hungry! Go lonely and unloved! Ungrateful wretch! Go!'

Rapunzel took to her heels and ran, ploughing into the depths of the dangerous forest, at the mercy of weather and wolves and weariness.

But Grizzel's temper was not yet fed.

Grizzel waited for the prince.

'Rapunzel! Rapunzel! Let down your golden hair!' called Prince Florian. Down snaked the shimmering plait. Up and up climbed the prince—above the treetops, up to the little window. Moss fell from under his scrabbling boots.

Suddenly, as he reached the sill, a face loomed out above him, and a pair of veiny, gnarled hands let go the rope of hair. As Florian fell he could hear Grizzel's cackling laugh. 'Thought you'd steal her, did you? My girl? My beauty? Well, you're too late!'

From top to bottom of the tower he fell, entwined in his lover's cut hair. He fell into the brambles, and his eyes were scratched, so that when he dragged himself away into the forest, like a wounded deer, Prince Florian was blinded—dark-blind.

On and on he wandered, hands outstretched, grazing his palms on the rough tree bark. For weeks he walked, dependent on the kindness of peasants and priests for a bite of bread, a drink of water, some shelter from the cold. Stumbling in winter snow, tripping in summer-tangling briars, he asked everyone he met: 'Have you seen a girl with a golden furlong of hair?' But of course no one had seen such a girl, for there was no such girl to see. He did not say he was a prince: who would have believed him? He did not even ask the way to his home or the comfort of his palace. He wanted only to find Rapunzel.

Then one day—one fine spring morning it was—he heard singing, and he followed the sound to a ramshackle hut in the midst of a stony garden. He could smell the scent of bell-flowers and hear washing flapping in the wind.

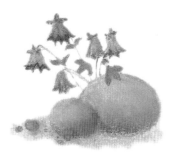

Then Prince Florian opened his mouth and joined in the singing of Rapunzel's song, and she heard him and came running.

Ragged and thin and blind, he looked such a piteous sight that Rapunzel thought her heart would break with pity and love. She took him in her arms and wept great tears of regret.

And the tears splashed his eyes—magic tears on a magic morning—and Prince Florian blinked once, blinked twice and saw his dear Rapunzel's face. She no longer had a golden furlong of hair, but then it was not her hair he had loved—not even her beauty. Like the bell-flower, her worth lay deeper down, sweet and healthful: the perfect makings of a princess and a wife.

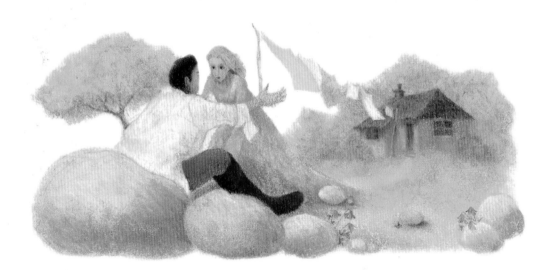

The Flower of Love

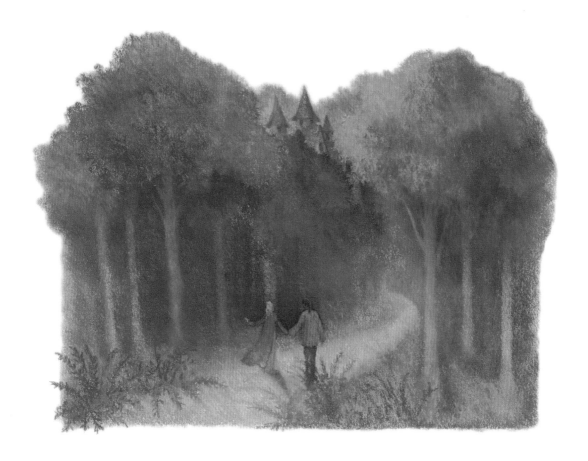

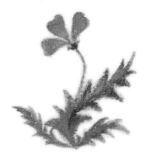

'Only one more day and we shall be married!' said Jim to Jemima. 'What man was ever as happy as I!'

'What girl was ever as happy as I?' said Jemima, and rested her head fondly on his shoulder.

They went for a walk in the wood—a last walk before their wedding day. And so entranced were they with each other's company that they walked deeper into the wood than ever before.

'They say there's a castle somewhere in these woods,' said Jim. 'A castle where an old witch lives.'

'Why would anyone build a castle in a wood?' said Jemima. 'Castles are built in the open, on the tops of hills.'

'Ah, but they say this old witch has terrible secrets to hide—prisoners, captives, pretty girls like you,' he teased. Jim could feel her hand trembling deliciously inside his own. 'They say she has taken seven hundred into that castle of hers, and not a one has ever come out again!' and he laughed at the silliness of the story. Jemima's hand slipped from his own, and he turned to see why.

The laugh froze on his lips, for there was no Jemima beside him now—

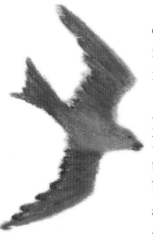

only a fluttering bluebird buffeting its little fragile body against his arm and shoulder and face. It sang the saddest song a bird ever sang.

Jim would have taken the bluebird in his palm and stroked her feathery little head, but he found he was frozen to the spot—powerless to move! His limbs were as heavy as the branches of the trees round about, his legs fixed as fast as the treeroots. In her distress, Jemima clamoured up against her motionless sweetheart, thrilling shrilly in his ear, but Jim could say nothing to comfort her, do nothing to help her.

Beyond her fluttering wings, he glimpsed a stark iron gateway in an ancient wall. Through it now came a bent old woman, rubbing her bony hands together with glee. 'Another little birdie for me? Good, good. Excellent. Very pretty. Here, my little chickadee. Here, my pretty wee creature.'

'Fly! Fly!' Jim wanted to say, but Jemima was too busy fluttering frantically against his face, trying to rouse him. The witch scurried up, birdcage in hand and, with a dreadful, cackling laugh, scooped little Jemima into the wicker prison.

'Another for my aviary!' she crowed, then snapping her fingers scornfully under Jim's nose, she turned and went back through the gate.

The rain rained on Jim, the wind blew on him and carried away his hat and neckerchief. Not until the sun rose next morning was he able to move again, to rattle at the locked gates, to pound with his fists on the high walls, calling, 'Let her go! Please let her go! She's my all! She's my everything! Jemima!'

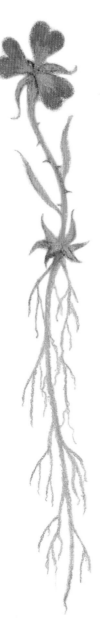

Guests gathered for the wedding, but no bride came to church, no bridegroom either. For on his wedding day, Jim was running distractedly round the endless castle wall, trying to find a way in. At last, exhausted and half mad with despair, he went home. Hoping he might wake to find it all a nightmarish dream, he threw himself on his bed and went to sleep.

He dreamed that night that he lay dead and buried under the ground. Out of his heart, bursting through flesh and soil, stones and slab, a small red flower pushed its way up into the sunshine. Its petals brushed the walls of a grim, gloomy castle, and the castle stumbled, tumbled, crumbled to ash. In his dream, Jim snatched the flower and tried to smell its perfume. But the scarlet petals turned to Jemima's face between his hands, and her scarlet mouth called, 'Find me, Jim! Find the Flower of Love! Save me!'

He woke with empty arms, her name on his lips, and he knew that if he could find that Flower, he would be able to enter the Castle of Birds.

He searched the cornfields, but though the poppies were scarlet, they were not the Flower of Love. He searched the meadows, but though he found speedwell and harebells, campanula and foxgloves, he could not find the Flower of Love. He searched the mountainside, but though he found

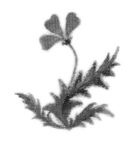

brave little flowers clinging to the bare rock through drought and rain, none were the flower in his dream. He searched gardens, but though he found forget-me-nots and love-lies-bleeding, he did not find the Flower of Love.

At last, where land meets sea, and east meets west, where high meets low, and diving birds meet flying fish, he spotted a single flower growing from a sheer cliff face. With no thought for his safety—reckless with desperate hope—he climbed the cliff. Skuas wheeled around him, the wind cracked his hair in his eyes. And when he reached it, the Flower of Love had three petals, a stem of thorns and roots as deep as the earth's core.

'O Flower of Love, let me pick you or let me fall into the ocean now and be lost!' he begged. 'Without Jemima, life is nothing to me.' As his fingers closed around the stem, the thorns withdrew, and the Flower of Love broke off as easily as a buttercup. It had given itself to him. Jim fastened it in his buttonhole, and climbed on up to the top of the cliff.

Back in the forest, the shadows did not seem so dark any more. When Jim reached the spot where the magic had paralysed him, no magic seized him and he was able to reach the castle gates unseen. At a touch of the Flower of Love, the gate crumbled to rusty dust, and Jim forged on up the winding driveway, through a maze of black-leafed shrubs, right to the castle door.

With the Flower of Love in his grasp, there was not a lock or bolt which could bar his way, and he was soon inside, climbing spiral staircases, feeling his way along dark, narrow corridors towards the distant twitter of birdsong.

At last he came to a string of rooms, one after another, crammed with shrieking, trilling birds. Tens and dozens of wicker cages hung from the ceiling, each one trembling with the violent flutter of the little bird inside. There were lyre birds, birds of paradise, macaws and canaries, owls and swallows. Orioles and blackbirds sang brilliant, thrilling songs, but all so sad, so heartbreakingly sad, beaks straining between the bars of their cages. The noise, in so small a space, was earsplitting. Jim whirled round and round, his hands over his ears, setting the cages swinging and bumping as he called, 'Jemima! Where are you? How shall I find you among all these?'

'That's right!' said a voice behind him. 'Call till your heart breaks. How will you ever find her among so many? Here are seven hundred of my little pets. Which one is your Jemima, eh? Now, by all the magic at my command, I command you: Stand still!'

Jim froze to the spot, moving neither hand nor head, neither lip nor eyelid. The witch gave a terrible cackle and skipped about among her cages. 'See, my pretty ones? I've caught an intruder. How did he get in, eh? A miracle! How will he get out, eh? An impossibility! Come, little Jemima, come and sing a last song to your foolish, reckless sweetheart before I turn him into a dog or a beetle or a worm!' And she lifted down one of the cages—one with a bluebird inside.

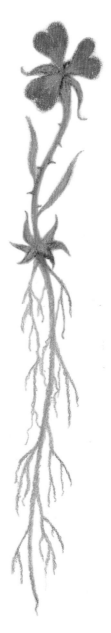

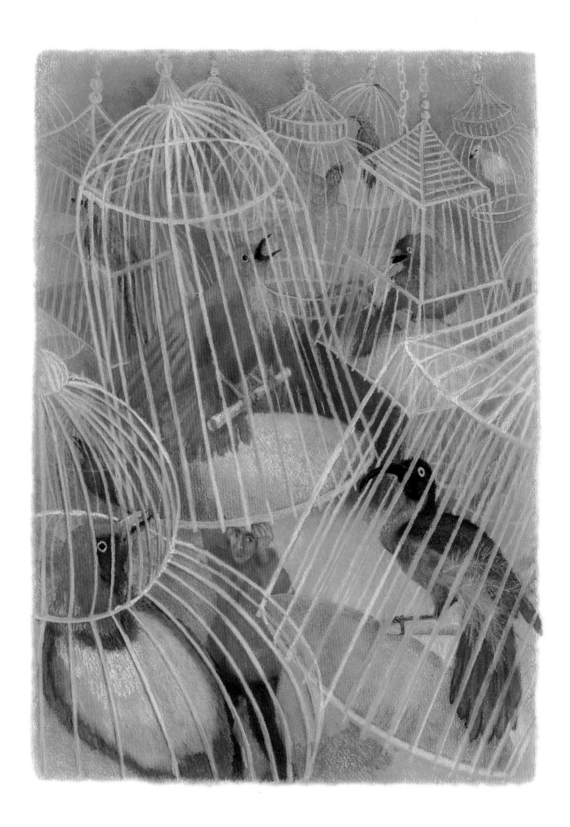

But bringing it close, to wag in Jim's face, she gave a sudden terrible cry and dropped the cage. For she had seen the scarlet flower in Jim's fingers, and the smile on his lips. He was not ensnared by her magic at all!

Out darted his hand and he struck the witch in the face with the Flower of Love. Pollen dusted her crooked nose. Her magical powers fell from her like leaves from a tree in autumn, and the Castle of Birds shook to its very foundations.

Quickly, Jim thrust the flower through the bars of the bluebird's cage, and brushed the pretty feathers with the scarlet petals. And there stood Jemima, her head thrown back in rapturous song! Moments later, twenty and thirty more maidens were dancing around Jim, thanking him, blessing him, as he moved from cage to cage, breaking the enchantment.

Clutching her moth-eaten shawl around her, the Witch of Birds scuttled like a rat towards the stairs.

'Quick! Stop her! She'll get away!' cried Jemima.

'Let her go,' said Jim softly. 'Her magic is all gone. Wherever she runs in the world, the birds of the air will mob her and people will shut their doors against her.' With the Flower of Love in his hand, Jim was powerless to hate even the witch.

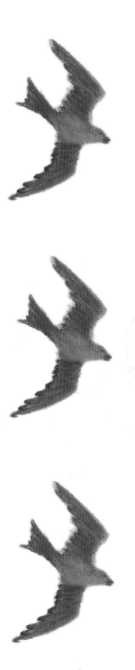

People say there was never a man and wife so happy as Jim and Jemima, and they put it down to the couple's great good luck. After all, not many newly-weds come by a castle to live in and a witch's treasure chest to make them rich. But I say it had less to do with castles and treasure than with what Jim and Jemima kept under their pillow. A little scarlet flower which never withered.

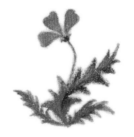

Cinderella

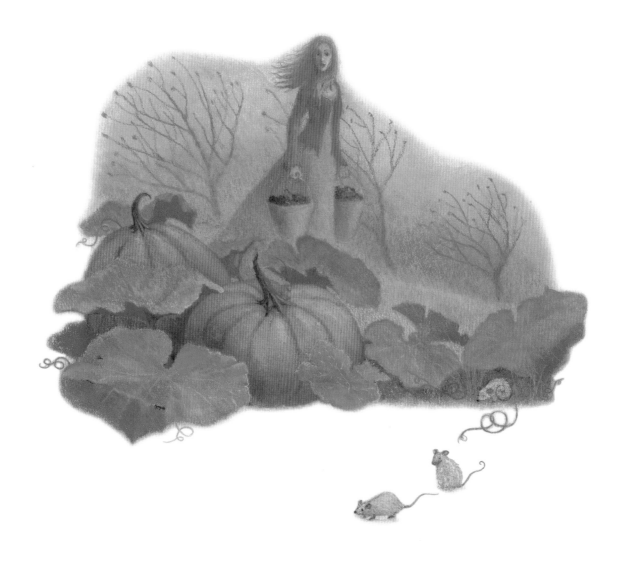

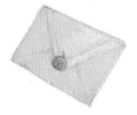

Cinderella was not her name. Once, long before, she had had another name. But her stepmother had forgotten it, along with her promise to Cinderella's father. Stepmother had promised, as he lay dying, to love his little daughter as much as she loved her own three, to treat her as kindly as she treated her own three, to share his money evenly between all four girls. But he was no sooner dead than the promise was forgotten. His daughter was turned out of her bedroom and made to sleep in the scullery, to clean the house and do the laundry, to cook and wash up and fetch in the coal. From dawn till dead of night, she had to work, to make life comfortable for Stepmother and her three lazy stepsisters, Raviola, Rigatona, and Linguina. No money was squandered on new clothes for her, no good food wasted on her. So her old clothes wore out into threadbare shreds. Then they called her Cinderella, because she slept among the cinders of the kitchen fire to keep warm.

But there was one thing Cinderella had which her stepsisters could not take away: her beauty. Their faces were like three plates of meatballs, but hers was as lovely as a bowl of creamed strawberries. They were as big and bulky as barrels and trunks and crates; she was as slender as a quiver.

Sometimes Cinderella wished she were not so pretty, for it made the sisters spiteful with jealousy. But mostly Cinderella wished for gentleness—for a smile, for a kind word, for someone to look her way without snarling a command:

'Scrub the steps, Cinderella!'

'Mend my shoes, Cinderella!'

'Wash my curtains, Cinderella!'

'Make my supper!'

Cinderella never complained. She was as sweet-natured as she was beautiful, and even they, with their bullying cruelty, could not stop her dreaming her happy daydreams.

One day, a letter was delivered to the door by a footman in a scarlet jacket. It was an invitation to a ball—to the Royal Ball. Up and down the street, windows were flying open, people were calling out to their neighbours:

'Did you get one?'

'Everybody got one! The king's invited everyone!'

'Every unmarried girl, anyway!'

'He wants Prince Boniface to choose himself a wife!'

Raviola, Rigatona, and Linguina twitched like hamsters at the sound of that word—'Wife'. This was what Fate had been saving up for them: marriage to a prince—riches, fame, luxury for the rest of their days. Each vain sister thought the same thing: he's bound to choose me! Each sister looked at her other two sisters and writhed with delight and hatred.

'You're so ugly, Raviola, the prince will never choose you!'

'You're so fat, Rigatona, he'll never choose you.'

'You're so stupid, Linguina, no one will ever choose you!'

They never even thought to look at Cinderella. Only their mother had the wit to know: pretty Cinderella must not be allowed to go to the ball.

Soon the day of the ball arrived. Stepmother kept Cinderella busy filling baths, fetching dresses, buying ribbons, cleaning shoes ... Raviola, Rigatona, and Linguina were in a frenzy to look their best, primping and prancing in front of the mirror, trying on one dress, trying on another. They painted their mouths, painted their cheeks; they even painted their eyebrows and coloured their hair. At last, when they stood in the hall on the evening of the ball, they looked quite ready for

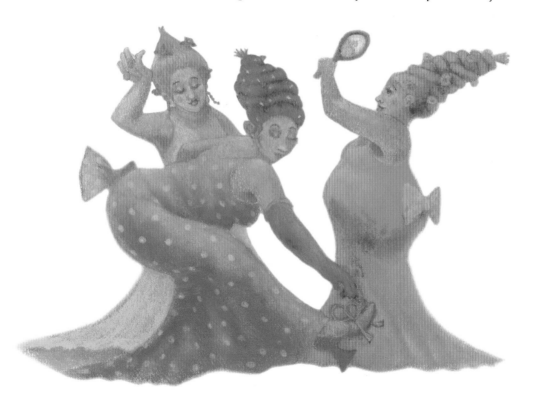

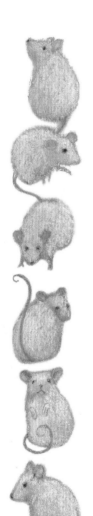

Christmas: a goose, a turkey, and a pork roast all trussed and larded.

'May I get ready now?' asked Cinderella, fetching them their velvet cloaks.

'YOU?!' Her stepsisters shrieked and twittered in horror.

'You?' said her stepmother, with a calm and chilling laugh. 'Do you really suppose the king wants a scullery maid eating off his best china?'

So saying, she swept her three daughters ahead of her out of the door and locked it loudly behind her. The sound of their carriage rattling away was almost drowned out by the three stepsisters squabbling and bickering:

'He'll marry me!'

'No, me!'

'No, me!'

Cinderella caught sight of herself in the hall mirror. Had she really thought to go to the ball? That unwashed, white-faced, half-starved waif in the mirror? Just because every young woman in the city was invited? Had she really thought her stepmother would grant her one glorious, happy night? Tears crawled like woodlice down Cinderella's grimy face, and she sank down just where she was, on the hall rug, hugging her knees, rocking to and fro. The seventeen clocks in the silent house ticked like clicking tongues: TICK TOCK TUT TUT TUT.

As the hall clock struck eight, the front door—the locked front door—swung open and in came a small, elderly woman, along with a flurry of dead leaves. She leaned on a silver-topped cane. 'Why are you crying, Cinderella?'

'Oh, it's stupid. I'm silly. Oh, but I did so want to go to the ball!' sobbed Cinderella, trying to dry her eyes on her apron.

'And so you shall, my dear. But jump up. There's work to do and it won't get done by sitting on the rug!'

Cinderella wondered if she was dreaming. But she got up and did exactly as the old lady said—'Wash your face. Comb your hair.'—It was easy: she was used to doing what she was told. 'Fetch me six mice from the traps, and a pumpkin from the garden.' It was soon done: she was used to heavy work and dirty, unpleasant jobs. 'Now set them down out there, in the road.'

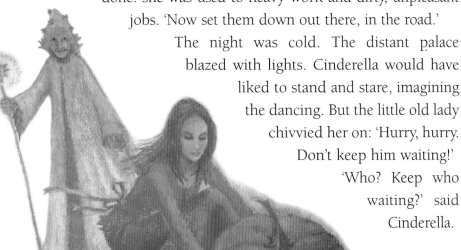

The night was cold. The distant palace blazed with lights. Cinderella would have liked to stand and stare, imagining the dancing. But the little old lady chivvied her on: 'Hurry, hurry. Don't keep him waiting!'

'Who? Keep who waiting?' said Cinderella.

'Well, the prince, of course!'

'Oh, but I—Look, I don't mean to be rude, but who are you, exactly?'

The old lady raised her silver-topped cane and flourished it three times in the air. There in the street, where the pumpkin and six mice had stood, a glass coach drawn by six white horses glittered in the starlight. 'I'm your fairy godmother, of course, child. Now hurry! The orchestra is just tuning up.'

'But I can't—' Cinderella began. 'A scullery maid can't . . .' Then she caught sight of herself in a puddle of rain. She was wearing a dress of white organza sprinkled with silver flowers. Her petticoats were of gold lace, and her hair was plaited with lilies. On her feet were glass slippers with heels like the stems of wineglasses, but so comfortable that she only noticed them as she climbed into the coach.

'One thing you must remember, child. On the strike of midnight, all magic fails and falters. Even mine. Be home by midnight, my dear, or you may never get home at all . . . Oh, my! Your dear father would be so proud of you tonight!'

'Did you know him, then? Did he send you?'

But the coach was already moving, the white horses leaping into a gallop without driver or whip. The little old lady standing on the road grew smaller and smaller in the distance, until she seemed small enough to have stood on the palm of Cinderella's hand.

At the palace, a marble staircase ran down like a white waterfall to the polished dance floor. Heralds blew fanfares to welcome each guest. Raviola, Rigatona, and Linguina were

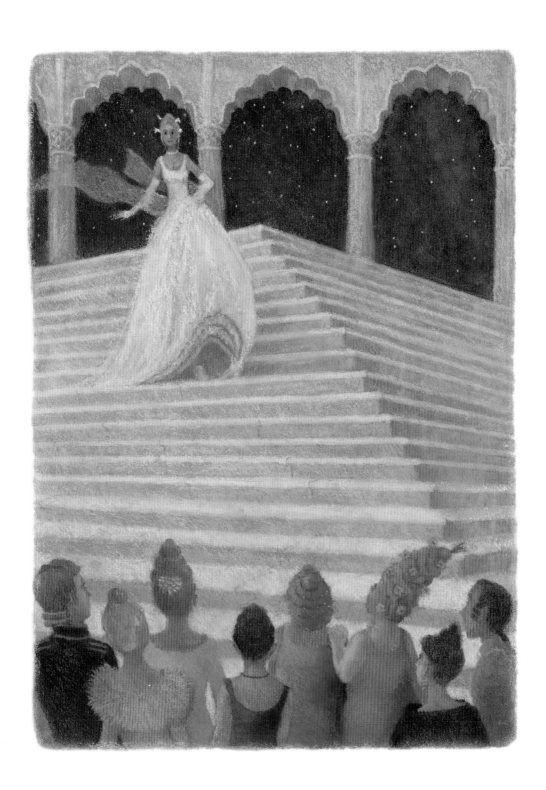

already dancing, with soldiers of the Royal Guard, but their eyes stayed fixed
on the prince, ready to wave or smile or wink if he glanced their way. The
prince was not dancing. He looked sad.

'Cheer up, m'lad!' said the king, slapping him on the back. 'Plenty of
handsome gals to choose from!'

'I just think it's a poor way to choose a wife,' muttered Prince
Boniface. 'I mean, what can I tell, just by dancing with a girl? How can
I get to know a girl in one evening?'

A last, late fanfare blew for one last, late arrival, and down the marble
stairs came a girl in white organza, sprinkled and plaited with flowers.
The dancers on the floor looked up and gasped. Such a dress! Such
petticoats! Such shoes!

But the prince saw none of that. He saw the blue of Cinderella's eyes,
her shy smile, her quick, skipping feet on the stairs. Hurrying to meet
her, he begged her to dance her first dance with him.

''Snot fair, Mummy,' snivelled Raviola. 'They didn't say princesses was
going to be here.'

'Who is she, Mummy?' snarled Rigatona. 'I could look like her if you
just bought me dresses like that!'

'Do something, Mummy,' whined Linguina. 'He's not even looking
our way!'

But for all her burning ambition, there was nothing their mother
could do. Prince Boniface had laid eyes on the love of his life, and now
no one else existed for him in the whole room.

They danced every dance together; they talked about everything in the world—except who Cinderella was and how she came to be there. Let him mistake her for a princess, she thought, otherwise he might wipe his hands on his jacket and turn away.

She saw her stepsisters, perched like plump cushions on the gilt chairs, sulking. She saw her stepmother scowling and scowling and cramming sweetmeats into her angry mouth. But they did not recognize her—did not see through her disguise, see through her magic-till-midnight finery.

Midnight! Oh!

The clock started to strike. ONE TWO.

'What time is it?' Cinderella gasped. 'Eleven o'clock?'

'Twelve,' said the prince. 'But we have the whole night ahead of us!'

THREE FOUR

'Let me go!'

'Why? Whatever's the matter?'

FIVE SIX

'I have to go! I must!' Cinderella broke away from him and started up the marble stairs.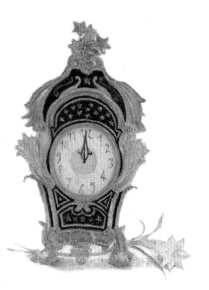

SEVEN EIGHT

Her legs were weary from dancing. The stairs seemed like a cliff. The prince called out behind her: 'Wait! You've dropped . . .' But she did not, could not wait.

NINE TEN

The cold night air broke over her like a seawave, unplaiting her hair. The six white horses were tossing their heads and pawing the ground, rocking the glass coach.

ELEVEN

As she sped away into the black of night—TWELVE—the coach burst apart around her like a snowball hitting a wall, and she went somersaulting over and over into a ditch. A pumpkin rolled in on top of her. Reaching to gather up her lovely skirts, she found no organza dress, no petticoats of gold . . . though on her left foot she still wore a single glass slipper, as if midnight had taken pity and spared her one shred of her happy, perfect evening.

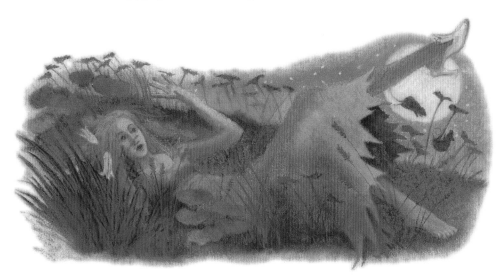

By the time the three stepsisters and their mother arrived home at dawn, Cinderella was asleep in her usual place, among the embers of the kitchen fire.

'Lazy, idle, good-for-nothing girl!' shrilled Rigatona. 'Get up and make me some breakfast. I've been dancing with the prince all night.'

'Liar!' snivelled Linguina. 'You didn't dance with him once. None of us did. We didn't stand a chance once he had seen that princess woman.'

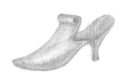

'Quiet!' snapped their mother. 'She ran away, didn't she? The game's not lost yet. How can he marry a girl who isn't there?'

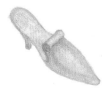

But next morning, the streets were noisy again with excitement. There were proclamations nailed to every tree, announcing that Prince Boniface had already decided on a wife. He would marry the girl with whom he had danced at the ball, and he would marry no other. Apparently, the lady had left behind, on the steps of the palace, a single glass slipper, and the prince had vowed to find the owner of that slipper. It would be carried from house to house, and every woman in the kingdom must try it on. Thus he would seek her out, hunt her down, the mysterious girl too shy to give him her name.

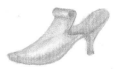

Raviola, Rigatona, and Linguina broke into howls of misery and rage, and beat on the breakfast table with their fists and foreheads. "Snot fair, Mummy! 'Snot fair!'

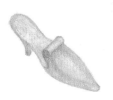

'Be quiet, you fools,' snapped their mother, her face set in grim determination. 'Cinderella! Fetch six buckets of ice from the ice-house! Be quick! If the prince wants a foot to fit his precious glass slipper, then that's what he shall have. We'll show him eight of the most delicate feet in Christendom!'

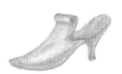

All morning they sat—stepmother and stepsisters—with their feet in buckets of ice. Though the girls whimpered and grizzled and complained—'So co-o-o-old, Mummy!'—and turned quite blue, their mother only glared and told Cinderella to fetch more ice. The cold would make their feet smaller, she said, three sizes smaller.

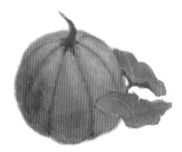

At last there was a knock at the door. The footman in the scarlet jacket stood once again on the step. This time he carried a crimson cushion and on it the single glass slipper. Pushing the buckets out of sight under the table, the four hobbled to the door. 'Come in! Come in!' said Raviola dragging him into the hall.

'Ah, you've brought back my slipper. So kind,' said Rigatona.

''Snot yours, it's mine. Let me try it on first!' shrieked Linguina.

While they squabbled, their mother calmly took hold of the glass slipper and tried to squeeze her own ice-cold foot into it. But try as she might—try as Raviola and Rigatona and Linguina might—all four had feet like shire horses. The cold had shrunk them, but not enough—not nearly enough to fit the tiny, magical glass slipper.

'Are you all the ladies in the house?' asked the flunkey.

'Yes, yes. Get out of here,' spat Stepmother in a frenzy of disappointment.

'Might I—' said Cinderella, peeping round the kitchen door.

'No! Certainly not! Get back to your work, impudent ragamuffin!' said Stepmother.

'My orders are,' said the flunkey, glimpsing a pretty face at last, 'that every lady in the land—'

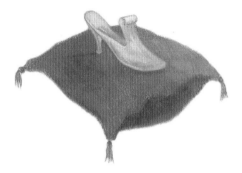

'She's no lady. She's the scullery maid!' cried Stepmother and laughed shrilly at the absurd idea of Cinderella trying on the slipper. 'She never even went to the ball! I know! I locked the door on her myself.'

'Even so . . .' said Cinderella, 'I should like to try on the shoe.'

And so she did. It fitted perfectly.

'Absurd! Ridiculous! She obviously wants to trick the prince into marrying her!' bayed Stepmother. 'She's had her feet in ice water to shrink them!'

But when Cinderella pulled from her apron pocket the matching glass slipper, its heel as fine as the stem of a wineglass, the flunkey blushed as red as his jacket and dropped to one knee. 'Begging your pardon, miss, but did you mean to break the prince's heart, running off like that?'

'If I had stayed, he would have found out who I was—what I was, I mean,' said Cinderella looking down at her rags.

'Begging your pardon, miss, but he knew that already. He knew you were the love of his life, and what else matters?'

Cinderella laughed shyly and kissed the flunkey on his bald, shiny head. 'If the prince's heart is broken, tell him I will gladly mend it for him,' she said.

And so she did. Cinderella and Prince Boniface were married within the week, and the wedding party went on for three days—three days of dancing and feasting, three days of music and fireworks. Even Raviola and Rigatona and Linguina enjoyed themselves.

Only their mother stayed at home, behind locked doors, and fumed like an old black cauldron as she stared into the embers of the kitchen fire.

As for Cinderella, she lived happily ever after, just as her father had always meant her to do when, at her birth, he named her. Not 'Cinderella', but Joy.

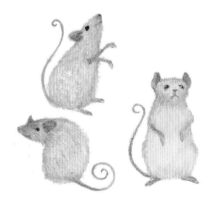

The Dancing Princesses

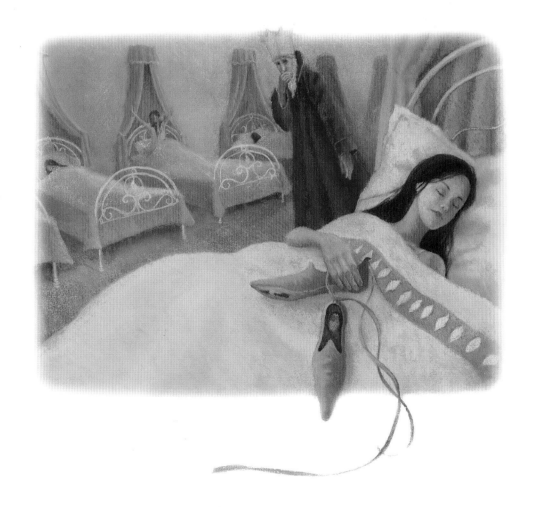

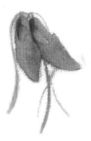

It was a time of war. Men thought only of fighting, and girls, left alone and afraid, wanted only to dance their worries away. The King of Terpsichoria did not want his twelve daughters to dance. He valued them like gold and silver and diamonds, and like gold and silver and diamonds he meant to keep them under lock and key where no one else could lay hands on them. So each night he locked them into their bedroom and each morning he found them sleeping there: still his.

But the king was baffled. The king was bewildered. The king was mystified. Every morning, at the foot of the twelve beds, were twelve pairs of satin slippers worn into holes. Twelve times he bought them new dancing slippers. Twelve times twelve! And twelve times twelve times the slippers were worn out overnight—as if the princesses had danced every hour that they slept. The king was baffled. The king was bewildered. The king was mystified. He made a decree:

'Let it be known that the king will give in marriage
the hand of a royal princess to the man who can solve
the mystery of the worn slippers!'

Every man in the land came running to the palace gates.

'I'll solve it!'

'I will!'

'I will!'

The king went on:

> *'Three nights the man may spend in the bedroom*
> *of the princesses. But if after the third night he has*
> *not solved the mystery, he shall die!'*

By the time he had said this, the queue had gone from in front of the palace gates. The princesses were beautiful, but not so beautiful that men would die to have them. War teaches people to cling on tight to their lives.

A few gallant princes came from foreign parts to attempt the quest; to discover the secret. But after three nights, none had even managed to stay awake, let alone find out how the princesses wore out their slippers. And so the princes died.

The princesses would not tell. What did they care if the princes who came never went home again?

Outside town, a wounded soldier sat with his back to a tree and wondered why the war had left him, Musgrave, alive. It had left him no

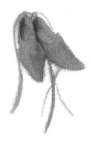

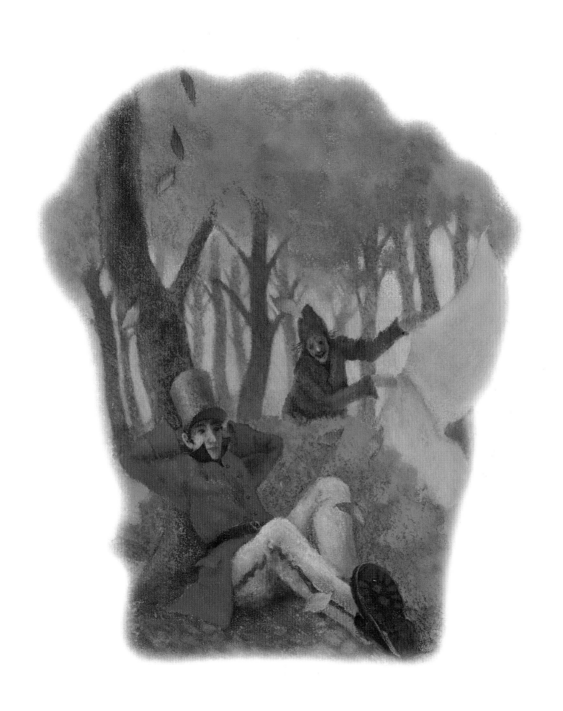

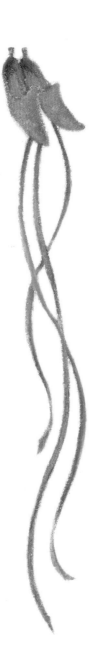

home, no job, and nothing to eat. So why had it spared his life? To sit in a wood with his back to a tree?

'I suppose you're on your way to the palace to solve the mystery?' An old woman, as wrinkled and brown as a fallen leaf, sat down beside him.

'What palace? What mystery?' said Musgrave. So the old woman told him. 'Why not? I've nothing to lose and everything to gain. I'll give it a try,' said Musgrave.

'Well said. Take this cloak,' said the crone, 'and take some advice, too. When the princesses offer you wine, don't drink it.'

'No one offers a wounded soldier a cup of wine in these heartless times, Granny,' said Musgrave, but he took the dirty rag she thrust into his hands, not wanting to offend her. The cloak looked none too clean, but then neither did Musgrave . . .

The king did not want this common, grubby soldier sleeping in his daughters' bedroom. But there were no princes left, and a hundred more pairs of slippers had been worn to holes since the challenge. So he let Musgrave try, comforting himself that in three days the impertinent young man would be dead like all the rest.

No sooner was Musgrave introduced to the

princesses, than they offered him a cup of wine, rich and red. 'Drink it! Do! You must be so thirsty after all that fighting.' Musgrave wanted it (more than any prince would have done), but he remembered what the old woman had said, and only pretended to drink, letting the luscious wine trickle out of his mouth onto his red jacket. (The stain did not show among all the others.) They showed him to a bed—soft and white and inviting. But many was the night Musgrave had had to stay awake on guard when he was dropping with fatigue. So he laid his head on the pillow, but he only pretended to sleep.

'Poor fool,' said the oldest princess. 'He hardly needed the drugged wine to make him sleep . . . Now! On with your slippers, sisters! Our partners are waiting!'

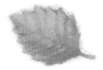

Eleven princesses leapt out of bed and ran to the great wardrobe where their dresses were kept. But the last little princess was slow to dress. 'So many young men are dead because of our dancing. Must this one die too? All is not well. My slippers are cold tonight.'

But her sisters only laughed at her and rustled into their gowns. Decking their hair and throats with jewels, they gathered together their huge skirts and squeezed into the wardrobe—and out again on the other side, into a secret passageway. A bitter draught spilled from the wardrobe into the room, making Musgrave shiver.

Wrapping himself round in the dirty rag of a cloak, he found, to his alarm, that his body suddenly disappeared! In a panic he clutched at his legs, at his arms. Phew! Still there. He was simply invisible.

Invisible! That meant he could follow the princesses! Creeping through the wardrobe, he closed the door behind him, click.

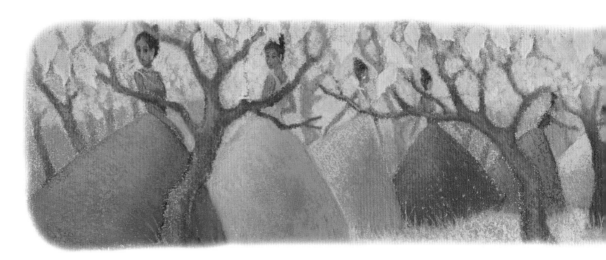

'What was that?' said the youngest princess. 'All is not well tonight. I feel it in my satins.'

But her sisters only laughed at her and ran on. The tunnel came out into an underground orchard whose trees glimmered with golden leaves. But the princesses did not stop there to dance. They ran on into an orchard whose trees scintillated with silver blossoms. But they did not stop there either to dance. They ran on into an orchard whose trees sparkled with fruits of diamond. Musgrave could not help but catch his breath at so many wonders.

'Who's there?' gasped the youngest princess. 'All is not well tonight. I feel it in my blood.'

But the sisters only laughed at her and ran on across the drawbridge of a subterranean castle. There, twelve princes with eyes of fire and hair of fur and suits of glistening jet took the princesses in their arms and danced with them till morning.

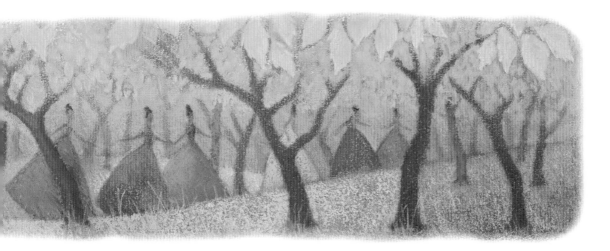

'So that is your secret, is it?' whispered Musgrave to himself.

'Who spoke?' said the youngest princess. 'All is not well tonight: I feel it in my hair!' But her partner only laughed at her and whirled her faster in the dance. The sulphur-yellow walls of the ballroom were lit with flickering red, and the flowers in the vases were not fresh but made of glass.

All night Musgrave watched. Then he followed the twelve princesses back through the three orchards and the tunnel, to their bedroom. Their slippers were worn to holes and they were pale with weariness. Musgrave could have gone then, and hammered on the king's door and told him the secret of the dancing princesses. But instead he ate the breakfast sent to him—and the lunch and dinner, too, and prepared for a second night in the bedroom of the twelve princesses.

Again he pretended to drink the wine they gave him. Again he pretended to sleep. Again the girls got up and crept, giggling and whispering, through their secret passage to their secret rendezvous. Again Musgrave followed. Although there was no sky overhead, the way was not dark, because of the shining of gold leaves, silver twigs, and fruits of diamond. All night Musgrave watched as the princesses wore their slippers to shreds dancing, then he followed them back to their beds.

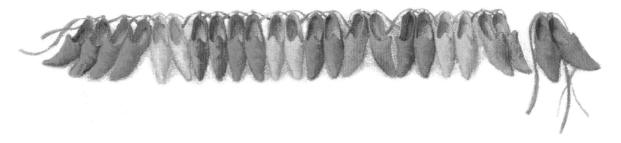

He could have gone then, and demanded to see the king, and claimed his reward for solving the mystery. But instead he ate the breakfast sent to him—and the lunch and dinner, too, and prepared for a third night.

On the third night he grew bolder. He followed the princesses so closely that he stepped on the train of the youngest's dress; she cried out in fright. Invisible in his magic cloak, Musgrave even joined in the dancing, tripping the princes with their hair of fur and their jet black suits, twirling the youngest princess around in his arms.

'Oh! Who touched me?' she said. 'All is not well tonight. I felt it in my arms—the ghost of one of those poor young men we have sent to their deaths!'

But her sisters and the princes laughed at her, and caught hold of her hands, and pulled her into their circle dance.

Back in their bedroom, the princesses kicked off their ragged slippers and fell on their beds, weary past words. The youngest looked with regret at the sleeping soldier in the corner and remembered that today was his day to die. But she too was powerless to stay awake. The nightly dancing was stealing away her strength, stealing away the roses in her cheeks, stealing away her soul . . .

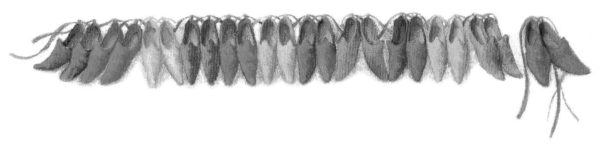

'Speak, soldier. Have you solved the mystery of the worn slippers?' asked the king, expecting to hear the same excuses: 'Please, Your Majesty, I could not stay awake. I tried—I really tried! Spare me my life!'

But Musgrave did not plead for his life. 'I have indeed solved the mystery, Your Majesty,' he said. 'Each night your daughters rise up from their beds and pass through a tunnel to an underground castle where they dance all night and every night with twelve princes. On the way, they pass through an orchard of golden trees, an orchard of silver trees, and an orchard of trees whose fruits are diamonds, to reach a castle with walls of sulphur-yellow and flowers of glass.'

'Lies! All lies!' said the oldest princess, choking down her amazement. 'He is making it all up to save his skin! Tell the liar to prove it!'

So the king went to the daughters' bedroom; so did Musgrave, and so did the executioner, busily sharpening his axe. The king blundered about among the satin dresses and silken petticoats, but could find no tunnel beyond the wardrobe. All he found were twelve pairs of ragged slippers with holes in their soles.

'The man was lying,' sighed the king. 'Take him away, executioner.'

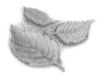

Musgrave put his hand inside his jacket. You may think he pulled out the cloak and disappeared. No. He pulled out instead a leaf of gold, a twig of silver, and a huge diamond shaped like a pear. 'These I picked in the three orchards,' he said. 'And this glass flower I took from a vase in the underground castle.'

Then the princesses burst into tears, knowing that their dancing days were over and they would see no more of the twelve princes. 'Choose your bride,' said the king. 'Choose the oldest and in time you shall inherit my kingdom and rule in my place.'

But Musgrave did not choose the oldest. He chose the youngest. 'I believe she has a little heart left to love me,' he said. 'The others have worn too many holes in their souls.'

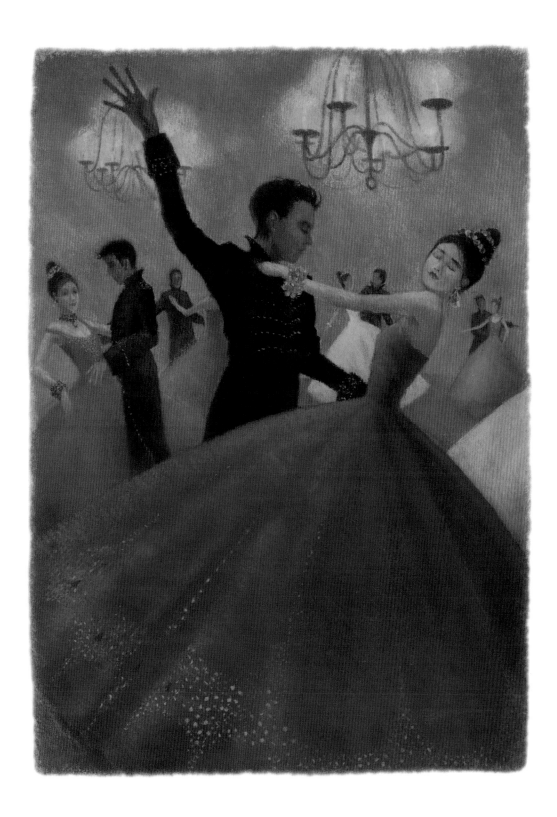

And because the king liked Musgrave's answer, and loved his youngest daughter best of the twelve, he shared his kingdom with the soldier anyway.

Which set Musgrave dancing until he wore his old army boots right through to his socks.

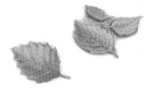

The Three Gifts of the North Wind

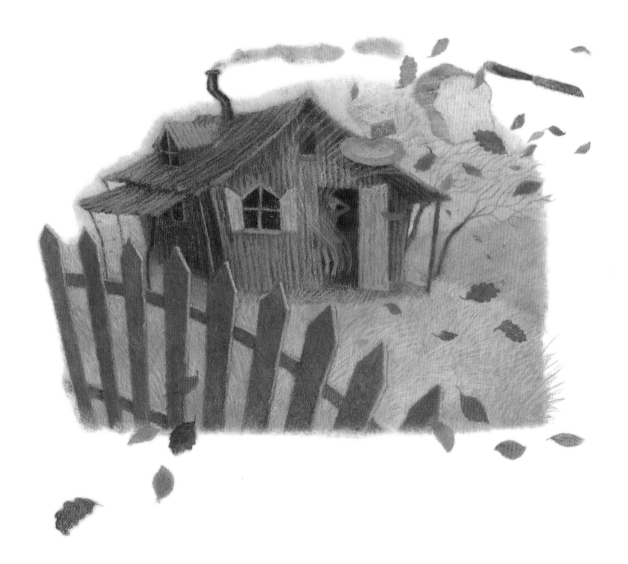

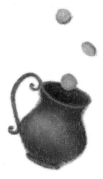

Times were hard—harder than the dry bread on Jack's table. There was nothing left in the larder but a slab of cheese, nothing in the jug but a swig of milk, no fuel to burn but the chair leg already crackling in the grate. And there wasn't a penny to buy more. But suddenly, with a roar that rattled the chimney, the North Wind blew over the hill, circled the cottage three times and, without even knocking, blustered into the kitchen.

It blew out the fire, spilled the jug of milk, and set the larder door banging. And when it swept out again, there was not a morsel of cheese in the larder, not a bite of bread on the table.

'Oho, very fine, very fine, I'm sure!' said Jack. 'Can't he pick on someone his own size?' And he was so angry that he put on his coat and went after the Wind.

Over the hill he went and through the woods. (He could see which way the Wind had gone, because the corn on the hill and the trees in the wood were laid flat.) Over the river he went and over the sea. (He could judge the course the Wind had steered, because there was wreckage on the waves and fish cast up on the rocks.) Over the horizon

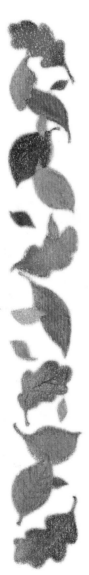

and under the rainbow went Jack, till he came to the home of the North Wind.

'All honour to your Mightiness, and all respect to your fame,' said Jack, 'but what is the world coming to when the strong steal from the weak? Give us back our supper, or my poor old mother will starve!'

The North Wind looked Jack up and down, down and up. 'The supper's eaten. Sometimes I am rash and sudden. I'm sorry.'

'Sorry won't feed my old mother,' said Jack, fists on hips.

'No, but this will,' said the North Wind. And he gave Jack a cow out of his own larder.

Now a cow is a very fair exchange for a meal of bread and cheese—especially since this cow was magic. When she was milked she gave not cream but a stream of gold coins. So Jack happily took the cow and led her homewards.

It was a long journey, so Jack had to spend the night at an inn. When the innkeeper asked him to pay for his supper, Jack simply held a tankard under the cow and milked her. Three gold coins jingled into the mug.

If the innkeeper was startled, he did not show it. 'That's a fine animal you've got there,' he said, and showed Jack to his bed.

But after Jack had gone, that innkeeper danced a jig on the floor, then went and hid Jack's cow in his own barn. In its place he led in a bull, painted it to look just

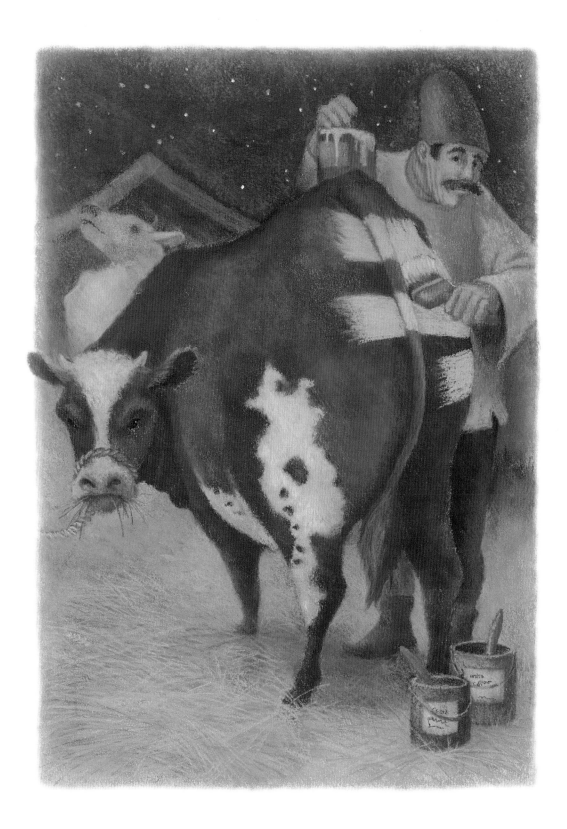

like Jack's cow, and left it tied up in the same place, saying, 'The lad's a
fool, and riches are wasted on a fool.'

So when Jack got home with his 'magic cow', he said, 'Mother,
mother, the North Wind gave me a cow that gives gold in place of milk!'

Well, when Jack's old mother tried to milk the cow, she got neither
milk nor gold, but a large hole in her cottage wall where the bull ran off.
'Oh, Jack, Jack, you're a gullible fool and I pity any wife that's fool
enough to marry you,' said Jack's mother. But he did not hear; he had
already gone . . . back to the home of the North Wind.

'All glory to your Mightiness and all sparkle to your fame,' said Jack,
'but what is the world coming to when the wise lie to the trusting? That
cow gave gold once and never again. She won't save my old mother
from going hungry!'

'I'm puzzled,' said the North Wind.

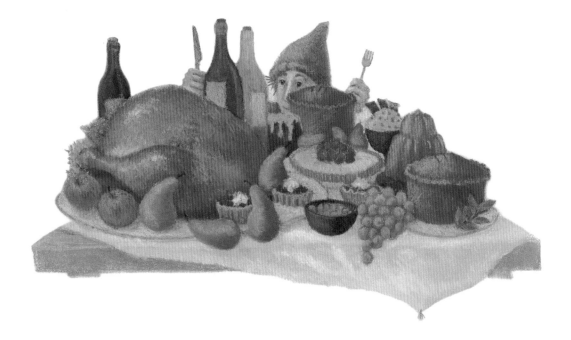

'Puzzled won't feed my old mother,' said Jack, fists on hips.

'No, but this will,' said the Wind. And he fetched a tablecloth out of his own linen basket, flicking it clean of crumbs.

Now a tablecloth may seem a poor exchange for a cow or a supper. But this cloth was magic. As soon as it was laid flat, and heard the words, 'Feed me food,' it filled up with all manner of wonderful things to eat. So Jack happily took the cloth and headed home.

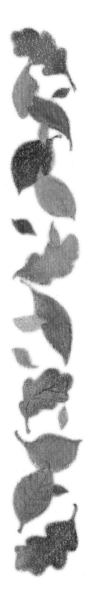

Once again he stayed overnight at the inn. But this time he ordered no supper. Instead, he laid the cloth on the table, said, 'Feed me food!' and—yum! yum!—there were pies and cold joints, tarts and fruit, jellies and bottles of wine enough to satisfy every hungry traveller in the inn.

If the innkeeper was surprised, he did not show it. But after Jack had gone to bed, he and his wife danced a jig on the messy tables, then fetched out the oldest pillowcase in the house. They stole Jack's magic cloth from under his snoring head, and put the pillowcase there instead, saying, 'The lad's a fool and fools don't deserve feasts.'

So when Jack reached home with his 'magic cloth', and spread it in front of his old mother saying, 'Feed us food,' nothing more nutritious than a bedbug and a flea appeared in front of them.

'Oh, Jack, Jack, you're a fool and a daydreamer, and I

pity the wife that's fool enough to marry you,' said Jack's mother. But Jack did not hear: he had already gone . . . back to the home of the North Wind.

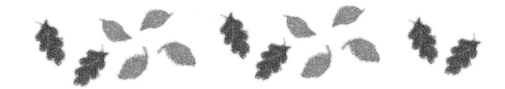

'Long life to your Mightiness and regards to your little ones, but what is the world coming to when the clever play tricks on the foolish? That cloth shrank to the size of a pillowcase before I even got it home, and my poor old mother hasn't had one bite to eat off it.'

'Ah, I think I understand!' said the North Wind.

'So do I,' said Jack (who was not the fool he looked). 'I was robbed by that fat blighter of an innkeeper. But what can I do about it?'

'Take this bag,' said the North Wind, 'and let it be heard by those with ears to hear, that the thing inside will do wonders for the man who asks it: Come out and do your worst!'

So Jack took the bag—it was long and thin and heavy—and travelled as far that night as the inn.

'And what wonder do you have with you tonight, Jack?' asked the innkeeper, all smiles.

'Oh, a marvellous thing, but not for strangers to see,' whispered Jack. (He put the bag under his jacket where it would not hear him.) 'If I were to say, "Come out and do your worst"—ah! then you would see a wonder!'

The innkeeper only polished a glass and shrugged.

But after Jack had gone to bed, he and his wife and his brother and his wife's mother all danced a jig on the stairs. 'The lad's a fool and fools don't deserve marvels,' they said, and stole the bag from the foot of Jack's bed.

'Come out and do your worst!' said the innkeeper.

'Come out and do your worst!' said his wife.

'Come out and do your worst,' said his brother.

'Come out and do your worst,' said his wife's mother.

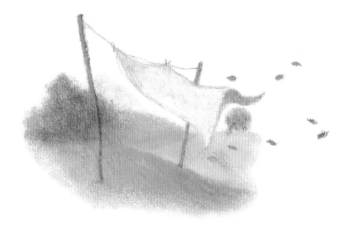

They were not left wanting for wonders. Out of the bag slid an enormous wooden club, and it began to swing and bat, thrash and clout for all it was worth. It chased the innkeeper and his family right out of the inn, over hill and fields, over the horizon, and under the rainbow.

So Jack and his mother left their draughty cottage and moved to the inn, where they found their magic cow munching hay in the barn and their magic tablecloth hidden in a drawer. 'Oh, Jack, Jack, you're a hero and a wonder, and the wife's not born who's good enough to marry you!' said his old mother fondly.

After that, the inn door stood open to any traveller who passed by. In fact the door was never shut—not even to the North Wind when he swooped and whistled out of a bitter sky and set the chimney rattling.

The Old Lady Next Door

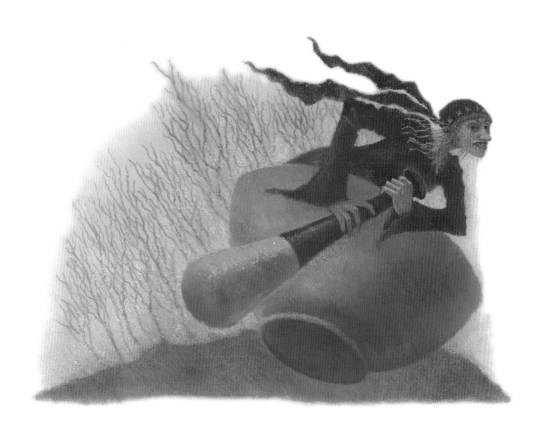

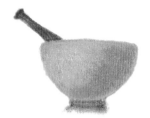

If it had not been for Vassia's doll, who knows what might have become of her? Vassia's doll was given her by her mother, and that made her special. But Kookolka was special in other ways, too. How many dolls can eat and talk, for instance? And Kookolka was clever— almost as clever as Vassia's mother when she gave the doll to her daughter, saying: 'Keep her always by you, Vassy. And if ever you are in trouble, ask her advice.'

Soon after that, Vassy was indeed in trouble, deep trouble. Her dear mother died, and her father married again—a fearful, cruel woman with two daughters more cruel and fearful still. Whenever her father was away on business (and that was often) Kasha and Masha and their mother did everything they could to make life unbearable. They ordered Vassy about like a slave, keeping her skivvying from morning till night.

'Oh, Kookolka, doll dear, share this food of mine and tell me what to do!' Vassy would say, breaking off a corner of hard black bread for Kookolka to eat. 'My sisters tell me I must dig the vegetable patch and paint the chicken run and wash the curtains and scour the stove—and all by sunset!'

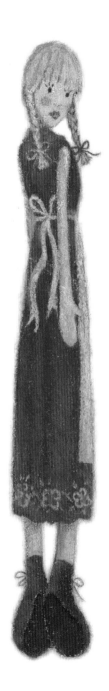

Then Kookolka would nod and nibble, nibble
and nod, and smile at Vassy with her red-thread
lips. 'I know a little bed of primroses in the wood.
Why don't you go and have a sleep there, my dear,
while I consider the problem.' So Vassy went and
slept on the primroses, dreaming golden dreams,
and when she woke—gracious and goodness!—the
chicken coop was painted, the vegetable patch dug,
the curtains were drying on the line, and the stove
was sparkling. Also Kookolka was back in Vassy's
pocket.

Every day Vassy grew more and more beautiful,
but not her sisters. They plotted such plots against
Vassy and they grew so furious when their plots did
not work that their foreheads were soon creased and
their mouths permanently puckered. Consequently,
the young men in town never looked at Masha or
Kasha. They only gazed in wonder at Vassia.

'That does it! The girl must go!' declared their
mother. 'And here's the way it shall be done . . .'

Kasha and Masha did as their mother told them
and snuffed all the lights in the house—the candles
and the lamps. They even poured water into the
stove to put out the glowing cinders. Then they
shouted, 'Vassia! Lazy girl! Light the lamps! Cook
the breakfast! Heat us water for our baths!'

'But there's no light in the house,' said Vassy. 'The
stove is cold and all the lamps are out.'

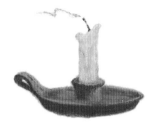

'Oh dear, oh dear, oh dear,' sneered her stepmother. 'Then you'd best go to our neighbour and ask for a flame. Well? What are you waiting for?'

Vassy was waiting for the beat to come back to her heart, for the sickness to go from her stomach, for the terror to drain out of her. 'Go next door? To Baba Yaga?'

Now the only other house for miles around belonged to Baba Yaga, the witch woman. The house itself was terrifying enough, for its garden fence was made of bones, its thatch of human hair, and it ran about on four chicken legs, up and down, to and fro, here and there. In place of bolts were two human hands, and in place of the latch a snarling mouth jagged with teeth. But Baba Yaga was far more fearful than her house, for she flew about in a giant mortar, punting her way through the air with the pestle and sweeping away all trace of her journey with a twig broom. And, of course, she ATE anyone who strayed too close to her house.

'Oh, Kookolka, doll dear, share this food of mine and tell me what to do! My sisters want me to go to the house of Baba Yaga to fetch a light. Give me a flame, won't you, so that I can light the stove again?'

Kookolka nibbled and nodded, nodded and nibbled her share of Vassy's dry black bread. But she would not give Vassy a flame. 'Put me in your pocket and don't be afraid. Who knows? Some good may come of a visit to Baba Yaga.'

Vassy was horrified, but she did as she was told, and with Kookolka in her pocket, she trudged into the dark wood which held Baba

Yaga's dreadful cottage. As she walked, a horseman overtook her—a horseman dressed in white on a white horse with white bridle and saddle, as darting as light. About noon, another horseman overtook her—a horseman all in red, on a red horse with red bridle and saddle, as hot as fire. All day it took her to walk to Baba Yaga's house, and just as she reached the bony fence, a third horseman shot by her, stirring up the leaves in clouds. He was all in black, on a black horse with a black bridle and saddle—and he appeared to ride straight through the wall of the cottage and disappear from sight!

Behind him came Baba Yaga!

'Oho! Oho! Supper on legs!' croaked the old witch in a voice like a roosting rook. 'What brings you here, girly?' Her mortar swooped so low over Vassy's head that it stood her hair on end.

'My stepmother sent me to ask for a light,' whispered Vassy, clutching the doll in her pocket, her eyes tight shut in terror.

But Baba Yaga did not club her with the giant pestle or tear her with her long nails. 'Very well. But I don't do favours. If you want a light, you must work for it. If your work is satisfactory, you shall have your flame. If not, I shall have you—and a tender little mouthful you'll make, for sure. Open, house!'

The house crabbed a few steps to the right, a few to the left on its chicken legs, then the bolt-hands unclasped and the latch-mouth closed, and the door

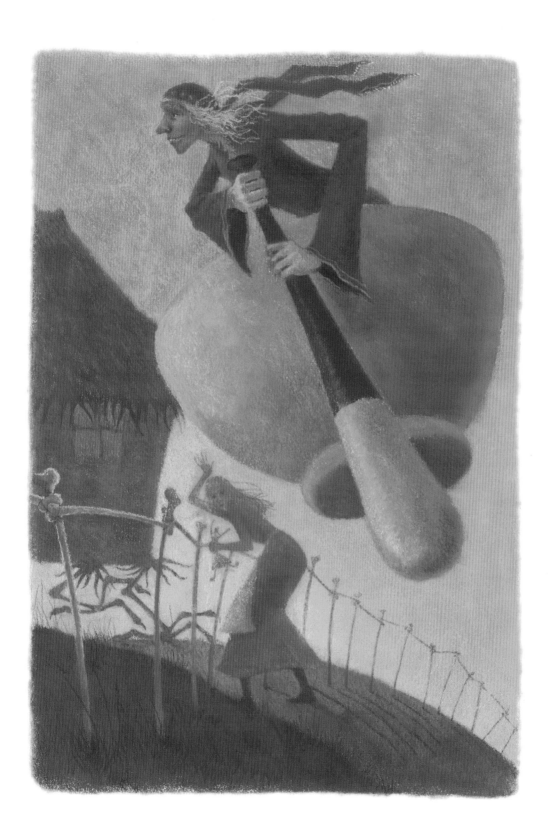

opened to Baba Yaga. 'Fetch me some dinner!' commanded Baba Yaga, and Vassy ran here and there, finding whatever she could. Everything she brought—salad, apples, cold meat, raw meat, porridge, and bread—Baba Yaga wolfed down, until the cupboards were bare. Then she ate the shelves from the cupboards and the coal from the fire, before wiping her mouth on her sleeve. 'Tomorrow you can clean all the wheat in that cornbin—sort grains from husks,' she told Vassy. 'And see it's done before I get home, or I'll EAT you. Hands! Hands! Come!'

Suddenly three pairs of hands—no bodies, no arms, just hands—appeared out of thin air, cleared the table, plumped the pillow on Baba Yaga's bed, and laid her gently down there. One pair of hands was white, one pair red, and one pair black. Then with a clap—one clap, two clap, three clap—all three disappeared.

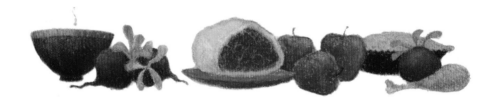

Next morning, away went Baba Yaga punting her pestle, and Vassy opened the cornbin. It stood as high as the ceiling and was full to the brim with wheat and husks, all mixed up together.

'Oh, Kookolka, doll dear, share these crumbs with me and tell me what to do! It will take a lifetime to clean this wheat!!'

Kookolka climbed out of her apron pocket and took the few crumbs from Vassy's palm. 'I saw a clump of bluebells in the garden. Go and pick some for the old woman—and don't worry.' So Vassy went and picked bluebells, and put them in vases all about the house. While she was outside, those horsemen rode up again—in at the gate and right through the house—first white, then red, then black. Vassy remembered the three pairs of hands. The third was no sooner past than dusk fell and Baba Yaga came speeding home, her mortar spinning, her pestle pushing, her broom sweeping away all trace of her passage through the forest. 'Open, door!' she screeched as she came.

Baba Yaga looked around her at the bluebells. 'And is it done? The work? Or am I to eat you for supper?' Heaving the lid off the cornbin she squinnied inside, and there— gracious and goodness!—were a dozen bushels of clean wheat. 'Oho, do I smell magic?' said the witch woman in a voice like a crooked crow. 'How came the impossible done by a young girl like you?'

'Please, ma'am, by reason that my mother loved me, I suppose,' said Vassy, curtsying. 'I'll just fetch your dinner.'

Once again the witch woman ate as much as an army of men, and again the three pairs of hands—white, red, and black—cleared the table and carried her to bed.

'Tomorrow your job is to part the poppy seeds from the gravel!' croaked a sleepy voice out of the darkness. 'Or I'll EAT you!'

On the second day, Vassy's doll sorted the million poppy seeds in the seedbin from a million grains of grey gravel, while Vassy cooked a delicious vegetable stew for the old witch. Again the horsemen thundered through the gate, through the garden, through the house—white, red, and

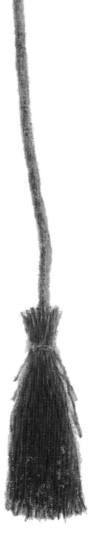

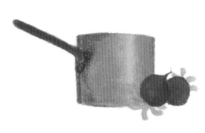

black. Again, dark fell and the witch was home again—push-swish, push-swish. 'Oho! Oho! I smell magic here!' she said, running the poppy seeds through her bony fingers. 'How came the impossible done by a young girl like you?'

'Please, ma'am, by reason that my mother loved me, I suppose,' said Vassy curtsying. 'I cooked you a special stew for dinner.'

Baba Yaga began to warm towards the young girl. 'Say, child, is there anything that puzzles you about this strange world?'

'There is,' said Vassy. 'Who are the horsemen I saw out there, in the forest—one white, one red, one black?'

'Oho! One is my bright dawn, one my red noon, one my dark knight!' said Baba Yaga and peered keenly into Vassy's pretty face. 'What else?'

'When I am older, I shall be wiser,' said Vassia politely. 'It would be rude to pester you with any more questions.'

'Oho! Oho! Well said!' cried the witch woman, leaping up and down with delight and shaking both her bony arms. 'If you had asked me one question about the inside of my house, I would have had to EAT you. As it is, you may have your light and go. But don't forget your old granny Yaga when your life changes for the better.'

She gave Vassia a tiny candle in a little candlestick, and sent her out into the night. Oddly enough, the light from the candle, small as it was, lit the forest path quite clearly. And though wolves howled, and owls hooted, after three days in the house of Baba Yaga, Vassia was not afraid of anything.

'Oh. It's you,' said Kasha, heartbroken to see her pretty stepsister safe home again.

'What took you so long?' said Masha, snatching the candle. 'You've been gone four days and here's us with no warmth, no light, and no hot water to wash in!'

But before Vassia could tell them everything that had happened, the flame of the little candle jumped off its wick and began to flit about the room. It grew bigger, too, until like a ball of lightning, it was rolling around the walls of the house, setting light to the curtains, the rugs, the bedding. Kasha, Masha, and their mother screamed and ran out of the house in their night clothes. Away they went through the forest, the flame splitting into three to chase them, three roaring fireballs which lit

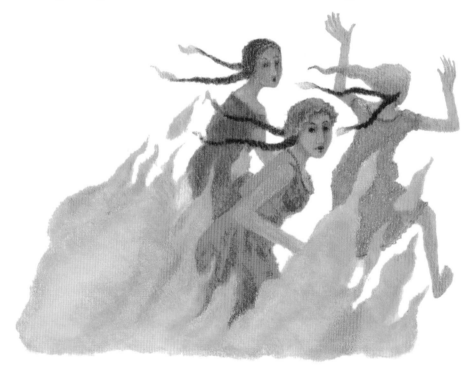

their flying plaits like the wicks of candles and drowned out their noise with incendiary crackling.

Vassia stood in the garden and watched her home burn down, enjoying the rosy silence, the scent of woodsmoke, savouring her freedom. She picked out of the ashes her few belongings (Kookolka was safe in her pocket, of course) and walked back through the forest to Baba Yaga's house, to tell her the news.

But instead of the chicken-legged house, she found only a little cottage, and living there a frail old lady with no one in the world to look after her.

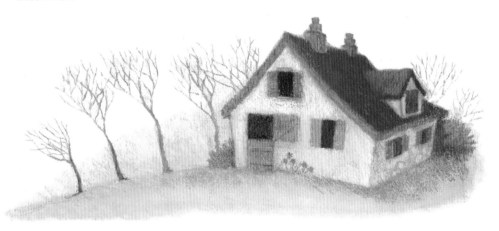

'May I lodge with you, Grandma?' said Vassia politely. 'If you buy flax, I can spin and weave it, and you can sell the cloth and keep the money. Like that, we may get by until my father comes home.'

The lady was very glad of Vassia's company and of her sensible suggestion. She went out at once and, with her last copeck, bought all the flax she could afford.

'Oh, Kookolka, doll dear,' said Vassy when she had the flax in her lap. 'Share this last crust of mine and then please help me spin my flax.'

Kookolka nodded and nibbled, nibbled and nodded. And of course Kookolka spun the flax far finer than any human hands could do, so that when it was woven into cloth, there was no softer, finer-woven piece of linen from Moscow to Petrograd.

'I'll take it to the Tsar!' cried the old lady. 'No one else in all Russia is good enough to wear such cloth on his back!' So the linen was presented to the Tsar, and he rewarded the gift with gifts of his own, saying, 'I have never seen cloth like it!'

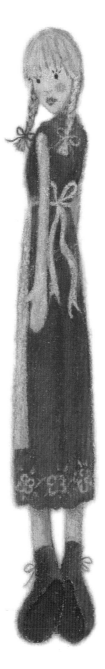

But—goodness and gracious!—the weave was so very fine that the Tsar's tailor had no needle sharp enough to sew it into a shirt! And though tailors were sent for from Kiev and Omsk and Archangel, none of them could sew the linen either.

So the Tsar sent for the old woman and said, 'Grandma, I'm afraid you will have to sew this for me. You have made it so fine that my tailor cannot pass a needle through it!'

'Bless you, Majesty, I didn't make it,' said the old woman. 'A young woman staying in my house spun it and wove it. And she is more beautiful than the cloth itself.'

'Then you'd better send her to me,' said the Tsar.

Vassia was sent for, and took back the linen, and asked dolly Kookolka to sew it into a shirt for the Tsar. Now whether Kookolka sewed magic into the seams, or whether the old woman was less ordinary than she seemed, or whether Vassy was more beautiful than I told you—when she placed the shirt in the Tsar's lap, he asked her to marry him, then and there—said he would have no other bride out of all Russia. And Vassia agreed.

Her father came home from business to a surprise or two—his house burned down, his wife and stepdaughters gone, his little Vassy betrothed to the Tsar. But he ran all the way to the palace and was there in time to see the ceremony. Vassia looked more beautiful than ever. And though many at the wedding wondered: 'Goodness and gracious! A wedding dress with pockets?'—Vassia said the pocket was for her doll and that she would go nowhere without Kookolka—not even to the altar.

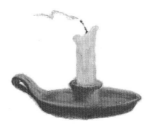

Snow White

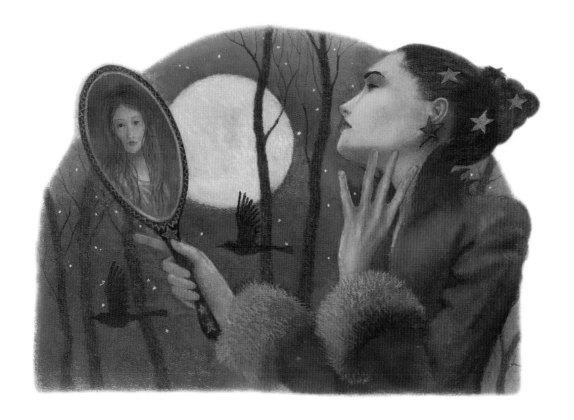

There was once a king who loved his daughter more than his kingdom, thought her black hair softer than night, her red lips more precious than rubies, her snow white skin lovelier than silk. But the child's mother was dead, and the king married again—a handsome woman named Grimalda—thinking his new wife could not fail to love Princess Snow White.

The new queen had a magic mirror, and every time the moon was full, she would ask the moonlit glass:

> *'Mirror, mirror in my hand,*
> *Who is the fairest in the land?'*
> And the mirror would answer:
> *'I cannot speak but what is true:*
> *No one is fairer, queen, than you.'*

But though the queen's face was beautiful, her nature was not. She envied Snow White her place in the king's heart, looked on her black hair, red lips, and white skin as fondly as coal and blood and sleet, and wished her away. Besides, she could not fail to see how every day Snow White grew more and more beautiful.

One day, when the moon was full, the wicked queen asked her moonlit magic glass,

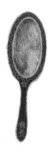

'Mirror, mirror in my hand,
Who is the fairest in the land?'
And the mirror answered:
'I cannot speak but what is true:
Snow White is fairer, queen, than you.'

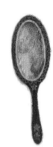

In her jealousy, the queen spat at the moon. 'Then she must die!' she cried, and the moon turned a little paler hearing it.

Summoning the royal huntsman, the wicked Grimalda said, 'Take Snow White into the forest, beyond paths, beyond tracks. And when you reach the darkest place . . . kill her. Bring me her heart, so that I may be certain you have obeyed me!'

The huntsman dared not refuse. But as he walked into the trackless forest, Snow White's little hand in his, he was glad of the shadows to hide his tears. At the centre of the forest, he pulled out his long-bladed knife with one hand while with the other he cupped Snow White's face. He saw her hair, black as the raven, saw her lips, red as the wild rose, saw her skin, whiter than the moon with fright. 'I can't do it, child. I can't kill you. The soul inside me forbids it. Run, child! Run and hide! Run, and don't stop running till you are out of this benighted land and into a better one. Run!'

Slipping and skidding on fallen leaves, Snow White fled. No hunted fawn, no songbird chased with nets ever fled as blindly as the panic-stricken princess. Through brambles and thickets, clearings and ditches, she ran on and on, the breath sobbing in her throat. The moonlight fell on her between the leaves like cold drops of water, and the mud plastered her skirts to her legs; her shoes filled up with stones.

Meanwhile, the huntsman killed a boar, cut out its heart, and took the heart to the queen, on a silver dish, to prove Snow White was dead. The queen believed him and laughed a strange, hooting laugh like a bittern booming on fog-bound marshes. The king believed it, too—believed his daughter had been killed by wild beasts in the forest. But though he searched and searched, he found no rag, no bone, no hank of black hair. It was as though Snow White had melted away.

All night Snow White wandered the deep, dark forests, lost and in despair. In the morning, she found a cottage—a wee building hardly bigger than a chicken shed and almost as ramshackle.

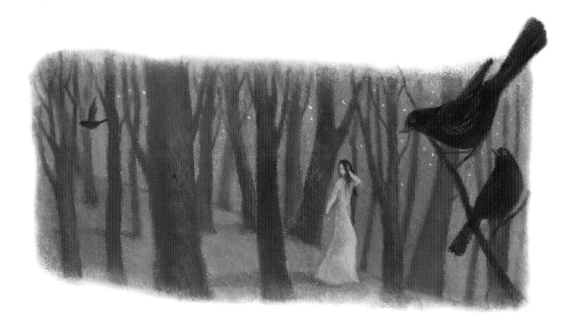

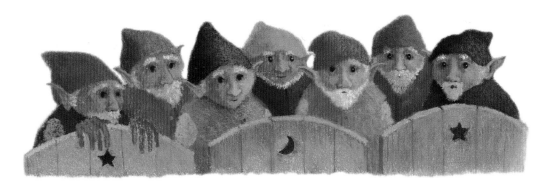

She called out, but no one answered. She knocked at the door, but nobody came. She ducked inside, and found seven little chairs round a table strewn with seven dirty bowls, knives, forks, and spoons. And she wondered, 'Are there other children like me in this forest?'

Upstairs, there were seven little beds, side by side. Chilled and exhausted, Snow White said to herself, 'Yesterday I was almost killed and if I die tomorrow, at least I have lived one more day.' And she lay down across all seven little beds and went to sleep.

When she woke, she thought she must have fallen into Fairyland, for seven small men were looking at her over the footrail of the bed. 'Is this your house?' she whispered.

'Just like it, and just where we left it this morning. But of course we could be mistaken, for there was no girl on our beds this morning.' Their ears were leafy and their hair like the tufts of sheep's wool that snag on briars.

When Snow White told them her name and her story, their eyes grew large as plums and filled with tears. 'You must stay with us, princess,' they said, 'and we shall love you as you should rightly have been loved all along. Only care for us a little, if you can.'

So Snow White stayed on in the little cottage, and cooked and sewed for the seven woodsmen. She mended their roof, too, when it leaked. And their boots. Before the moon had waned and waxed once more, she had grown very fond of her seven friends.

Each morning, as they set off to work, they warned her, 'Lock the door and don't open—no, not to knocking or calling. One day the queen may find out you are here, and if she does, she won't come with kisses in her pocket.'

They were right. One night, when the moon was full, the wicked Queen Grimalda asked of her magic glass:

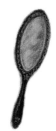
'Mirror, mirror in my hand,
Who is the fairest in the land?'
and the mirror replied:
'I cannot speak but what is true.
Snow White is fairer far than you.'
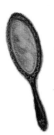

At that, the queen spat at the stars. 'Not dead? Then where is she? Tell me! I must know!' And, because it had no power to lie, the mirror told the queen the way to the cottage in the woods.

First the blackbirds stopped singing. Then there came a knock on the door. 'Greetings to the lady of the house! Won't you open to an old tinker woman and see my tray of pretty things?'

Snow White remembered the words of the seven woodsmen, and peeped cautiously out of the window, to see if it was the queen. But it was only a ragged gypsy, peddling ribbons and buttons and belts. So she opened the door and gazed in delight at all the colourful things on the tray. Prettiest of all was a belt plaited from white leather. 'How much is the belt?' she asked.

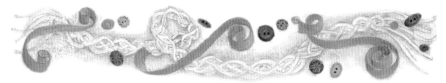

'Because your skin is just as white and soft, you may have it for nothing,' said the gypsy. 'Let me put it on for you.' And she put the belt round Snow White's waist and pulled it tight.

Tight and tighter she pulled it, sharp and cruel and fierce. 'Oh! I can't breathe!' cried Snow White, but the gypsy only pulled harder and harder, until the princess fainted for want of air and fell to the ground.

Then the wicked Queen Grimalda threw off her ragged disguise. 'Dead at last!' she crowed and swaggered back to the palace.

When the seven woodsmen came home, they found Snow White lying across the threshold as white as death. At once they cut the leather of the belt, and with a cry like a woodcock, she drew in a great breath. And when she saw the seven anxious faces looking at her, she laughed and said, 'I may die tomorrow, but at least I have lived another day!'

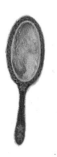
'Mirror, mirror, in my hand,
Who is the fairest in the land?'
asked the wicked queen
when next the moon was full.
'I cannot speak but what is true;
Snow White is fairer far than you,'
replied the mirror.
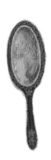

In her fury, the queen spat at the sky. 'Not dead? Then I must try harder!' she cried, and wanting a better disguise than before, conjured herself the face and body of an old lady.

First the thrushes stopped singing, and then there came a knock at the door and a voice at the keyhole. 'Pretty trinkets! Lovely things for a lovely girl! Open and see!'

Snow White remembered the words of the seven woodsmen, and peeped down from an upstairs window. But when she saw the grey hair, the stooping back, the weather-beaten ugly face, she knew it could not be the queen and opened the door. 'How much is that pretty comb?' she asked.

'Because it shines like your glossy black hair, dearie, you may have it for nothing. Let me comb out the tangles.' And she began to comb Snow White's jet black hair.

But with every stroke of the comb, the princess felt the strength drain from her arms, from her legs, from her heart—'Stop, please!'—until with a sigh she crumpled to the ground. The wicked Grimalda laughed aloud and snarled the comb deep into Snow White's hair. 'Dead at last!' she crowed and, throwing off her magic disguise, straightened her

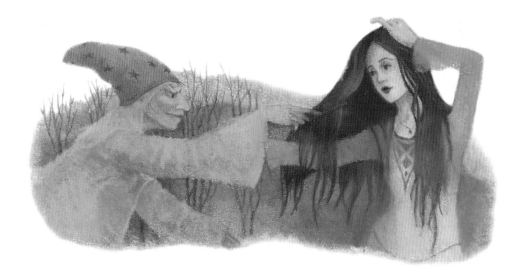

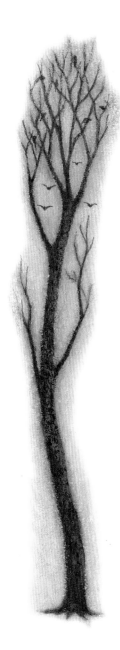

willowy back. Still, some of the magic clung to her, and she walked back to the palace more slowly this time, aching, as if a grain of old age had lodged in her bones.

When the seven woodsmen came home, they found Snow White sprawled across the threshold, white as death, though with no sign of a hurt. They searched for many minutes before they found the comb tangled in her hair and pulled it free. With a cry like a gull, she opened her eyes and drew in a great breath. Then seeing the seven anxious faces leaning over her she smiled and said, 'I may die tomorrow, but at least I have lived one more day!'

'Mirror, mirror in my hand
Now who's fairest in the land?'
asked the wicked queen when
next the moon was full.
'I cannot speak but what is true;
Snow White is fairer far than you,'
replied the moonlit mirror.

In her rage, the queen spat at the mirror, but only succeeded in dirtying her own reflection. She saw her mouth twist as it formed the words: 'Next time I shall not fail!'

First the larks stopped singing. Then there came

a knock at the door and a voice at the keyhole and a rattling of the lock. 'Fine juicy apples! Buy my fine juicy apples!'

'No,' said Snow White through the locked door. 'I never open the door to strangers.'

'Quite right, quite right,' said the deep, dark voice outside. 'Won't you open the window and just see my apples?'

Snow White remembered the gypsy and the old woman and the words of the seven woodsmen. But when she looked out of the window and saw a handsome young man with a basket of rosy apples, she could see no harm in the world. 'How much is one apple?'

'Because your lips are as red as any apple, take one and welcome.'

So Snow White reached down and took an apple . . . then she put it back. No, no. It may be poisoned, she thought.

'Do you fear it's sour, lassie? Do you fear it's wormy?' chuckled the young man, and took a great cracking, juicy bite from the green of the apple. 'See? Quite safe to eat.'

So Snow White laughed with relief and took the apple from the young man's hand and bit into it—bit into the rosy red side . . . bit into the side painted with scarlet poison.

With a cry like a swan shot from the sky, Snow White fell to the floor. 'Dead at last!' cried the wicked queen, shrugging off her magic disguise. Rushing home to the magic mirror, she at once pulled it out and began to ask:

> *'Mirror mirror in my hand . . .'*

But the reflection in the mirror was so ugly, so lined by hatred and cruelty and jealousy, that Grimalda could not bear to look at it and thrust the mirror away, deep under her pillows.

When the seven woodsmen came home, they found Snow White lying on the floor of the cottage. Though they searched her hair, her hands, her pockets, they could find no reason for her death, but could only cry and keen and sorrow at the loss of their dear, dear princess.

They could not bear to bury her in the dank, wormy ground, so they made a glass coffin, and placed her inside it, in the full face of the sun. At first they could only sit and gaze at her pale, lifeless loveliness. But after a time there was work to be done, and they would visit her each evening with flowers and fresh tears.

So Snow White's body in her glass coffin was quite alone the day the prince rode by. Lost in the forest he stopped at the cottage to ask the way. Seeing the coffin in the garden, he stopped to look at the young girl inside. Stopping to look, he found he could not look away, for she was the loveliest girl he had ever seen. He was still there, gazing and gazing, when the seven woodsmen came home that evening.

'Her name was Snow White,' said the oldest, startling the prince who had not heard them coming. 'A princess and as sweet-natured as she was beautiful.'

When the prince heard her story, he was filled with such a passion of grief that he struck the coffin with his fist, and cracked it clean across. When he saw the breeze ruffle Snow White's clothes and stir her raven-black

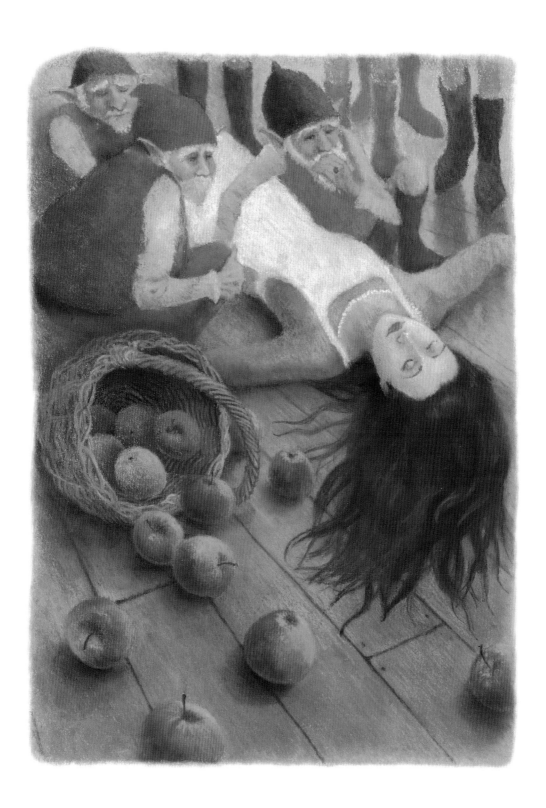

hair, he struck his chest as though to break the heart inside. Then he gathered Snow White up in his arms and kissed her full on the mouth.

The piece of poisoned apple lodged in her throat was shaken loose, and Snow White woke up with a cry of happiness. When she saw the prince's face close up to her own, she smiled and said, 'I may die tomorrow, but at least I have known what it is to be in love.'

The queen dreamt that the moon rose blood red and that the stars were falling on her. She thrust her hand under the pillow and pulled out her magic looking-glass.

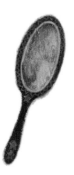 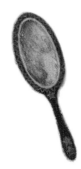

'Mirror, mirror in my hand
Who is the fairest in the land?'
And the mirror answered:
'Lovely Snow White, happy bride
Is the fairest far and wide,
But fairer still will be her heir—
The little daughter she will bear.'

The queen's rage knew no bounds, no depths, no end. She smashed the mirror against the moonlit wall—and in that very instant, fell dead.

But her soul? Oh, her soul was in that mirror—had been for many years. And that lived on, trapped for ever within a thousand broken shards of glass, and a magic circle of ebony.

Meanwhile, Snow White dreamed that the moon leaned down from the sky to kiss her. But when she woke, she found it was only the prince, her husband. So she smiled, kissed him back, turned over and went back to sleep.

The Three Oranges

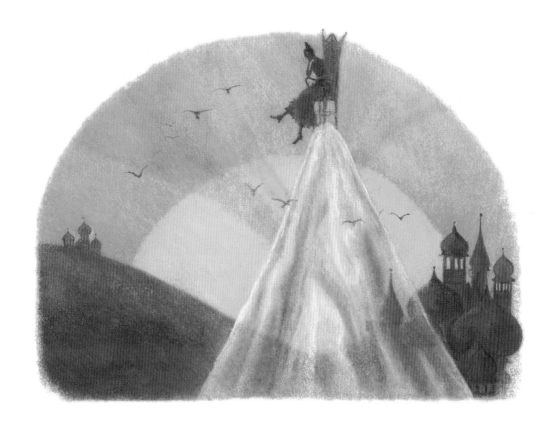

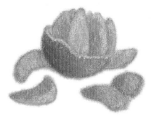

There was once a king who wanted, and did not want, his daughter to marry. So anxious was he to take care of her that he would have kept her in a box if he could and taken her out only to dust. Instead, he built a crystal mountain—a pyramid of steeply sloping glass, a transparent icicle one hundred feet high. And there at the top he placed a throne, where Princess Purity could sit and watch the world without any danger of it harming her.

'If any man can climb to the top of the glass mountain,' he decreed, 'and take the three oranges lying in my daughter's lap, he may marry her, and I shall give him half my kingdom!'

Each morning and evening, the rising or the setting sun shone through the glass mountain making rainbow flickers. But Princess Purity was lovelier even than the flickering rainbows. And so suitors came from all over the world to try for the three oranges she held in her lap.

They went up barefoot and in boots. They rode up on horseback and in chariots. They brought axes to cut hand-holds, and ladders to climb. But their feet and boots slipped, their axes broke, their ladders toppled

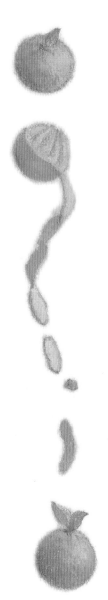

and their horses and chariots tumbled off the glassy cliff on top of them. No one got so much as head-high off the ground.

The crowds who gathered at the bottom of the mountain clouded the glass with their breath. But Princess Purity had to go on sitting, in lonely splendour, like an angel on a spire of ice.

*   *   *

'Another night like this and we shan't have any hay to sell,' said Farmer Herbert to his three sons.

They stood in Home Meadow and looked around them. All the tall, lush, green grass which had waved in yesterday's wind was cut as short as a shaver's beard.

'What did it, Dad?' asked Bigg Herbert, the oldest son.

'That's for you to find out,' said his father. 'Keep watch in Near Meadow tonight and make sure the thief doesn't come back for more. . . . And mind you don't fall asleep!'

So Bigg Herbert spent that night in Near Meadow, under the apple tree there. And he did not fall asleep—or so he said. 'No, I saw the moon rise, and the stars come out. I felt the wind get up and the tree sway. But then the ground began to rumble and the earth began to shake . . . so I ran for my life!'

Next morning, Near Meadow was cut as short as a monk's hair. 'Another raid like this and we shan't have enough hay to last the winter,' said Farmer Herbert.

'Who did it, Dad?' asked Lessor Herbert, the second son.

'That's for you to find out,' said his father. 'Keep watch in Middle Meadow tonight, and make sure the thief doesn't come back for more. And mind you don't fall asleep like your worthless brother. Earthquakes and rumblings, indeed!'

So Lessor Herbert spent that night in Middle Meadow, under the chestnut tree. And he did not fall asleep—or so he said. 'I saw the moon rise and the stars come out. I felt the wind get up and the tree sway. But then the ground began to rumble and the earth began to shake . . . so I ran for my life, or it would have got me, it would, whatever it was!'

Next morning, Middle Meadow was cut as short as the hair on an egg. 'Another disaster like this and we shall be ruined,' said Farmer Herbert. 'Earthquakes and rumblings, bah!'

'I'll keep watch tonight,' said Scruffy Herbert, the farmer's third son. Scruffy's job on the farm was mucking out, so he was always smelly and filthy. His father and brothers had quite forgotten what he looked like underneath all the muck and grime.

'You?!' sneered his brothers. 'You're no use in the daytime, let alone at night!'

But Farmer Herbert did let Scruffy Herbert keep watch in Far Meadow, sitting under the oak tree there. And he did not fall asleep.

No. He saw the moon rise, the stars come out. He felt the wind get up and the tree sway. He felt the ground tremble and the earth quake, and he saw the great white horse whose hooves were making all the din.

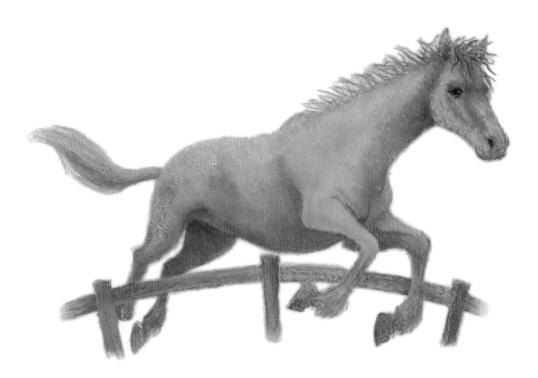

It leapt the fence and began to eat the grass in Far Meadow.

Scruffy Herbert did not run away. He climbed up the oak tree and, when the horse came to graze beneath the tree, dropped down on to its back, knotting his fingers in the mane. At once the horse raised its head and cantered away, carrying Scruffy over field and hill—as gentle and obedient as if Scruffy had always been its master.

In the morning, Scruffy went home on foot. 'You shan't be troubled any more, Dad,' he said.

His brothers jeered and sneered. 'Why? Did you scare off the evil magic with your ugly face?' Scruffy said nothing. He took no notice. He did not mention the little matter of the horse.

With only one field to reap and bale and stack, the Herbert boys finished harvesting early that year. 'So can Lessor and me go to see the Glass Mountain?' said Bigg. 'Everyone's going. They say the princess is real beautiful and princes are coming from all over to try the climb.' Farmer Herbert said they could go.

'Can I come?' said Scruffy, but they only threw a bale of hay at him: 'If the princess caught a whiff of you, she might fall off her mountain! Go and spread muck.'

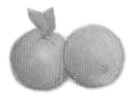

Bigg and Lessor joined the crowds around the base of the glass mountain, and gazed and gawped at all the princes in their armour, the pedlars selling things, the jugglers performing, and, of course, the suitors sliding helplessly down the glassy slopes on their faces, horses, bottoms, and chariots. It was quite a circus.

Suddenly, cantering through the crowd came a young man on a huge and beautiful white horse. He was dressed in green velvet, with felt boots and a belt of red copper, and he set his horse right at the mountain. It fairly leapt up the glass precipice. Halfway to the top, though, the horse stopped.

Princess Purity, who had sunk into a kind of sleepy misery on her mountaintop throne, stared in amazement. The most handsome face she had ever seen was looking up at her. So much did she like the face that she threw one of her oranges to the young man, who caught it, before his sure-footed horse slithered back down the glass slope on its hocks.

'You should have seen it!' said Bigg and Lessor at home that night.

'I wish I had,' said Scruffy.

But his brothers threw rotten sprout-tops at him and jeered, 'Sorry: no dogs allowed in the palace grounds.'

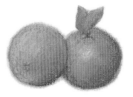

Next day Bigg and Lessor went back. There were no princes left among the watching crowd: they had all tried and failed to win the princess. Bigg stood on Lessor's shoulders. But as soon as he set one foot on the glass, he slithered down again, squashing his brother.

Suddenly, through the crowd came a young man on a huge and beautiful white horse. He was dressed in blue velvet, with felt boots and a belt of silver links, and he set his horse right at the mountain. It fairly leapt up the glass precipice.

Princess Purity, who was still thinking about the face she had seen the day before, heard the clatter of hooves on glass and looked down to see the same face. Higher and higher it came. A reaching hand brushed the tips of her shoes. She slipped an orange into the hand. Then horse and rider slithered back down the glass mountain, though the horse kept its feet and galloped away uninjured.

'You should have seen it!' said Bigg and Lessor at home that night.

'I wish I had,' said Scruffy.

But his brothers only threw rotten mangelwurzels at him, and said, 'Sorry, no pigs allowed in the palace grounds.'

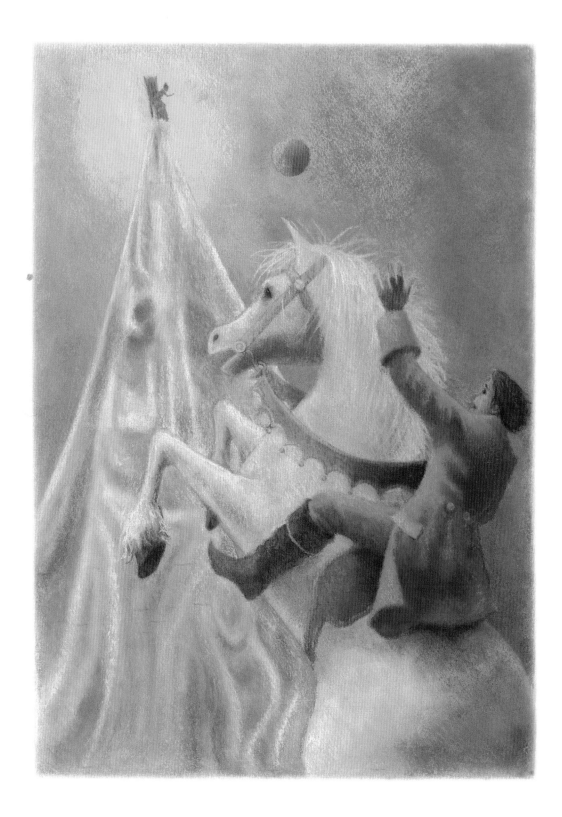

Next day, Bigg and Lessor went back to the glass
mountain. Lessor stood on Bigg's shoulders. But
though he jumped as high as he could, he only slid
down, like a monkey on a greased pole, and squashed
his brother flat.

Suddenly, through the crowd came a young man on a huge and
beautiful white horse. He was dressed in scarlet velvet, with felt boots
and a belt of gold coins, and he set his horse right at the mountain. It
fairly leapt up the glass precipice.

It was him again! Princess Purity stood up to urge him on. Her
fingers dug deep into the third orange, and juice ran down her silken
skirts. Up and up the sure-footed horse ran—Purity could feel the
clatter of its hooves on the glass, see its nostrils flaring, feel the heat
from its flanks. The young man loomed up over the peak of the glass
mountain. She held out to him the last orange, but he swept up both
her and her orange in his arms and, in one bound, launched his horse
off the mountain and down to the ground. Pausing only to set the
princess down at the palace gate, the young man in red velvet galloped
away into the evening gloom.

The king came running out, the crowd milled about, the mountain
crazed, cracked, and tinkled into a thousand fragments.

'Oh, you should have seen it!' exclaimed Bigg and Lessor
that night.

'I wish I had,' said Scruffy.

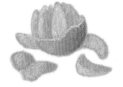

But his brothers threw handfuls of broken glass at
him and said, 'Fine guest you would make at a
royal wedding, dung beetle!'

Even so, the whole family went to the

palace park next day. Everyone in the world seemed to
be there. For the king had called on the Chevalier of the
Three Oranges to present himself and claim his bride.

'Come forward, whatever prince has achieved those
three oranges and the love of my daughter!' cried the
king. But no prince came forward (though there were
dozens there) because no prince had the three oranges.

'Well then, come forward whatever knight has
achieved those three oranges and the love of my
daughter!' cried the king. But no knight came forward
either (though there were hundreds there) because no
knight had the three oranges.

'Well, somebody must have it!' said the king, rather
desperately. 'Come forward whoever you are, or my
daughter will never forgive me!'

Scruffy edged forward through the crowd.

'Where do you think you're going?' said his brothers.

'I just want to see the princess,' said Scruffy.

Then all at once he was at the front of the crowd and
walking towards the king, and kneeling down on one
knee.

'What's the fool up to?' said Farmer Herbert.

The king held his nose, then forgot to hold it. For out
of the pockets of Scruffy's stinking clothes came first
one, then two, then three oranges, the third rather
squished and spoiled. Then Scruffy threw off his work
clothes, and underneath he was wearing . . . red velvet.
But not until he had washed his hands and face in the

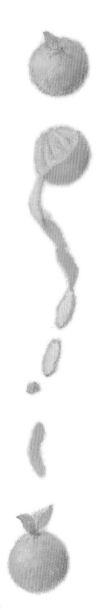

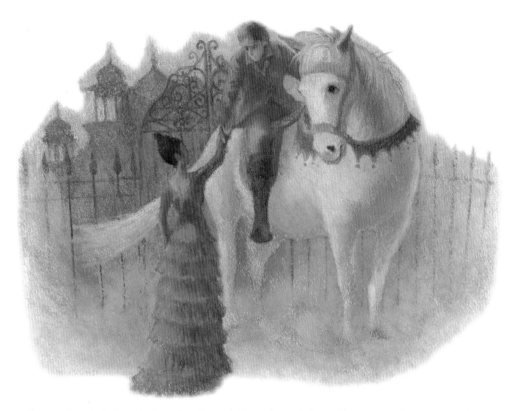

fountain did he shake the king's hand and kiss Princess Purity, to the cheers of the crowd.

When he whistled softly, his magic horse (who had eaten up three meadows and run three times up the glass mountain) came cantering through the crowds, bowling over Bigg and Lessor as it came. Lifting Purity into the saddle, Scruffy mounted behind her, and together they rode to the cathedral to be married.

Shocking to say, the king ate oranges all through the ceremony, and got sticky right up to his elbows.

The
Thirteenth Child

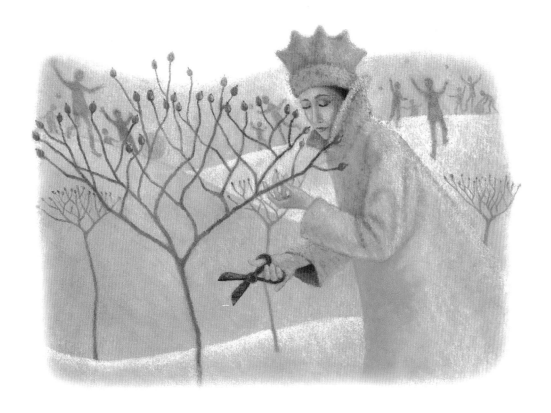

When the queen had a baby boy, the king was delighted and gave him a silver spoon on a cord to wear round his neck. The queen, too, was happy, thinking the next child might be a girl. When the second was a boy, he too was lovely. He too was given a spoon. But the queen did hope her next child would be a girl. Or the next. Or the next. At last, king and queen were blessed with twelve sons—big-boned, bonny boys, bold as bears, each wearing his spoon like a battle medal. The king was hugely happy, but the queen's wish had become a desperate longing.

One winter's day, when the princes were particularly noisy and rough playing snowballs, the queen went, for peace and quiet, to prune her rose garden. A thorn pricked her finger, and blood fell on to the snowy ground.

'If only I had a daughter with skin as white as snow and lips as red as blood,' said the queen to herself. A snowball hit her on the back. 'If I had a daughter like that, those boys could fly away, for all I care.'

It was a terrible thing to say—not meant, hardly meant. But the words hung in the air as a frosty smoke, while her blood dripped on to the snow. Soon the queen was expecting another child—the thirteenth. And the thirteenth was a daughter.

The baby's first cry pierced the air like a thorn, and in the same instant, all the windows of the palace blew open. At first, the twelve princes thought they had been smothered by an avalanche of snow. Then each looked down and found himself . . . transformed: in place of boots, webbed feet, in place of a face, a beak, in place of arms a pair of wings, in place of skin, feathers. All twelve had turned into wild ducks. Through the open window of the palace they flew away—a chevron in the sky, an arrowhead of migrating ducks.

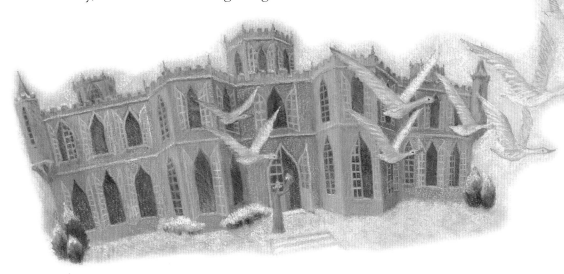

The queen finally had her daughter, and the daughter was as lovely as any rose garden, with blood-red lips and snow-white skin. She too was given her silver spoon. Princess Snow-Rose was a dear, loving child. And yet never a day passed but she felt some dark and terrible sadness haunting the palace, which no one would talk about. She was lonely, too.

'If only I had brothers and sisters to play with,' she began to say one day—and her mother promptly burst into tears! The whole terrible story came out—how her twelve brothers had been turned into wild ducks and had flown away.

'And all because of me,' she whispered, chilling outside and in. 'I wish that I had never been born. I must go and find them, and save them, even if it costs me my life.'

Nothing the king or queen said could change her mind. She took no purse and she took no carriage, but walked through the world till she was ragged. For three years she walked.

One woodland morning, a skein of twelve ducks flurried up into the sky ahead of her. At just the spot where they had taken off, she found a little cottage, and in the cottage twelve chairs round a table, and on the table twelve silver spoons.

I have found them! she thought, dizzy with excitement and hunger. Now all I have to do is wait for them to come home. Porridge was cooking on the stove. She ate a bowlful, using her own silver spoon, then lay down on one of the twelve beds and fell asleep.

With a rattle of wings, the twelve brothers flew home at nightfall. As the last ray of sunlight left the sky, their feathers dropped down in a snowy moult, and they were themselves again—twelve handsome young men (who looked a lot like the king). Sitting down to supper, they picked up their spoons to eat. And there, glittering on the table, lay a thirteenth spoon!

The oldest boy knocked over his chair with a clatter. 'Up and search, brothers! Who can this spoon belong to but our sister—our curse and our sorrow—the cause of all our misery!'

They tore open the cupboards, they overturned the table. They slashed at the curtains and ripped the covers from the beds. But as, at the twelfth bed, brothers and sister came face to face for the first time, and daggers were drawn, the youngest prince raised his voice.

'Stop! Don't kill her! How can she be to blame for what happened to us? She was not three seconds old when the enchantment fell on us.'

Snow-Rose stood up on the bed, her face streaming with tears, her shadow dancing in the lamplight. 'For three years I have searched for you. If killing me will free you from this enchantment, please— kill me now. Otherwise, tell me how to lift the spell and I will do it!'

'Impossible,' said the oldest brother.

'You couldn't,' said another.

'We shall always be ducks by day and men by night.'

'No remedy.'

'What? Weave shirts from nettles?'

'Weave twelve shirts from nettles?'

'And not weep?'

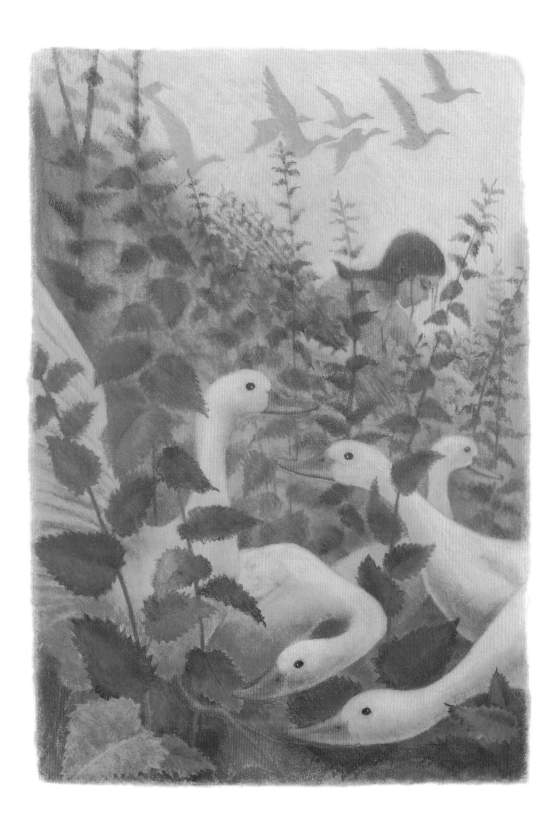

'And not speak, all that while?'

'Impossible.'

'No. We shall always be as we are,' said the youngest prince.

Snow-Rose said nothing in reply, only nodded her head, unsmiling, dry-eyed. Tomorrow she would begin work. Twelve shirts for twelve ducks. And not a word or a tear or a laugh till the last shirt was made.

Each morning she left the cottage at the same time as her brothers flew off into the cornfields to feed. But Snow-Rose waded, instead, waist-deep into the nettle patch, and gathered up swaithes of nettles in her arms.

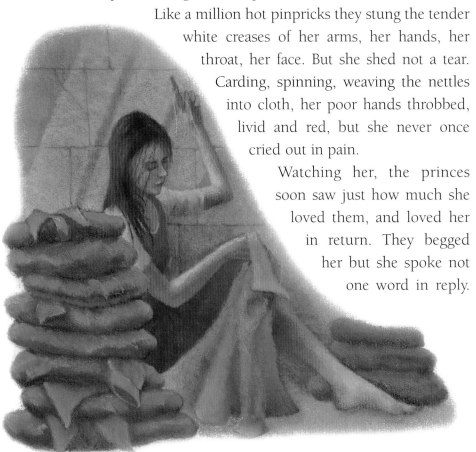

Like a million hot pinpricks they stung the tender white creases of her arms, her hands, her throat, her face. But she shed not a tear. Carding, spinning, weaving the nettles into cloth, her poor hands throbbed, livid and red, but she never once cried out in pain.

Watching her, the princes soon saw just how much she loved them, and loved her in return. They begged her but she spoke not one word in reply.

For then it would all be for nothing.

Weeks turned to months, months to a year. The nettles were all gone from round the cottage— gone throughout the wood. And Snow-Rose had to fetch nettles home miles, in bales on her back. And she worked all day and half the night. Soon all that remained was to sew the woven pieces together.

By noon there were only four more shirts to sew. By nightfall the princes would have their shirts, and her ordeal and theirs would be over . . .

Suddenly hoofbeats clamoured through the forest, riders with plumed hats and quivers of yellow arrows.

Arrows!

Snow-Rose thought of her brothers winging home over the treetops. She imagined the hunter's arrows piercing them one by one.

Sweeping together her sewing, swinging the bundle over her shoulder, she pelted after the hunters. She could not call out to them, could not shout a warning to her brothers! In the distance, she could hear the whirr of wings, the creaking cry of her brothers singing out to her for their supper . . .

As the lead huntsman raised his bow, a ragged girl rushed out of the trees and grabbed his bridle, almost unseating him. His arrow flew wide. The ducks flew by overhead, unhurt.

The king whose aim she had spoiled was only angry for a moment; he had rarely seen such a pretty girl as the one now standing in front of his horse. He smiled and asked who she was.

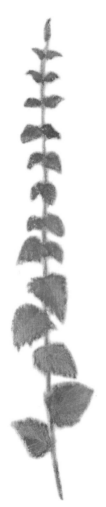

Snow-Rose did not answer.

'Don't be shy. Why did you stop me shooting?' he asked.

But Snow-Rose did not answer, could not answer.

'Come back to the castle with me, won't you, and tell me all about yourself?'

And Snow-Rose had to go—could not tell him how vital it was to get home, to take the shirts home.

* * *

This dumb, ragged, unsmiling beauty intrigued the king, and he soon found himself falling in love with her. It was annoying that she never laughed at his jokes, but something noble and sorrowful spoke to him out of her eyes, so that he was content to sit in silence with her for hours.

But the king's love for Snow-Rose made the ladies of the royal court seethe with jealousy. 'Look at her—all spotty red!' they sneered. 'She probably has some disgusting disease!'

'She never cries when I pinch her at table.'

'Never cries out when I kick her under the table.'

'She's probably a witch. Witches never cry.'

Snow-Rose could not defend herself. When they began to make up lies about her, blame her for everything bad, accuse her of witchcraft and sorcery, Snow-Rose could say nothing in her defence. At last, blood was found on the snow beneath her window, and she was accused of murder. At that, the king's love turned to horror, and he condemned Snow-Rose to death.

'See! See! She doesn't even cry!' jeered the ladies of the court. 'We told you she was a witch!'

As Snow-Rose was led away to a prison cell to await her death at dawn, she made signs that she wanted her bundle of sewing. The prison warder brought it—ooching and ouching—flung it in after her and went away sucking his stinging fingers.

All night Snow-Rose sewed, while outside a bonfire was built of branches and benches and brooms. At the heart of the bonfire was a stake of wood, and round the stake a golden chain. Anyone else would have wept for sheer fear, but Snow-Rose only sewed and stitched, stitched and sewed. Panic swept over her when, at the last moment, she found one sleeve missing: it must have dropped from the bundle as she ran through the woods! Perhaps the magic would fail, for want of that one sleeve. But there was no time to replace it. Morning spilled in at the barred window. The warder's key rattled in the lock.

'Time to die, miss,' he said.

As Snow-Rose walked to the bonfire, she dropped behind her, one by one, twelve coarse and rather odd-smelling green shirts. No sooner did they touch the ground, than wild ducks settled out of the sky, picked them up in their beaks, and flew off with them.

'One last time, I beg you, girl,' said the king. 'Speak and defend yourself against this terrible charge!' But Snow-Rose would not speak, could not speak. So they tied her to the stake and lit the fire around her.

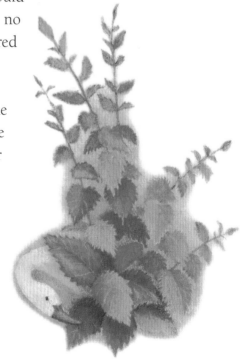

Suddenly hoofbeats clamoured over the castle drawbridge, and into the yard rode twelve princes leaning forward in their saddles, shouting themselves hoarse. They came on at the charge, forcing courtiers and ladies to jump aside. 'Let our sister go, or die on our swords!' they yelled. 'She is innocent of any crime but love!'

The fire was doused, the golden chain snapped, and Snow-Rose leapt down from the bonfire to hug all her twelve brothers. 'You're safe! You're saved!' she cried, and her tears of joy intermingled with sobs of laughter.

Now everything could be explained to the king, and the ladies of the court were put to shame for their lying. The blood on the snow, they admitted, had been nothing more than the blood of a pet duck.

With a shudder, the youngest prince held his cloak tight around him and said to Snow-Rose, 'Let's leave this place and go home.'

'Yes, but I may return here. I have grown rather fond of the king,' said Snow-Rose, 'and I may well marry him . . . But tell me! Did you find the lost sleeve, or was my work enough to recover you all completely?'

'Not completely,' said the youngest brother, and his cloak fell open. In place of his left arm was a duck's wing.

Still, I never heard that he was loved any the less for his strange appearance. Nor, when they returned home to their mother, did she prize her boys any less than her girl—no, not by the breadth of a rose stem, not by the weight of one snowflake.

Tamlin

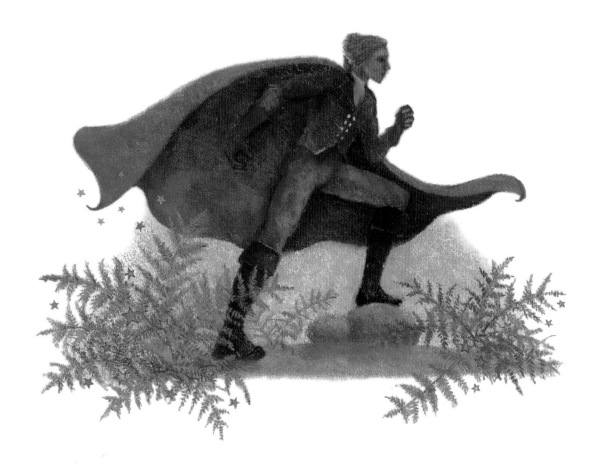

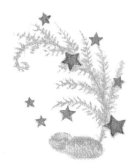

One day and one week and one year, in the parish of Melrose, Young Tamlin fell from his horse while riding. He fell into the Land of Fairies, and into the power of the Fairy Queen, who dressed him in green velvet and silks but locked up his soul in Fairyland.

When he did not come home, Tamlin's sweetheart Janet wept for him. And after that, she searched for him, asked after him from Melrose to Selkirk. But no one had seen so much as one red hair of Tamlin.

All they had seen was a highwayman dressed in green, a robber with red hair, who stopped maidens by the holy well at the crossroads and demanded their cloaks or rings or dresses. The maidens said that the robber's eyes were blue as the sea but seemed to be full of tears.

So Janet went to the crossroads, well-dressed in her finest clothes. And there the highwayman leapt out at her, with a 'Stand and deliver! Your green cloak or your finery!'

'Shame on you, Tamlin! Come you home at once,' scolded Janet. 'Do you call this honest work for the Master of Carterhaugh? Come home with me, this instant.'

'Ah, Janet, Janet!' sighed the young man. 'I fear I can never come

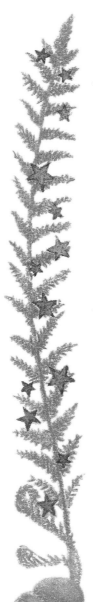

home. For I kissed the queen of the fairies, and now for seven years I must obey her every command.'

'Kissed her? Then I'm sure you deserve your fate!' said Janet, flaring up. And she turned her horse and rode back home, her nose sniffy-tilted in the air.

But when her temper cooled, Janet sat down and thought. She sat and thought from Harvest till Hallowe'en, and then she saddled her horse and said goodbye to her mother.

'I must go and rescue Tamlin, for you know how helpless men are to save themselves.'

'Oh, but you'll not go out tonight!' protested her mother. 'Not when the wind is so keen.'

'I have a warm cloak to keep off the wind, mother,' said Janet.

'Oh, but you'll not go out tonight!' begged her mother. 'Not when the rain is so teeming!'

'I have a hood to keep off the rain, mother,' said Janet.

'Oh, but you'll not go out tonight, of all nights!' pleaded her mother. 'Not on All Hallows Eve when all the powers of Hell and Fairyland are out and roaming the world?'

'No other night will do,' said Janet, and kissing her mother she mounted up and rode into the wild, wet, windy night.

She rode to the crossroads where the gallows stood. She braved the ghosts who floated in the misty hollow. She braved the demons who snatched at her skirt out of the long grass. She braved the witches who flitted and twittered across the stormy moon. And she braved the graveyard where dead souls hooted in the trees.

Hiding behind the well, at the crossroads, Janet waited for midnight, when the gates of Fairyland would open and loose the troops of the Fairy Queen to fly about and make mischief.

At last they came, the queen leading the way. Her horse's mane was knotted with silver bells, and her stolen silk petticoats swept the muddy ground. Her company of men was huge—each one young and handsome, each one kidnapped from the sunlit world. Last of all came Tamlin, on a milk-white mare, and the moon glinted on the teardrops in his eyes.

Out sprang Janet, and dragged him from his horse, pulling him to the ground, knotting her white fingers in his rust-red hair. 'Come with me and stay with me,' she said, 'for you are my true-love, Tamlin!'

But the thing in her arms was not Tamlin. In moments, he had changed into a slithering snake which knotted and coiled and writhed all around her.

'Now will you let him go, foolish Janet?' laughed the Fairy Queen.

'Never! You may change him, but my love for him never changes,' and she clung on tight to the snake, though it made her skin crawl with horror.

But the thing in her arms was no longer a snake. Suddenly it had put on feathers and claws, and was slashing at her with a sharp, hooked beak.

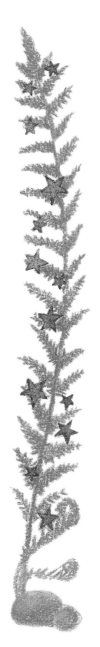

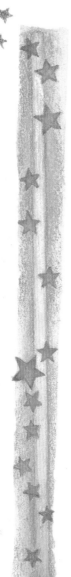

'Now will you let him go, foolish Janet?' sneered the queen.

'Never! You may change him, but my love for him never changes!' and she gripped so tight to the vulture that tufts of black feathers came away in her hands.

But the thing in her arms was no longer a vulture. Suddenly it had put on fur and grown into the towering figure of a bear. It hugged Janet to its furry ribs with a strength which all but wrung the life out of her.

'Now will you let him go, foolish Janet?' called the queen.

'Never! You may change him, but my love for him never changes!' and she sank her fingers deep into the bear's fur, so that they looked like two dancers whirling in the moonlight.

But the thing in her arms did not remain a bear for long. It became a lion, a conger eel, a wolf, and a boar. It became a skeleton, a goblin, a dinosaur, and a cackling witch. Even so, Janet refused to let go.

Last and worst of all, the thing in her arms lost all living shape—lost arms and claws and tusks and tail. It thinned to the girth of a spear—cold and rigid—though soon it grew warm in her grip. Tamlin had turned into an iron bar, almost too heavy for Janet to carry. And as she staggered under its weight, the iron bar grew hot, red hot, white hot, singeing her cloak and her hair.

'Drop him! Let him fall, foolish Janet!' shrieked the Fairy Queen. But Janet would not let go her grip on the enchanted Tamlin. Instead she walked with the white hot bar to the brink of the well, and threw it down into the holy water.

There was a mighty hiss of steam.

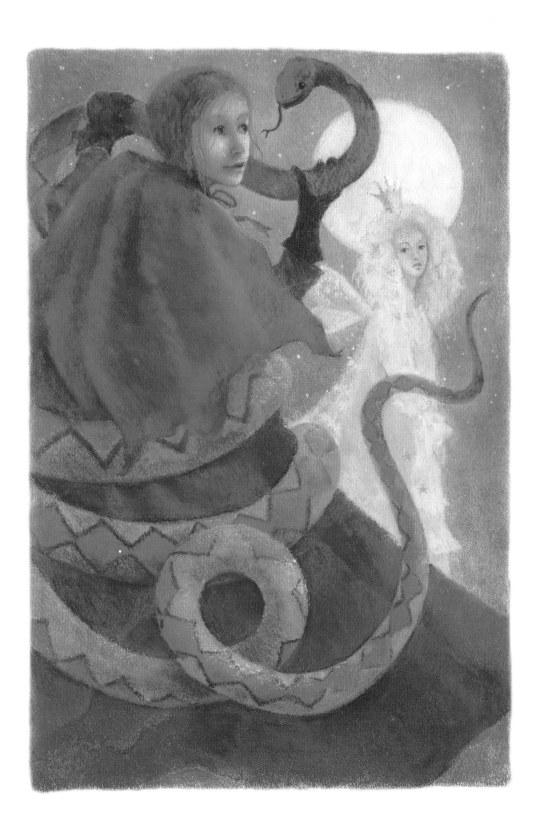

'Away! Away, your Majesty!' cried Janet. 'Dawn is almost here—the feast of All Hallows—when the angels ride out to hunt the likes of you!'

With a howl of vexation, the Fairy Queen gathered up her reins. 'A curse on you, brave Janet. For you have robbed me of the finest man in my whole company! . . . Away, men! Away!' And the ground shook to the thunder of their galloping hooves as the Enchantress and the Enchanted fled back to Fairyland.

Janet reached down and took her sweetheart's hand. Shivering and sodden, mossy and with frogs in his pockets, Tamlin climbed out of the well. His fairy clothes had fallen into rags, but his hair was still as red as copper and his eyes were still as blue as ever they had been.

'I'll still marry you, though I'm probably a fool to myself,' said Janet, looking him up and down, her hands on her hips. 'But if ever I hear you've been kissing fairies again, I swear I'll take the broom to you and sweep you out of doors! Now, let's get you home before you catch your death of cold.'

And sharing her horse, they rode home.

Now when the young men of Melrose heard what Janet had been ready to do for her sweetheart, they came round her door as eager as bees round a pot of honey. A prince and a chieftain both asked to marry her.

But Tamlin rolled up his sleeves and spat on his hands and said he would fight every man in Scotland before he let his Janet go. For the love he harboured in his heart now would never change—no, not till Fairyland fell into ruins and the hills wore down to sand.

The Four Friends

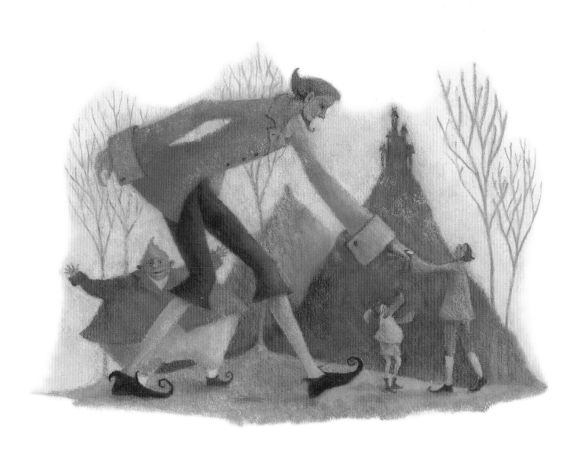

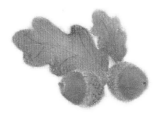

I am old,' said the king to his son. 'Before I die, let me see you married, Boy.'

Well, Boy had never thought of marrying before, but he had nothing against the idea. 'All right, father. Who?'

'Go into my art gallery,' said the king. 'There hang portraits of all the unmarried princesses in the world. Choose one, and I will arrange everything.'

It seemed a good way to buy a carriage or a house; not such a good way to choose a wife. But Boy was an obedient son. He took the key from its rack, unlocked the Long Gallery, and walked the length of the room, to and fro, all afternoon. Some were whale-fat, others beanpole-thin. There were ugly, pretty, and pretty ugly princesses; tall ones whose ankles showed, squat ones like pink meringues. There were even some handsome, elegant girls whom the prince studied hard.

But at the end of the room one portrait had been covered—hung with a dust sheet—and there was a notice beneath it which read: LOOK NOT HERE. What would you have done?

So did Boy. He gave the cloth a tug, and down it fell. Then he looked and he looked again. 'You are the one for me,' he said. And the girl in the picture covered her sad face with her hands and turned away. With a series of bangs, all the other portraits fell from the wall, face-down on the carpet.

Boy's father was not angry.

He was heartbroken.

'Why did you have to look where you were forbidden to look?'

'Because she is my Fate, I suppose,' said Boy. 'Who is she?'

'The Princess Perdita—stolen away by the evil sorcerer Chornoy, and kept prisoner by him no-one-knows-where. They call him Sborshchik—The Collector.'

'He collects princesses?'

'He collects the souls of those who try to rescue her and fail! . . . But if Perdita is your Fate, nothing I say will sway you. Take my blessing and go in search of her.' He looked his son fondly up and down—short, short-sighted, and rather short of brains. 'If only you were a boy better framed for Adventure.'

Boy set off. But he did not get far. Before he was out of the palace grounds, he got lost in a wood. Suddenly he fell over the long legs of a man sleeping on the ground.

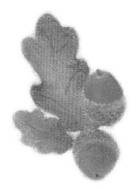

'Hello,' said the stranger. 'You look like a good man. Will you give me a job?'

'Why, what can you do?' asked Boy.

'Ooo, polish high windows, clear gutters, ford rivers, and so forth.'

'For the right master, I'm sure you would be just the man,' said Boy politely. 'But all I need right now is to get out of this wood.'

'Oh, no prob',' said Long (for that was his name), and he stood up. When he stretched he was so tall that his head stuck up high above the trees.

'The road is that way,' he said. 'I can see it . . . I suppose you wouldn't have a job for a friend of mine?'

Out of his pocket, he drew a small, round man like a football.

'Why, what can he do?'

'Ooo, fence fields, stop draughts, mop up spills and so on,' said Long. 'Show him, Wide.' Wide grinned, broadly.

'To the right master, I'm sure he—' began Boy politely. But Wide was breathing in, growing as he did so.

'Run!' said Long, and without knowing why, Boy ran. Behind them, the empty landscape began to fill up as Wide grew.

First Wide's chest swelled, then his belly, then his head and legs and arms, until just by breathing in, he had grown to the width of a small mountain. With a sigh which blew off Boy's hat, he shrank back to normal size, saying, 'It's an honour to work for you, sir. I suppose you wouldn't have a job for a friend of mine?' Out of his pocket he took a diminutive man in leather shorts and an alpine hat.

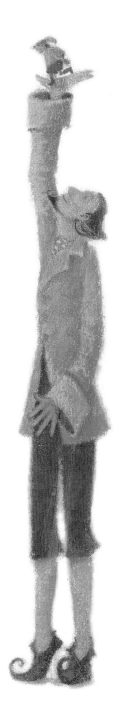

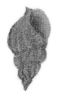

'Why is he wearing that blindfold?' asked Boy. 'Is he blind?'

'Not exactly,' said Wide.

'Well, I'm sure to the right master he would be just the man. But all I need right now is to find the Princess Perdita.'

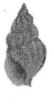

'Easy-peasy,' said the diminutive man (whose name was Quick-Eye). Long stretched up tall and held Quick-Eye in one hand above his head. Quick-Eye took off the blindfold and looked in every direction.

'Without this blindfold, my gaze is so piercing that I tend to set light to things,' Quick-Eye explained. 'Ah yes. There she is. In the Ebony Fortress, among the Hills of Coal, beside the Black Sea. Oh dear, she's crying, poor soul.'

Then Wide put Quick-Eye back in his pocket, and Long put Wide into his pocket and, taking Boy by the scruff of his jacket, set off in the direction of the fortress. His legs were so long that they got there in no time.

A notice was tacked to the door. It said:

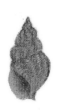

Let him who would have her, keep her.
Let him who would take her, hold her.
Let him who would try, succeed or DIE!

'Go in! Go in! Do!' urged a voice behind them. 'The door is not locked.' It was the sorcerer, Chornoy! 'Permit me to show you round my humble home.'

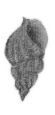

Warily the four friends went inside, and Chornoy led them through his fortress. In every room, on every stair stood strange ebony statues.

'What carving!' exclaimed Boy. 'They could almost be real!'

'They were,' said Chornoy, 'before, like you, they tried to save the princess. There is a forfeit, you see. If you cannot keep the princess by you till morning, you must pay a forfeit.'

Boy gulped. He could see now: the stone figures were frozen in the very act of running or falling, drawing their swords or cowering in fear.

Princess Perdita was even lovelier than her portrait. Her skin was peachy-soft, her mouth as luscious as watermelon, her eyes grape-blue. . . . But she did not move a muscle. Round her waist were three bands of iron without clasp, without padlock, without hinge. And bound by the iron, the princess could neither speak nor move. She looked at Boy with large, imploring eyes which seemed to say, 'Hopeless! It is impossible.'

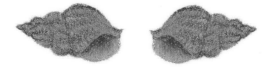

'Guard her well, young man,' said Chornoy with a heartless snicker. 'Unless I find her here with you in the morning, your soul is forfeit to me, and your body to my collection!'

As night fell, they were left alone in the topmost room of a coal-black tower. As soon as Chornoy was gone, Long took Wide from his pocket, and Wide swelled to the size and shape of the door, to block it. Long wound himself around the tower, to guard it. Boy took hold of Perdita's hand, and they all agreed to keep awake.

Ah, but there was magic at large! By midnight, they were all sound asleep—all except the princess, whose eyes could not close, but whose lips could not speak a warning.

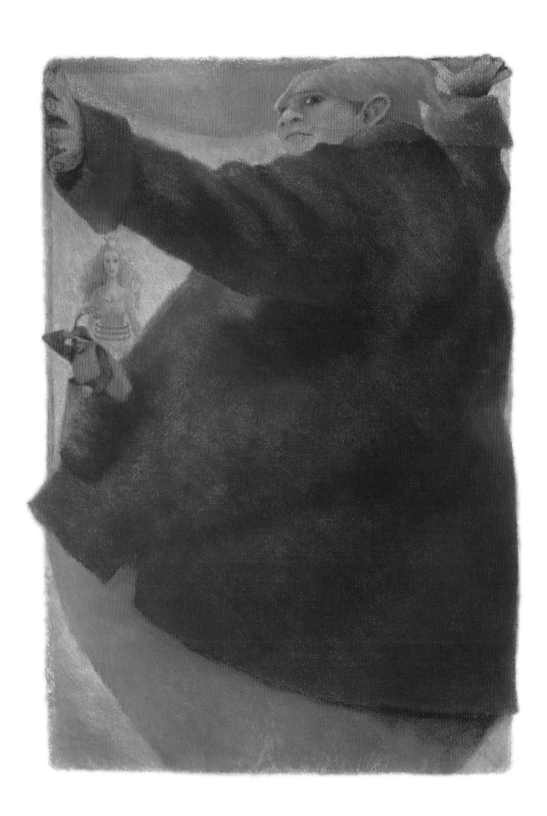

In the morning, to Boy's horror, she had gone! He sat down on the floor and wept. 'I'm done for, and there's nothing to be done.'

'Quick! Quickly, Quick-Eye!' said Long. 'Look and tell us where she is!'

The littlest of the four friends took off his blindfold. There were four windows in the tower, one looking north, one south, one east, one west. From the northern window Quick-Eye could see Chornoy coming, hurrying to claim his forfeit. From the east, Quick-Eye saw the princess.

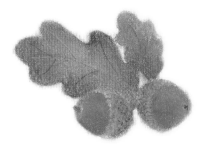

'Easy-peasy, master. One hundred miles from here is a forest, and in the forest is an oak tree, and in the oak tree is an acorn, and in the acorn is the princess.'

'No prob',' said Long. 'I'll just go and fetch her back.'

And so he did, his long legs covering the ground faster than thought. By the time Chornoy had climbed the winding stair, the princess was hand-in-hand once more with Boy, a sprinkling of oak-leaves in her hair. Chornoy could hardly believe his eyes. With a dull clank, one of the iron bands round the princess's waist fell to the ground, and she was able to move her hands.

'Two nights more you must endure!' raged the sorcerer, then recovering himself he gave a slow, leering smile. 'In the meantime,

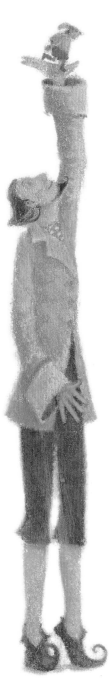

gentlemen, do please enjoy the comforts of my home.'

Next night Boy once again sat by the princess and held her hand. Wide stuffed up the doorway, Long encircled the tower, and they all vowed to stay awake. But there was magic afoot, and by midnight they were all snoring (except for the princess whose eyes could not close but whose lips could not speak a warning). In the morning, she was gone.

Boy sat down on the floor and wept. 'Then I'm done for, and there's nothing to be done!'

'Quick! Quickly, Quick-Eye,' said Long.

Quick-Eye ran to the northern window. He could see Chornoy coming, hurrying to claim his forfeit and turn Boy into another statue for his collection. From the east window, Quick-Eye saw nothing, but from the west, he saw the princess.

'Easy-peasy, master. Three hundred miles from here is a mountain, and in the mountain is a rock, and in the rock is a ruby, and in the ruby is the Princess.'

'No prob',' said Long. 'I shall walk there and fetch her back in no time!' and stretching his long legs to the full, he strode off across countryside and moor.

Up the stairs came Chornoy, grinning an evil grin. 'Look your last on the world, fool, for now you have failed—Urghuh!?' He stared in amazement at Boy who sat hand-in-hand with Princess Perdita. With a dull clank, a second iron band round the princess's waist broke and fell to the ground, and she was free to blink her eyes.

'You shan't be so lucky a third time!' Chornoy threatened. 'Enjoy my hospitality while you still may, young man. Tomorrow you will be dead— stone dead!'

That night they tried even harder to stay awake, but there was magic in the air. They nodded, they dozed, they slept. And in the morning the princess was gone.

'Quick! Quickly, Quick-Eye!' said Long. Quick-Eye ran to the northern window. He could see Chornoy coming, skipping and hopping along, laughing and rubbing his hands. But from the east window and the west window, Quick-Eye saw nothing.

Then Boy sat down on the floor and wept. 'I'm done for, and there's nothing to be done.'

'Aha!' said Quick-Eye leaning out of the southern window. 'One thousand miles from here there is a country and in the country is a sea, and in the middle of the sea is a shell and in the shell is the princess.'

'No prob',' said Long, but this time he stuffed Wide into his pocket before striding off across field and moor and mountain with his long legs at full stretch. He reached the sea in no time. But the

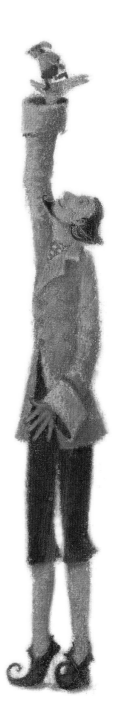

sea was so deep! Even Long, at full stretch, could not wade out to the middle without the water closing over his head. 'This is a problem for you, Wide my friend,' he said, and taking the round little man out of his pocket, set him down on the beach.

Wide got down on his hands and knees, put his lips into the rippling waves, and began to drink. He drank till his chest and belly swelled up as big as cathedrals. He drank till his head and his arms and his legs swelled up and he filled the beach like a great, wibbly-wobbling mountain, full of seawater. The sea was now much emptier than before, and Long was able to stride out to the very middle and pick up the shell with the princess inside. It was a long way. Wide began to grunt and groan and turn slightly blue in the face. 'Hurry! Hurry!' said Quick-Eye peeping out of his pocket and beckoning Long. 'He can't hold his breath much longer!'

Long hopped ashore and Wide opened his mouth with an enormous spluttering gurgle.

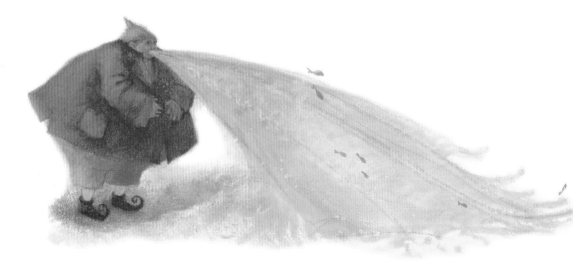

Out came the seawater, sinking moored boats, scattering shoals of fish, frightening the mermaids. The sea returned to its normal level, and the three friends set off for the Hills of Coal and Chornoy's Ebony Fortress.

But emptying the sea had taken time, and they were one thousand miles from Boy! Peering ahead from amid Long's hair, Quick-Eye said, 'We are never going to get there in time! Chornoy is already climbing the stairs! I do believe we have failed our friend!'

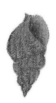

Boy heard the wizard's feet on the stairs and shuddered. He ran to the southern window, but there was no sign of his friends, no sign of the princess. Now he would have to pay the price of failing. Now Chornoy would turn him into a statue.

Chornoy entered, looked all round the room and grinned. 'I did not think you would get her back from there,' he chortled. 'And now the princess is mine, your soul is mine, and your body may join my collection!'

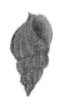

There was a tinkling of glass. Through a pane of the southern window came a tiny sea shell, to land at Boy's feet. It broke open—and there stood . . . the princess! The third iron hoop was already gone from round her waist, and she flung her arms round Boy's neck and kissed him tenderly.

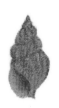

Throughout the Ebony Fortress, the statues stirred and stretched and grumbled sleepily. Scores of princes—angry, vengeful princes—came charging up the stairs of the tower to lay hands on Chornoy. Outnumbered, defeated, Chornoy leapt from a window of the tower and fell into the moat—

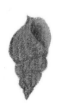

just as Long and Wide and Quick-Eye got back from their day out at the seaside.

'When I saw we would not get here in time,' called Long, 'I threw the shell (with Quick-Eye's help). I hope our aim was true?'

'It was, it was!' said the princess, hanging out of the window and blowing kisses to the band of friends. 'Your aim was perfect.'

She had her choice of husbands now, for so many princes had come to try to rescue her from Chornoy's black fortress, and all were now restored to life. Some were very handsome indeed. But she chose Boy, of course, even though he was rather short, rather short-sighted, and rather short of brains. 'You have such nice friends,' she said. 'And you make me laugh.'

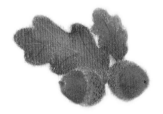

The Chase

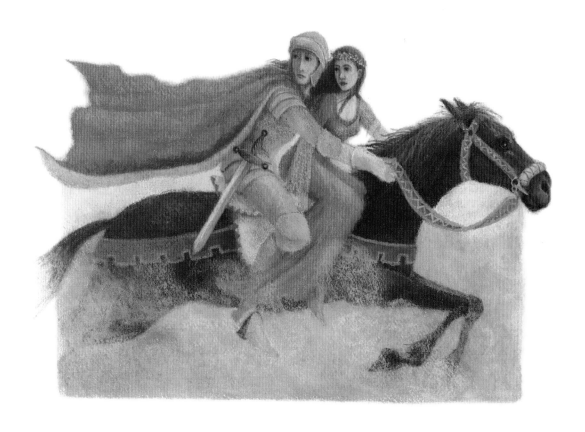

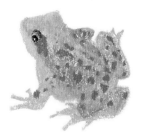

A wizard (as wizards will) took prisoner a beautiful maiden, wanting to marry her. A young hero (as heroes will) came to rescue her. And with both sharing the one saddle, the two escaped.

But the wizard came after them. Faster and faster he gained on them, closer and closer he came, his purple cloak cracking in the wind, his mouth shouting curious curses.

'I shall stand and fight him!' said the knight boldly.

'Don't be silly. He would turn you into a frog,' said the maiden. 'Seven years I was a prisoner in that wizard's lair, and do you think I sat twiddling my thumbs all that while? I've learned a thing or two about magic.'

So saying, at the next fork in the road, the maiden turned herself into a bucket and the horse into a well. The knight took off his armour, threw it down the well, and leaned over the well wall, so that his head was out of sight.

Up came the wizard in a clatter of hoofbeats and whirl of dust. 'Churl, churl, did you see a knight and a maiden sharing a horse? Which road did they take?'

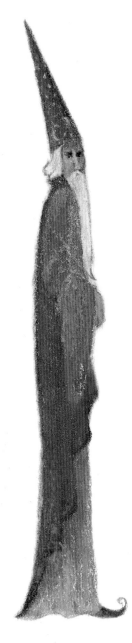

'Yes, I saw them. They took that road,' said the man with his head down the well, his voice all hollow and echoing.

Away went the wizard. The well changed back into a horse, the bucket into a maiden, and away went they down the other road.

By noon, the wizard realized he had gone wrong somewhere, and doubled back. He picked up their trail at the fork in the road. And being only one-in-the-saddle, he soon caught up with them. Faster and faster he gained on them, closer and closer, his purple cloak cracking in the wind, his mouth mumbling imprecations.

'I shall stand and fight him!' said the knight boldly.

'Don't be foolish. He would turn you into a rat,' said the maiden. 'Seven years I was a prisoner in that wizard's lair, and do you think I sat knitting dishcloths all that while? I've learned a thing or two about magic.'

So saying, at the very next crossroads, she turned the horse into a church and herself into the church bell. The knight (climbing down carefully off the church roof) rummaged in the vestry and found a priest's habit with a big hood.

Up came the wizard in a clatter of hoofbeats and a cloud of dust. 'Priest! Priest! Did you see a knight and maiden sharing a horse? Which way did they go?'

'Bless you, my son, I did! They went north,' said the priest, his face hidden inside his deep hood. Away went the wizard, to the north, and behind him a church bell began to peal out happily.

Then the church turned back into a horse, the bell into a maiden, and the knight took off his priest's habit. Away they went down the road to the south.

By tea-time, the wizard realized he had been tricked, and turned back, picking up their trail at the crossroads. He was angry now, and only one-in-the-saddle. Their horse, by contrast, was feeling not quite itself.

Faster and faster the wizard gained on them, closer and closer, purple cloak cracking in the wind, vowing to be avenged on the knight.

'I must stand and fight him!' said the knight.

'Don't be daft. He would turn you into a Christmas turkey,' said the maiden. 'Seven years I was a prisoner in that wizard's lair, and do you think I sat embroidering tea-cosies all that while? I've learned a thing or two about magic. Get off and lie down on the ground.'

So saying, she turned him into a meadow. Herself she turned into a poppy growing in the meadow.

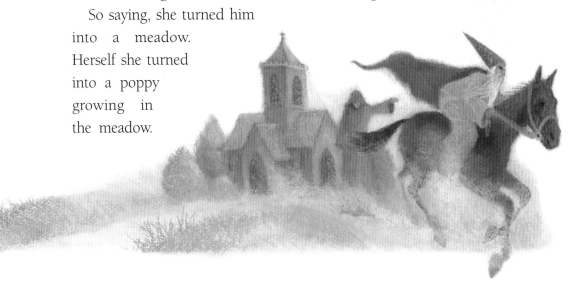

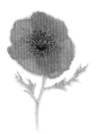 And the horse she turned into a river of chocolate flowing through the meadow.

Now the wizard was very partial to chocolate. The maiden had not lived seven years in his lair without discovering that. As soon as he saw the river, he jumped down from his horse and began scooping up runny handfuls. Soon his beard was sticky brown, his hair clarted, and his purple cloak smeared with chocolate.

Once or twice he thought of the escaping knight and maiden and got up to leave. But the chocolate was so delicious that he could not resist going back. At last he lay down on the bank and let the chocolate ripples lap into his mouth. He got full and fuller, fat and fatter.

Meanwhile, his horse cropped the grass of the meadow, grazing closer and closer to the blowing red poppy. The poppy trembled in the breath from its snorting nostrils. In a moment, the maiden would have to change herself back or be eaten by the wizard's horse!

Suddenly the wizard gave a groan of pain and pleasure and died of eating too much chocolate. The poppy turned back into a maiden (to the great surprise of the wizard's horse). The meadow turned back into a knight (although his hair had been grazed extremely short) and the river turned back into their own trusty steed.

Now, they had all the time in the world to get home, and they had two horses to ride. That was just as well, mind, because the knight found that his chocolate-brown horse was a good bit smaller than before: his feet trailed along the ground when he mounted up, and the creature's tail was only as long as a bootbrush.

The Frog at the Well

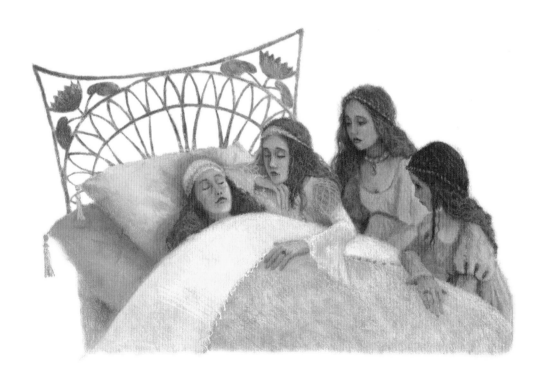

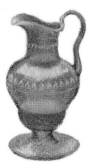

The queen is sick!'

'The doctors fear for her life!'

'They say she will be dead by morning!'

The queen dead by morning? It was unthinkable. Never had the Highlands seen such a rare and lovely woman as the queen who now lay stretched at the threshold of death.

'Her foot is in the stirrup; she will ride away before morning on Death's black horse,' said the royal physician.

'Her black sail is hoisted; she will sail away before morning to the land from which none return,' said her priest.

'Go? And leave not one word for us?' said her three daughters as they sat and wept by the bed.

The queen opened her eyes and smiled. 'I had a dream just now: it's still so bright before me and loud in my ears. A man all in green . . . "A cup of water from the True Well would heal your sickness," he said.'

'Then I'll go at once to the True Well and bring some back!' exclaimed Prudence, the eldest daughter, jumping to her feet. 'You'll see,' she told her sisters. 'Our mother will be all right after all!' At the bedroom door

she turned back: 'How shall I
find the True Well, Mama?' she asked.

'Follow the great white gull!' whispered
the queen, and spoke not a word more.

As Prudence passed out of the castle
gate, she looked up—and there in the sky
was a big white herring-gull crying as
though its red heart were broken. She
followed it. Over land and brook and
shore and sea she followed it, till, on
an island, she heard the croaking of
a frog.

The frog was seated on a rock
beside a pool of green water which
shone like an emerald. Though
both frog and pond were green, it
has to be said, the frog was not as
pretty as the glittering pond.

'I hoped you'd come,' said the
frog. 'I'm waiting here for a
wife.'

'You'll wait a long time,
with a face like yours,' said
Prudence. 'Would you let
me get by? I need water.'

'Will you marry
me?' asked the frog,
not moving.

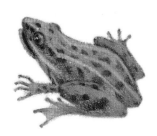

'I've no time to spare for fools or frogs. Of course I won't marry you!' said Prudence, offended that such an ugly creature should even ask.

'Then you won't get your water,' said the frog and jumped into the pool with a ploop.

Prudence took no notice. She knelt down on the bank to scoop up water in her blue-glass pitcher. But the water would not be drawn. It soaked away down into its bed until there was no more than a mud-wallow swarming with beetles and snails.

> *'Marry me! Carry me!*
> *Love me or go thirsty!'*

sang a small, cracked voice from somewhere beneath the earth.

But Prudence flung down her blue-glass pitcher and smashed it, saying, 'Never!'

Back at the palace, the queen lay closer to Death than ever. Her eyes were closed, her cheeks were as sunken as a dry pond. Her two younger daughters were frantic for their sister's return—and yet when she came, she had no water—not a drop.

When she told them what had happened, Patience, the second daughter, jumped up. 'I'll go. It takes more than a slimy frog to keep me from what I want!'

Following the great white gull, she crossed land and brook, shore and sea until she too came to the island and the spring, glittering as green as envy. The frog (though it was uglier than she had expected) did not take her by surprise.

'I hoped you'd come,' said the frog. 'I'm waiting here for a wife.'

'So I hear, and here am I, the very wife for you. Just let me draw some water and then we'll be married.'

The frog was so delighted that it somersaulted into the pool crying, 'Marry me, carry me! Marry me, carry me!'

Patience stooped down and filled her red-glass pitcher. This time the magical water did not soak away, but glugged, clear and cool, into the jug. No sooner was it full than Patience leapt up and set off to run, her skirt hitched up into her belt, laughing and yelping with triumph: 'Did you really think I'd marry you, you piece of green slime? Now I've got what I want, you can whistle for a bride—if frogs can whistle. Ha ha ha!'

Back at the palace her sisters were delighted to see her. The queen was more sick than ever, her eyes as circled with dark as the day is, her breathing as hard as if she were under water. 'Don't worry, mother!' cried Patience, darting into the room. 'I've brought you water from the True Well! You'll be singing and laughing again before long!' And she poured the water into a cup and held the cup to the queen's lips.

'Tip it higher!' said Prudence. 'Her lips are not wet.'

'Tip it higher!' said Charity. 'Her lips are not wet.'

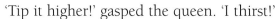

'Tip it higher!' gasped the queen. 'I thirst!'

But though Patience tipped the cup higher and higher, the water shrank down and down in the cup and would not wet the queen's lips. Even when Patience held the cup upside down, not a drop dripped down. She ran to the red-glass pitcher for more water, but when she tipped it up, instead of glug-glug-glug came only the gurk-gurk-groak of a frog's croak. The pitcher was dry.

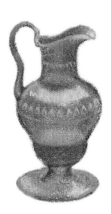

The queen turned her face to the wall.

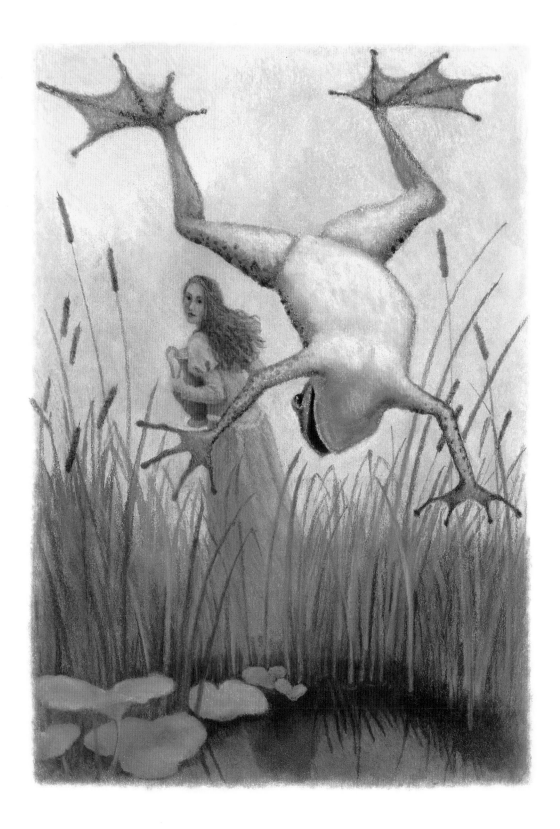

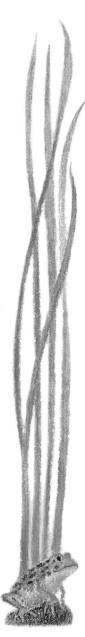

'Now I must go to the True Well,' said Charity, the youngest, 'and fetch back some water for Mama. Her wings are spread and she will fly away from us before morning unless I do. Please, Mama! Stay alive until I come back!'

Following the great white gull, she ran across land and brook, shore and sea, until she came, breathless, to the island and the pool as green and shining as a mermaid's eye. There sat the frog on its rock.

'I hoped you'd come,' it said. 'I'm waiting here for a wife.'

'And I will be that wife, if you will have me,' said Charity. Picking up the frog in both hands, she ran with it to the nearest kirk, where a minister (much against his will) declared they were married.

Filling her green-glass pitcher at the pool, and carrying her husband in her apron pocket, Charity ran back over sea and shore, brook and hillside as fast as legs would carry her. But oh! how the tears crammed her throat as her home came into sight. A black flag hung from the flagpole: the queen was already dead.

'Too late! You're too late!' sobbed her sisters, as she set down the pitcher beside the bed. The queen lay there, as white as a gull, no breath between her lips.

From Charity's pocket came the gurk-gurk-groak of a frog's croak. 'Give her the water, wife,' said the frog.

So Charity filled a cup and tipped it against the queen's lips. This time the water did not draw back, but

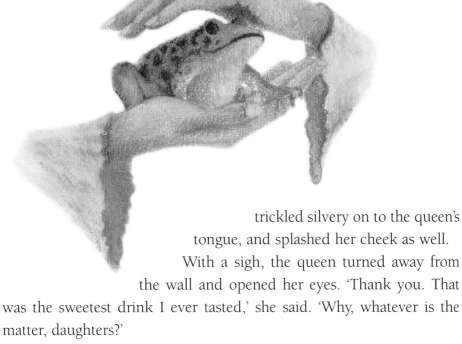

trickled silvery on to the queen's
tongue, and splashed her cheek as well.

With a sigh, the queen turned away from
the wall and opened her eyes. 'Thank you. That
was the sweetest drink I ever tasted,' she said. 'Why, whatever is the
matter, daughters?'

Prudence gulped and Patience hiccuped, and Charity was filled with
such joy that she took the frog from her apron pocket and kissed it on
its ugly green nose. 'Forgive me, Mama, but since you took ill I have
married without your permission. Will you give your blessing to me and
my new husband?'

'You didn't!' said Prudence.

'Urgch!' said Patience. 'How could you!'

'Of course,' said the queen sitting up. 'You chose well, my dear. I don't
believe I ever saw a more handsome or pleasant-looking gentleman in
all my days.'

The sisters stared. It was true. Instead of an ugly green frog, there stood a dashing young man in green velvet, with green eyes, and an emerald in the hilt of his sword.

'I am Prince Ranine,' he said, bowing low to the queen. 'I was enchanted by a witch for ten long years, but your daughter married me and carried me and brought me out of magic. And for that I love her and will do all the days of my life.'

Which pleased Charity, for though she held her mother's life dearer than her own happiness, she had always secretly dreamed of marrying a young and handsome prince.

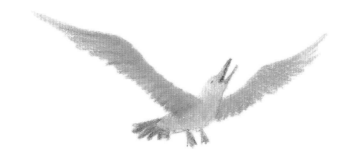

The Little Mermaid

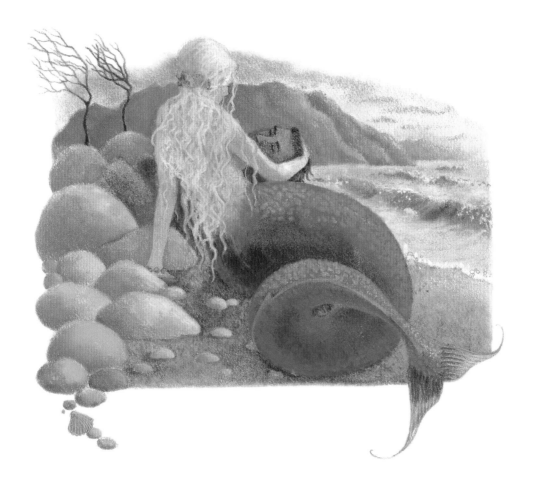

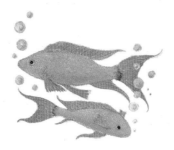

The waves heaved themselves into the air and fell on the ship like the black flukes of a whale, smashing the aftermast to matchwood. False fire gathered round the mizzen, and the cargo in the hold slid from side to side, like the clapper in a bell. With a dreadful splintering crack, the ship broke its back.

'Abandon ship! She's going under!' called the captain, though his words were snatched away like fish by gulls.

Down on the sea bed, the bells of drowned ships rang a knell for the wreck of another, and the mermaids were stirred from their sleep by the flicker of lightning on the roof of their ocean world. Marina swam to the surface, to sing to the music of the storm. No one sang like Marina.

It was there that she saw him—a young man clinging to a broken spar, eyes shut, hair awash in the creamy foam. She thought he was the most beautiful soul she had seen in all the tides of her saltwater life. Water washed over his face, in and out of his mouth, and she knew that he could not live long in the cold and the violence of the pounding sea. As a wave dragged him off the spar and sank him, she caught him in her gleaming arms and carried him, his head on her breast, away from

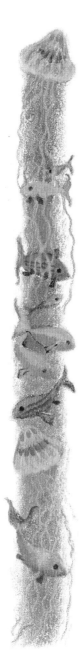

the foundering ship, away from danger, all the way to shallow waters and a beach.

With her tail thrashing the soft sand, it was all she could do to roll the young man out of the sea, where he lay, half dead with exhaustion. Waiting for his eyes to open, she planted a single fervent kiss on his lips and said, 'I love you.' Then voices on the cliff path sent her darting under the cover of the waves. Unwilling to leave, she stayed to eavesdrop.

'Look! A sailor lost in the storm!' It was a girl's voice. Running feet crunched down the beach. 'No, not a sailor! Look at his clothes. A prince, surely!'

'Dead?'

'No! No, look! His eyes are opening! Lie still, sir! You are safe! Safe from the sea! Lie still.'

Marina told herself she was glad—that she had saved a prince's life, and that those who loved him would be happy past words. But how could she go back to the bottom of the sea, having seen this sun-kissed land-man, having held him in her white arms, having given her heart to him? He did not even know she existed! With a storm raging within her fiercer than the one which had sunk that ship, Marina swam out towards the morning horizon.

But she returned, time and time again. She returned to the shore where she had left him and, listening to the fishermen working there, mending their nets, learned the name of her prince and the name of his homeland. Time and again she swam to the marble foundations of his seashore castle, to gaze at its fountains, its grand guests. She asked her sisters: 'How can I leave the sea and go to him?'

But her sisters said, 'It's impossible. Forget him. These humans are born and dead in a matter of years. Not like us mer-people.'

'All the more reason I must hurry!' said Marina. 'I must be with him. I would give my hair to be with him!'

'It would cost you more than that,' said her sister unkindly. 'Fishes die out of water.'

But Marina could not forget the prince. She took her courage in both her white hands and swam to the lightless deep-sea trench, to the lair of the Great Sea Witch.

'You come here out of love for a man,' said the Sea Witch, fanning herself with a purple frond of sea coral.

'I do,' said Marina. 'Can you make me a human girl, with legs to run to my love?'

'At a price,' said the Sea Witch. 'Give me your voice, and I shall give you legs.'

Marina put her hand to her throat. In lagoons and reefs, on the backs of turtles and in the wake of whales, she had sung her sweet, mellifluous songs for a century—sung to the strains of harp seals and birds' cries. Her singing was loved and admired by everyone. And without her voice, how would she . . .

'Well? That's the price. Your voice for a human form.'

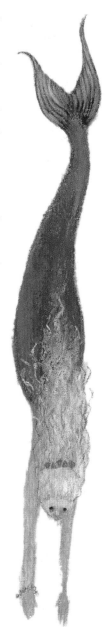

'I'll pay it,' said Marina. And the next moment she felt a pain in her throat of a crab gouged from its shell, and saw her iridescent tail dissolve in a shower of scales.

'Be sure and win his love, mind,' said the Sea Witch, with a cackle like the crackling of dry seaweed. 'The day he marries another and gives his body and soul to her, yours will dissolve like that tail of yours, into white sea foam.'

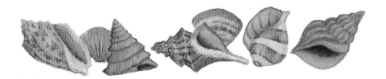

The prince was intrigued by the strange girl he found sitting on the harbour steps. Just where he moored his rowing boat and where he liked to fish for dabs, this beautiful, naked girl suddenly appeared one morning, and no one knew where she had come from. She looked at him with such large, affectionate eyes that he felt he must know her from somewhere—could almost remember her from somewhere. And yet, when he asked her her name, where she came from, what she wanted, she said not a word. It was all very mysterious.

Naturally, he took her in—gave her clothes and food and a room in the palace. She was extremely beautiful, and walked with the swaying elegance of a sea flower, and danced more lightly than anyone at court. But not knowing her story, her background, or what she wanted . . . it was a little baffling.

Marina watched her prince like a fish imprisoned in a tank of water, looking out through the glass, gaping soundlessly. She could not tell

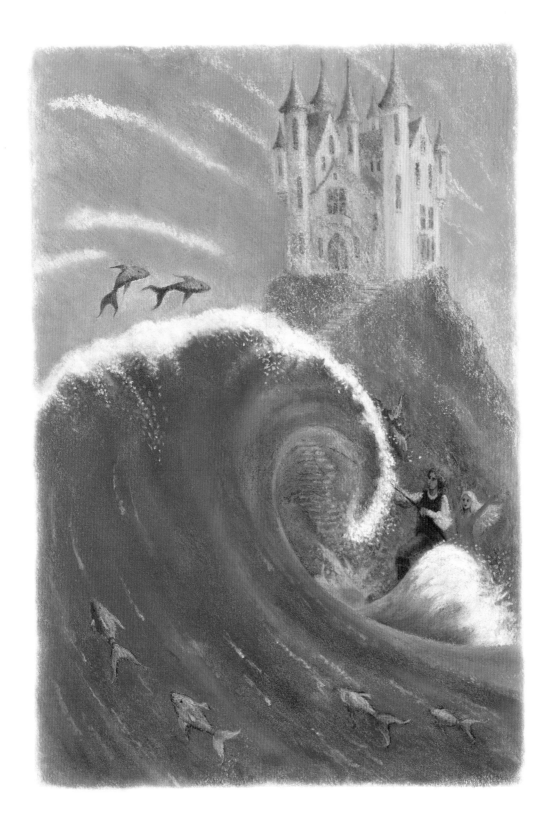

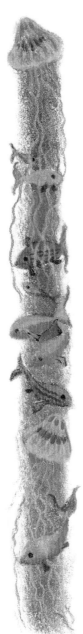

him that every step she took burned in the hollow veins of her legs like fire. Instead she smiled and smiled, and hoped that somehow, in time, her love would show in her eyes as clearly as a lighted lamp at a window.

Marina and her prince became inseparable friends. They did everything together, because there was nothing she was not prepared to do. Unlike most of the other young ladies he knew, this one loved to fish, to be out on the water, to climb mountains and to walk in the rain. She also listened when he talked and never did—never could—interrupt.

'I hope our son is not becoming too attached to that strange young woman with the long hair,' said the king.

But the queen reassured him. 'Of course not, my dear. After all, she is only a poor dumb thing. A playmate.'

Sometimes, dangling the fiery agony of her legs in the cool water by the harbour steps, Marina felt a deadly home-sickness for the sea. But she told herself that she had the friendship of her prince, and that was more than voice and tail and sea.

Then he told her of the wedding. 'We're cousins, though we've never met. She was sent to school overseas. Our parents have always wanted the match.'

Marina felt the scream struggle in her throat, powerless to escape. 'You have me!' she wanted to say. 'Marry me! Why not me?' But her voice was tightly sealed in a clam-shell on the barnacled shelves of the Sea Witch's cave, and she could not make him understand.

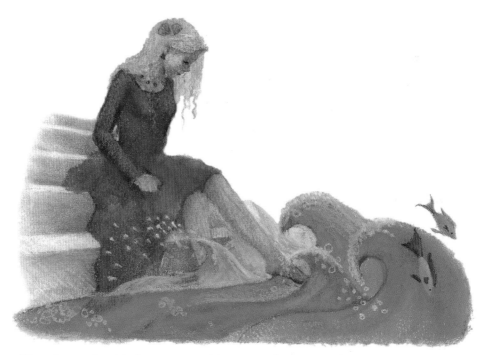

'You know,' said the prince, 'there's only one girl I shall ever love, whoever they find me for a bride.'

Marina's heart swelled and ached with happiness. It was enough. She was loved. And the souls of those who love one another are together for ever when they die, aren't they?

'Yes,' said the prince. 'It was before you and I met. I was shipwrecked one stormy night, and when I woke on the beach and opened my eyes, there was a girl looking down at me—a beautiful girl. She cared for me until I was fit to travel home—but who she was I'll probably never know . . . Oh! Whyever are you crying, little friend?'

It's not fair. It's not fair. It's not fair. The words beat at her brain like a hammer. If he had woken a moment earlier, the face he saw would have been hers. Marina felt robbed, cheated—as though the girl on the beach had deliberately stolen away her every hope of happiness. Marina drew a deep, trembling breath. But *I am here, and she is not,* she thought. *And that makes it all worthwhile.*

As the wedding came closer, the prince became more and more uneasy. 'I do declare,' he said, 'if I can't love this cousin of mine, I shan't go through with the marriage. I shan't. I shall marry you, instead!'

They even travelled together by ship to the wedding. And in the ship's wake, Marina saw her sisters swimming, beckoning, begging her to leap overboard and join them. Their song came over the water, as sharp as starlight in Marina's ears: 'Come away! Come away! Leave the world of men! Before it's too late!'

But Marina knew that it was already too late. She belonged to the world of men because her heart belonged to a man-of-the-dry-land. It was live or die, love or perish.

Die, she thought, when she saw the prince's face. He had just glimpsed

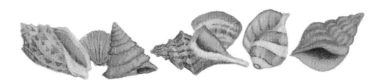

his bride—and the bride was none other than the girl on the beach; the one who had won his love with nothing more than a smile. Marina had to admit, the princess was very beautiful. She was ashamed of the words hammering against her brain: *It's not fair. It's not fair. It's not fair.*

That night, Marina stood on the deck of the ship, her legs on fire, her heart ragged with regret. So. She must die with the sunrise. The prince's heart was given to another girl, and Marina's must dissolve into sea foam. For this she had deserted her own kind. For this she had given up the turquoise pools, the whalesong, the halls of pearl and scarlet coral. For this the Sea Witch had gashed her tail into feeble little legs, silenced her singing.

The bridal tent stood billowing on the deck, golden pennons stirring, small silver bells jingling in the breeze. Inside slept the prince and his bride. The sea kissed the hull of their ship.

Up through the waves came five strange, seal-like heads, whitely grotesque in the moon. It was her sisters, their heads shaved, their eyes big with shock. Something glinted in the moon: a long knife with a curved blade. 'We sold our hair to the Great Sea Witch to buy this! Kill the prince before morning and you needn't die! You shall have back your tail! There are centuries more life waiting for you in the sea. Hurry, little sister!'

Their kindness moved her to tears. 'Oh thank you! Thank you, my

dear, dear sisters!' she mouthed into the wind. The long knife arced through the air and rattled on the deck at her feet. She snatched it up and ran—oh, the pain of running!—to lift the flap of the bridal tent.

There lay the prince, his bride's head on his chest, his hands full of her hair. One blow, and Marina would be free of her disastrous bargain, free of pain, free to live! The sharp rim of the sun was just cutting the wire of the horizon. Her blood seemed already to be turning to sea foam. She folded her two hands round the hilt, kissed the blade . . .

. . . and flung the knife away over the ship's rail. Kill her prince? Not for a world of sea treasure, not for a million years of joy. Climbing a short way up the rigging, she threw herself headlong into the sea, feeling, even as she fell, her heart and body flaking into foam.

And yet she never touched the waves. Her sisters, clutching each other in horror as they saw the precious knife thrown overboard, looked in vain for the droplet fragments of their dead sister; the sea was as smooth as gunmetal and there was not one fleck of foam. Then one mermaid shouted, and the others looked where she was pointing. There in the brightening sky, above the rosy clouds of morning, was the flicker of white wings. Gulls? No.

On board ship, the prince woke with strange misgivings and began searching for his little friend—calling, growing anxious. Fearing she had fallen overboard, he gazed down into the sea, not up into the sky, of course, or he might have glimpsed the angel, new-made by God to watch over him and his bride and his unborn children and his children's children. Wherever such a quantity of love is found in one heart— whether it is a mermaid's or a human heart—there are the makings of an angel. So before the long-bladed knife had even fallen to the ocean bed, Marina had regained her voice and was, to her great astonishment, singing among choirs of angels in the turquoise steeples of the sky.

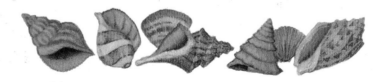

Hansel and Gretel

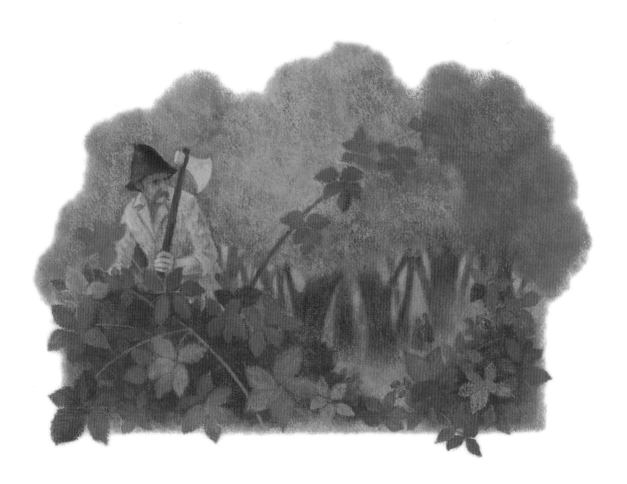

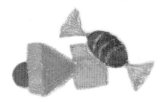

Their father loved Hansel and Gretel very much. Perhaps that is why their stepmother hated them so, wanting all his love for herself. But since she ruled the household with her nagging tongue, she knew she could find a way to be rid of them. When the famine began she said to her husband, 'There's not enough food to keep us two alive, let alone those worthless children of yours. Take them into the forest with you tomorrow, and see to it that they . . . lose their way there.'

Luckily, little Gretel was lying awake, too hungry to sleep. She heard what her stepmother said. 'Wake up, Hansel!' she whispered. 'Our mother means to kill us!'

When Hansel heard about the plan, he soothed his sister's crying and crept out of bed. In the moonlit garden he filled his pockets with all the white stones he could find, then crept back to bed and tried to sleep . . . though who could sleep with such a day ahead?

Their unhappy father was a woodcutter and each day went deep into the forest to work. That day he took his children with him and led them, down mazes of tangling pathways, to a clearing in the very middle of the woods. 'Wait here for me,' he said, kissing them and wiping tears from his eyes. 'I'll come back for you at home-time—God forgive me if I don't.' They could hear his axe-blows—thud, crack—echoing further and further off. Then silence settled on them like leaves.

When night fell they were all alone—abandoned, lost. Gretel began to cry. 'Don't fret,' said Hansel. 'You know those stones I gathered last night? As we came here this morning I dropped them one by one. All we have to do is wait for the moon to rise.'

And sure enough, the rising moon, like a lighthouse casting its beam across a black sea, shone on the forest and lit the white stones Hansel had dropped. They shone out like gems, guiding the children to the very front door of their cottage. Knock knock. The look on their father's face when he opened the door was like Christmas morning. The look on their stepmother's face was Hallowe'en.

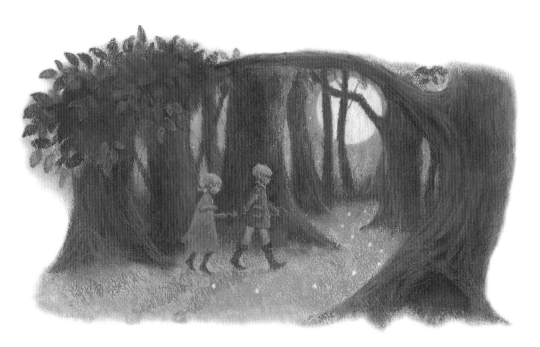

When the children were safely tucked up in
bed, they could hear the bark and snarl of her,
as she nagged her husband. 'You fool! Trust
you to let them find their way home! You'd
better make a better job of it tomorrow, or we'll
both starve!'

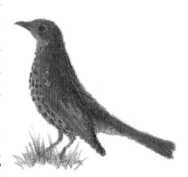

Gretel clutched her brother's hand in terror,
but he soothed her sobbing. Instead of eating
the crust of bread given him as supper, Hansel
pushed it deep into his pocket.

Next day, as the woodcutter led them down miles of tangling
pathways into the very middle of the woods, Hansel picked from the
crust crumb after crumb of bread, dropping a trail of breadcrumbs,
marking the way they had come. In the heart of the forest their father
kissed them and dried his eyes. 'Wait here for me. I shall come back for
you at home-time. God forgive me if I don't.' They could hear his
axe-blows—thud, crack—echoing further and further off. Then
silence fell, and Gretel began to cry.

Hansel was not worried. He even whistled as he waited. He
knew their father would not come back for them. But he
also knew that the white breadcrumbs would shine out in
the white moonlight, and show them the way home to
their front door.

Daylight faded. The woodcutter did not come.
The moon rose . . . And all the little birds of the
forest went home to their nests with white bread
in their beaks for their hungry chicks. When
Hansel and Gretel began to look for the path

home, every moonlit path looked the same; there was no way to tell them apart. The birds had eaten every crumb. Hansel and Gretel searched and ran and called, but they were alone in the heart of the great forest, lost, hopelessly lost.

Huddling together for warmth, the children slept. And the birds, realizing what they had done, dropped a blanket of leaves over the sleeping pair, a quilt of green and yellow.

Next day the children began walking aimlessly through the forest, searching for berries to eat. They were fearfully hungry. So both thought they were dreaming when, in a sunlit clearing, they saw a funny little cottage.

Its walls were made of gingerbread, its roof of marzipan. Its shutters were wafers, its door chocolate, each chimney a twist of barleysugar. Hansel and Gretel rushed up a path cobbled with sugared almonds and raced around the delightful house, sniffing and stroking the walls, trampling flowerbeds of parma violets without even realizing. Hansel broke a piece off the roof and crammed it into his mouth.

'Oho! Rats in the eaves, eh? Nibble my house, would you! Well, you'll be sorry . . . !' Out of the house scuttled a bent, gnarled old woman, her face as crumpled as a ball of paper. But peering short-sightedly at the visitors, she showed her yellow teeth in a twisted smile. 'Children, is it? Well, how nice. Help yourselves, little ones. Do! There's better inside. Won't you come in and dine?'

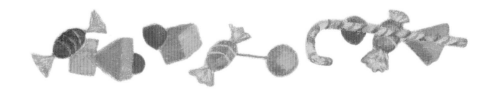

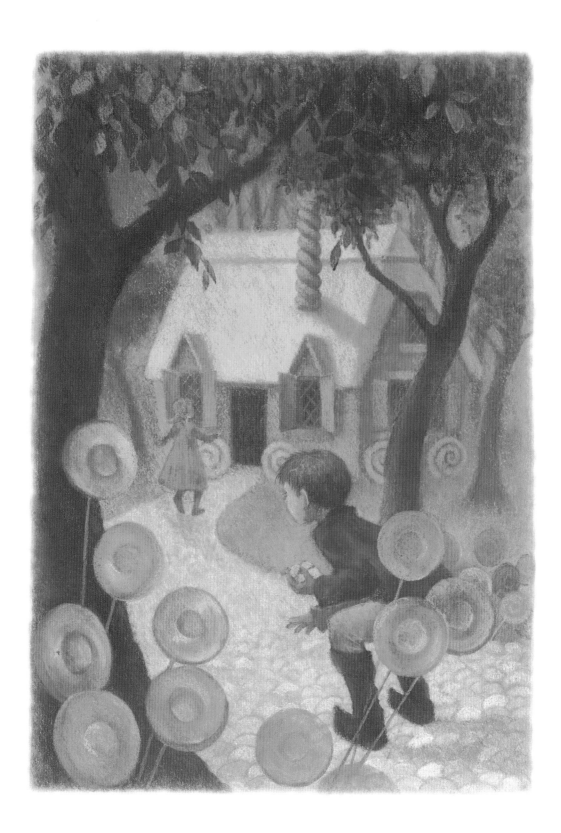

In went Hansel and Gretel: 'We're very sorry! We were just so hungry, and all those delicious—'

'Not another word,' said the old lady, sitting them down at table. 'Here's caramel for you, boy, and limedrops for you, my dear.' And she brought so many plates of sweets to the table that the children groaned with pleasure.

It was a strange kitchen, with a big stove and table, the rest of the room bare but for a large cage in one dark corner and a large locked chest in another. 'Now who's good at housework?' asked the old lady, as they sat loosening their belts. At once Gretel jumped up.

'I am! Shall I wash up, Grandma?' she asked.

'You will!' Suddenly, with a cackle that shattered the water jug, the old woman knocked over Hansel's chair, spilling him on to the floor. With a twig broom, she pushed him into the cage and clanged shut the door before throwing the broom at Gretel's head.

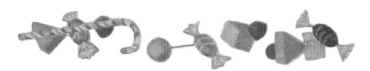

'And when you've done the dishes you can sweep the floor and make my bed—scrub the step and feed the chickens! From today onwards, you're my slave! House-breakers! Roof-nibblers! You're the lucky one, girl! Your brother won't live as long!'

Hansel rattled the bars of the iron cage. 'Why?! Let me out! What are you going to do to me?'

The old witch hobbled over to him and peered through the bars. Her lips drooled. 'Well, EAT you, of course, boy!' she croaked. 'As soon as you're fat enough!'

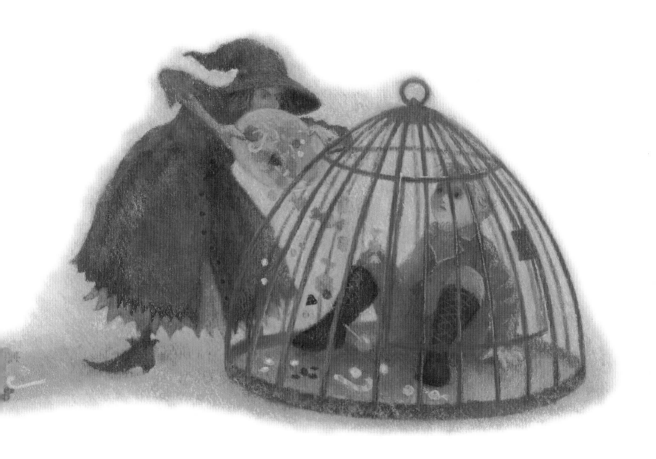

Naturally, thanks to the famine, Hansel and Gretel were about as thin as two children could be. But the old witch (who liked only meat, and plenty of meat on the bone) had a remedy for that. Every day she served Hansel a delectable meal of sweet things, fattening him up for the day she would roast him and eat him with a sprig of parsley in his hair.

Being short-sighted, she bumped about the house breaking off pieces of candy and fumbling them on to a plate which she tipped through the bars of the cage, showering Hansel with sugar. Then, 'Put out your finger, boy!' she would yelp, and squeezing his finger fiercely between her toothless gums, she would spit with disgust and say, 'Too thin! Too thin! Not ready yet!'

Oddly enough, Hansel's finger grew no fatter. Shall I tell you why? It was Gretel's idea. 'Whenever the witch says, "Put out your finger!"' she whispered to him one night, 'hold out this stick instead.' And she gave him a thin twig from the kindling beside the stove. So no matter how much the witch fed Hansel, the 'finger' she mumbled each day between her toothless gums grew no fatter than a twig, and away she would go, saying, 'Too thin! Too thin! Will this boy never be fat enough to eat?'

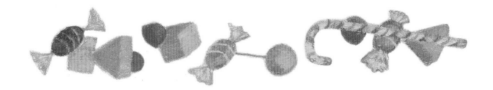

Inside his cage, plump, round Hansel sat and watched his sister work her fingers to the bone doing the witch's housework while he ate and slept and thought of the day when the trick with the twig stopped working.

'Enough!' screeched the witch one morning. 'I've waited long enough. I haven't eaten roast boy now for a year, and I have a mind to eat some today! Gretel! Light the stove!'

Now the stove was huge—a cast-iron cave of a cooker, with a grate deep at the back which had to be lit by hand. The witch gave Gretel a lighted spill and told her, 'Crawl inside and light the stove, girl, and be quick about it!'

'I don't know how,' said Gretel.

'Just crawl inside and light the kindling, you stupid child!' said the witch.

'I don't understand, ma'am,' said Gretel.

'Why not? It's as easy as spitting!' raged the old witch.

'I'm very stupid,' said Gretel. 'Stepmother always said so.'

'Must I do everything myself!' exclaimed the witch in exasperation, and snatched the spill from Gretel. Stretching her scrawny neck and poking her goat-like head in at the door of the oven, she reached forward and lit the kindling.

With a single blow of her broom, Gretel whacked the witch's black behind with all her might, toppling her into the oven and slamming shut the cast-iron door. The fire in the oven blazed and roared. The witch burned with a purple flame. The gingerbread ceiling softened and sagged in the heat, and both chimney pots fell to the ground outside.

Meanwhile, Gretel fetched the keys from under the witch's mattress, and freed Hansel: he could barely squeeze through the cage door, he was so fat. Inside the locked chest they found a fortune in pearls and jet and gold—none of it made of sugar.

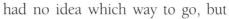

So with one sack full of gingerbread and one of treasure, the two children set off back through the forest. They had no idea which way to go, but came soon to a wide river where swans as large as Venetian gondolas cruised up and down, up and down.

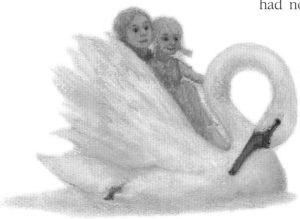

'Will you carry us over?' called Gretel, and one swan drew close to the bank, allowing the children to nestle down between its folded wings.

Down the river, riding the current, went the great white swan until, at last, Hansel recognized the countryside around him. 'I know where we are! We could be home in an hour!'

The swan set them ashore, and Hansel and Gretel walked the rest of the way to their own front door, dragging their heavy sacks. But there was something strange about the ramshackle old cottage, something different. It was silent. No shrill carping or complaining disturbed the birds from the roof-ridge. No noise of nagging unsettled the butterflies from the flowers. Their stepmother was nowhere around.

When their father opened the door, he hugged his lost children so close they could not speak. 'I thought you were dead! I thought I'd killed you! I haven't had a minute's peace since I gave in to that cruel, wicked woman! I should never have listened to her! Can you ever forgive me? She's gone now! Dead and gone, and good riddance, I say! Come inside, come inside! I'll find you something to eat—something, somehow . . .'

But there was no need for the woodcutter to sacrifice his last bite of bread. For Hansel and Gretel had brought a sackful of gingerbread to eat, and gold to buy meat and bread and more. And with the death of the witch, deep in the forest, the famine left that part of the world—spread its wings and flew away like a great black crow, leaving the fields full of grain once more and the cows as brown as gingerbread . . . and almost as fat as Hansel.

The Tinderbox

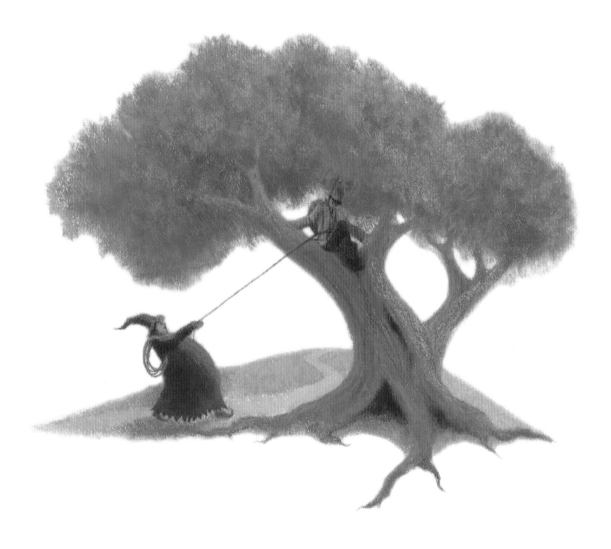

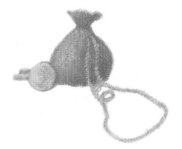

There was once a leaf trembling on a twig, the twig on a branch, the branch on a tree, the tree by a road, and under the tree—a big fat witch in an apron.

Along the road came a soldier, as thin and sharp-nosed as the bayonet on his rifle. 'Hoi! Young man! How would you like to be as rich as now you are poor?' called the witch.

'What must I do? Marry you?' said the soldier. His mother had warned him not to speak to strange women, and this was as strange as any he had ever met.

'This tree is hollow. But it's thin, too, and I am fat,' said the witch. 'Now you, you're as thin as a hair; I could thread you through the eye of a needle and mend my socks. So climb down the tree and fetch me something from the cavern below.'

'Why? What's down there that you want so badly?' asked the soldier, whose name was Tommy.

'I want a tinderbox that lies in the third room. Bring me that and you can help yourself to anything else you find down there. Here, tie this rope round your waist and I'll lower you down. Take my apron, too.'

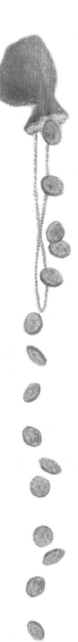

'I have to cook?' said Tommy, holding the apron at arm's length between finger and thumb.

'The three rooms are guarded by three dogs. No, don't worry. They won't hurt you if you sit each dog on this apron. Hurry now! Or do you want to be poor all your life?'

Tommy was curious to see inside the tree. More out of curiosity than greed, he jumped into its branches and slipped down inside the hollow trunk, knapsack on his back and the witch's apron and rope round his waist.

It was a long way down, and dark. A ferocious barking came up the narrow flue and, as his feet touched ground and he struck a match, he was confronted by a dog.

Did I say dog? It was as big as a lion, with eyes as large as saucers. Quickly Tommy whipped off the apron and laid it down, then—'Steady now—I've got you!—Don't wriggle!'—sat the dog on the apron. Quiet as a tea cup, the dog sat and stared at Tommy with its huge eyes, while Tommy stared around him, his eyes almost as big. Everywhere he looked, he saw the red glint of copper. There were copper coins spilling out of barrels, chests, and baskets.

This is some robber's lair, he thought, cramming his pockets and knapsack with such a weight of coins that his knees bent. Nudging the dog off the apron, he went on into the second room, just as the match between his fingers fizzled out. He had no sooner struck a second match than he was confronted by a second dog.

Did I say dog? It was as big as a horse, with eyes as large as dinner plates. Tommy laid down the apron then—'Oof!—If you'd just—shift over—ow, my back!'—got the dog on to the apron. Quiet as a dinner table, the dog sat and stared at Tommy with its gigantic eyes, while Tommy stared around him, his eyes almost as big. Everywhere he looked he saw the thin gleam of silver. There were silver coins spilling out of crates, vases, and panniers.

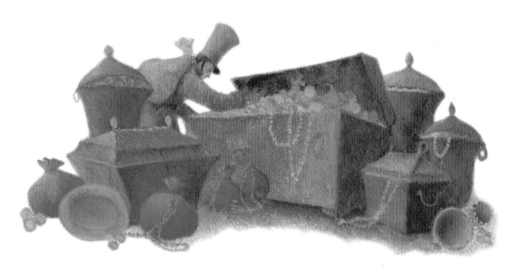

This is some pirate's treasure, he thought, emptying his pockets and knapsack of copper to fill them with silver. He picked up such a weight of silver that he bowed at the knees. Then, leaning against the huge dog, he got it off the apron and went on into the third room, just as his match went out.

He had no sooner struck another than he backed straight out of the room again. For it was almost full of dog. Wall-to-wall dog: a beast as vast as an elephant, with eyes as large as cartwheels and a bark like a thundercrack. Tommy waved the apron at it like a flag of surrender, then—'Go on!—uugh!—move yourself!—Ooof!—Go on, you brute!'— barged and shifted the monumental dog on to the apron.

Quiet as a wagon, the dog sat and stared at Tommy, its vast eyes slowly revolving, while Tommy stared around him, his eyes nearly as big. Everywhere he looked, he saw the sunny sparkle of gold. There were gold coins covering the floor, piled against the walls, spilling out of sacks and trunks and troughs.

This is some wizard's fortune, thought Tommy. No ordinary man carried all this here. And he emptied his pockets and knapsack of silver, to refill them with gold. Just before his match went out, he noticed a cheap tin tinderbox lying on the floor and picked that up, too.

The witch's rope was tugging at his waist now. Her fat voice came oozing through the darkness: 'What's keeping you? Where are you? Hurry up! Have you found it?' Tommy let her pull him up from the cavern; up the hollow tree until he could wriggle out on to a branch. 'Did you get it?' she demanded. 'Did you get the tinderbox? Did you?' Jumping up and down in a frenzy.

'What can it do? Why do you want it so much?' asked Tommy.

'Give! Give it! Give! Give! Give!' screamed the witch, clawing at his dangling boots. Unfortunately, she pulled so hard that she dislodged him from the branch. He fell, knapsack and all and, like a rock falling on a beetle, squashed the fat witch flat.

She was quite dead. There was nothing for Tommy to do but go whistling on his way into town.

What a popular man he was when he got there! He bought drinks,

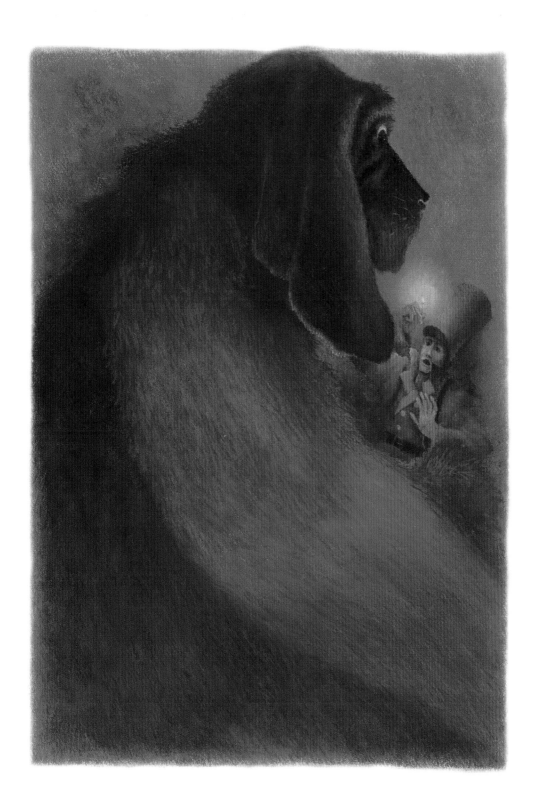

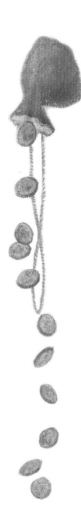

he lent loans, he gave gifts, he kept open-house, inviting everyone to dinner who cared to come. He bought the most fashionable clothes, saw the most fashionable plays, betted on the prettiest horses at the racetrack. In no time at all he had a thousand dear friends who loved him like a brother.

Every day they talked about the same thing, those fine gentlemen. They talked about Princess Blaise— whom no one had ever seen—guessing what she looked like, guessing her age, guessing whom she might marry. It did not seem very likely to Tommy that Blaise would ever marry anyone. For she lived in a tower of copper, safe from spying eyes, by order of the king. 'What I'd give to see that princess!' said Tommy, but then all his dear friends said the same.

And then the money ran out.

In no time, Tommy's stomach was as empty as his knapsack. His landlord turned him out of his luxury lodgings, and his dear friends melted away like the morning frost. He found himself back in the wood, sheltering under a tree, with nothing to his name but one fashionable suit, a gun, a knapsack, and a cheap tin tinderbox. Breaking twigs from the dead trees, he built himself a fire to keep warm by, and struck his last match to light it. The match went out.

Now, the right and proper purpose of a tinderbox is to strike sparks and light fires. So that's what Tommy did. At least that is what he started to do.

No sooner did he strike a spark than through the wood came bounding and barking the dog from the cavern, its eyes as large as saucers. 'Whaadawaant, master?' it barked.

'Oho, is that how it goes!' said Tommy and struck the tinderbox twice. Two sparks, and through the woods came bounding and barking the dog with eyes as large as dinner plates.

'Whaadawaant, master?' it barked.

'So that's why the fat witch wanted the tinderbox,' said Tommy and struck three times. Three sparks, and through the wood came bounding and barking, felling trees like a stampede of elephants, the dog with eyes as big as cartwheels.

'Whaadawaant, master?'

'I see now that I am the richest man in the kingdom,' said Tommy to the dogs. 'Let's start with a sack of gold, if you would be so kind.' The dogs fetched what he wanted instantly.

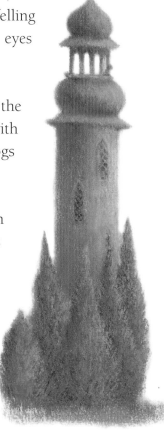

* * *

Rich once more, Tommy took fine lodgings again in town. But this time he did not think of parties or fashionable clothes, of making himself popular or making himself famous. He just thought of the Princess Blaise. Striking the tinderbox once, he summoned the dog with eyes as large as saucers.

'Whaadawaant, master?' barked the dog.

'I wish to see the princess from the copper tower,' said Tommy. 'Is that possible?'

Away went the dog, as fast as thought, and back it came. Stretched out along its back, sound asleep and dreaming, lay the Princess Blaise, her coppery hair hanging down. Tommy stared and stared. She was so beautiful that he could not help but kiss her. Then, ashamed of himself, he told the dog to carry her safely back to bed before she woke.

* * *

'I had the strangest dream last night,' said Princess Blaise to her parents. 'I dreamt a dog with eyes as big as saucers carried me down to the town, and there a soldier with eyes like stars kissed me.' And she sighed, as if to say, 'Sweet dreams.'

'How nice, dear,' said the queen. But her fist tightened on her teaspoon and her teeth ground on her toast. 'I don't care for such dreams,' she told the king later. 'Let's set a maid to keep watch over our dear darling daughter.'

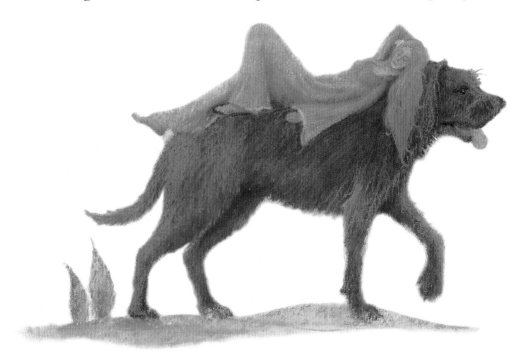

All day, Tommy could think of nothing but the princess. Next night he struck the tinderbox and asked the dog with eyes as large as saucers to fetch the princess to him again.

Away went the dog, as fast as thought, and home it came, the sleeping princess on its back. This time Tommy gave her two kisses, and stared till his eyes felt as big as dinner plates.

Little did he know that a maid had been keeping watch over the lovely princess. What a fright that dog had given her! But she was a brave girl, and when the dog carried the princess away through the open window, she hitched up her nightdress and ran after it, all the way to town.

Seeing the house to which the dog ran, the maid said to herself, 'All these houses look the same. How will the king's soldiers find this one in the morning and arrest this vile kidnapper?' Clever girl that she was, she took out a piece of chalk and drew a cross on Tommy's door.

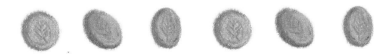

Later that night, Tommy sighed one more sigh and told the dog to carry his beloved princess back to her bed. Luckily, the dog's huge eyes gave it the sharpest sight. As it looked to left and right, it saw the chalk cross on the door. And just as if that dog had gone to school all its life and learned the alphabet up to X, it took out a piece of chalk and drew crosses on every other door in the street—every other door in the town.

* * *

The king's troopers came back from town glum and empty-handed. 'Well? Did you arrest him?' demanded the king. 'Did you find the house with the cross on the door?'

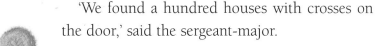

'We found a hundred houses with crosses on the door,' said the sergeant-major.

Well, the poor maid almost lost her head. 'If you please, your Majesty,' she begged, 'give me one more chance and I'll find him out for you, the kidnapper! I know how it can be done! Just sew a silk purse to the princess's nightdress— a purse with a little hole in it—and fill the purse with buckwheat.'

When, on the third night, Tommy sent his dog to fetch the sleeping princess from her bed, no one followed his bounding down to town. There was no need. The buckwheat trickled, grain by golden grain, down from the silk purse, and left a trail on the moonlit ground. Though Tommy took from the princess no more than three kisses, and though he soon returned her unharmed to her bed, the royal guard came pounding on his door at dawn and dragged him away to prison in his nightshirt.

'He shall hang in the morning!' vowed the king.

* * *

Through his prison bars, Tommy could see the scaffold. He could see, too, the distant glimmer of the copper tower, could see the stars setting on the last night of his life. He was very afraid.

A little boy kicked a fir cone across the prison yard. Tommy knew by the sharpness of his nose that the boy was hungry. 'Psst! Psst, boy! How would you like to be as rich as now you are poor? Run to my lodgings and fetch me the tinderbox lying on the table. You can help yourself to anything else you find there.'

Behind him a key rattled in the lock, and in came the jailer holding a noose of rope. 'Yer wanted, sir,' he said. 'At the gallows.'

The king and queen were there to see the execution. Drums rolled, people stared, their eyes as big as gold coins, as the prisoner was led out to the scaffold. At the last moment, a little boy darted through the crowd and thrust a cheap tin tinderbox into the hand of the condemned man.

'May I smoke a last pipe before I die?' said Tommy to the king. 'It's not much to ask.' The king nodded.

One—one two—one two three times, Tommy struck a spark.

Bounding and barking, over market and river, over coaches and platoons of soldiers, over houses and shops, came all three dogs, eyes whirling and blazing in their heads, their steamy breath clouding the cold morning air. They bit through the gallows, they tossed the executioner over the church. They licked the queen and picked up the king by his gown.

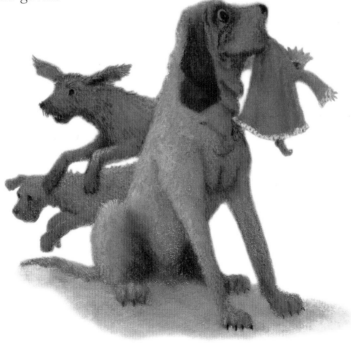

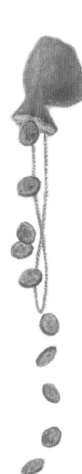

And if Tommy had been a worse-tempered man, who knows what his dogs might have done at his command.

You have no idea how popular Tommy became all of a sudden. 'Hurrah for Tommy!' shouted the terrified crowd, as the three dogs tore round and round them. 'We want Tommy for Prince! Three cheers for Tommy!' All thoughts of hanging him were forgotten, and the king and queen vowed they had never met a more suitable bridegroom for their dear, darling daughter.

But Tommy did not use his magic dogs to scare the princess into marrying him. He did not need to. She said, 'You remind me of someone I met in a dream. It was a sweet dream. I liked you then and I like you now.'

It is lucky she liked dogs, too, because all three came to the wedding, bounding and barking ahead of the golden coach, then lolling on the church steps, staring and staring and staring.

Cap-o'-Rushes

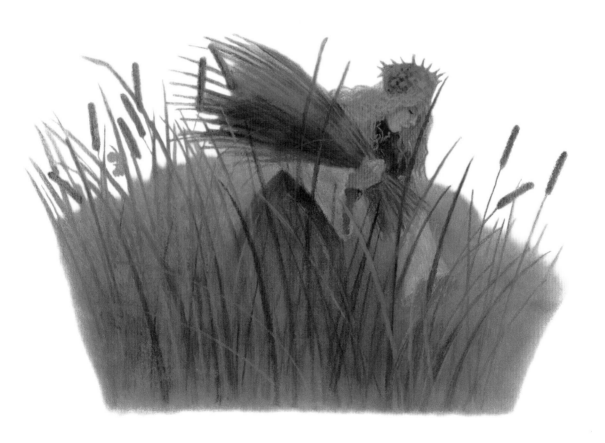

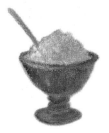

A weary old king took it into his head to retire and to split his kingdom between his three daughters. But which of them should have the fat green lands to the south, which the bare bleak mountains to the west, which the purple wilds of the north? He could have tossed a coin to decide. But being a vain man he asked each girl instead: 'How much do you love me?'

'More than gold and silver,' said Goneril, his oldest daughter, wanting the best share.

'More than diamonds and rubies,' said Regan, trying to outdo her.

The king purred with pleasure. 'And you, Cordelia?' he asked his favourite daughter. 'How much do you love me?'

'As much as meat loves salt,' said the little princess.

'What's that supposed to mean?' said the king scowling. 'Speak again.'

But the youngest would say nothing more. The king, who had always thought she loved him best of all, threw a terrible tantrum, tossing furniture about and shouting: 'If I mean so little to you, you can just get out! Go on! Get out! And don't come back! I'll split my kingdom between Goneril and Regan. As for you, you can walk the world and starve for all I care! Meat? Salt? Heartless, thankless child!'

So Cordelia went out into the stormy world, taking with her only three dresses of her dead mother's, as remembrances. She picked rushes from the river bank and wove herself a cap and cloak, such as beggars wore to keep off the rain and cold. And she threw her name into the river, so afterwards people had no name to call her by but 'Cap-of-Rushes'.

If she was ever to eat again, she had to find work. So she knocked at the door of a royal castle in the kingdom next door. 'I would work hard for no pay and only a bite to eat and somewhere to lay down my head,' said Cap-of-Rushes.

'Then you may scrape pots and shine pans in the kitchen,' said the housekeeper, 'and sleep by the stove at nights.'

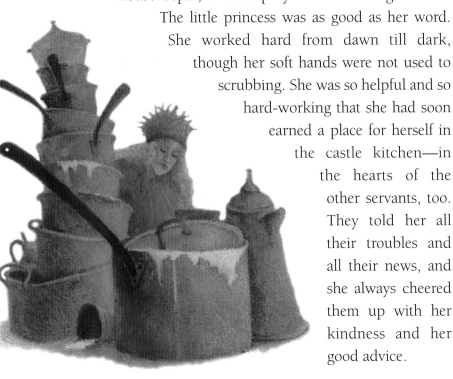

The little princess was as good as her word. She worked hard from dawn till dark, though her soft hands were not used to scrubbing. She was so helpful and so hard-working that she had soon earned a place for herself in the castle kitchen—in the hearts of the other servants, too. They told her all their troubles and all their news, and she always cheered them up with her kindness and her good advice.

So when the king announced that he was to give a party, with dancing and feasting and orchestras and a hundred guests, the word soon reached the little scullery maid.

'Oh, Cap-of-Rushes! Cap-of-Rushes! It's going to be such a grand affair! Three days of dancing! One, two, three!'

'The king and the prince and all the dukes and duchesses will be there!'

'Everyone in the kingdom is invited! And we shall serve the food and take the cloaks and wait at table and see it all, Cap-of-Rushes . . . though you'll have to find something better to wear than that cape of yours!'

'It sounds grand,' said Cap-of-Rushes, nothing more.

But on the day of the first ball, she said she was too tired to go upstairs and watch the dancing. So the other servants left her asleep in front of the stove and went without her.

As soon as they were gone, Cap-of-Rushes opened her eyes, fetched out her bundle, and took off her coarse cape and cap. She put on a dress of her mother's—a white dress stitched all over with pearls—and brushed her hair until every tangle was out. Then she ran upstairs to join in the dancing.

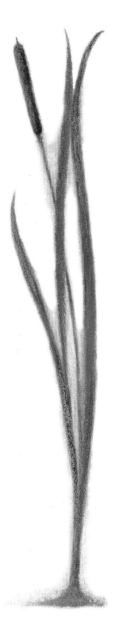

* * *

'Cap-of-Rushes! Oh, Cap-of-Rushes, you should have been there!' The servants and footmen and maids and cooks all tumbled into the kitchen, noisy with excitement. The little scullery maid asleep in front of the stove blinked her eyes and sat up.

'There was this princess—oh! she was lovely!'

'A white dress . . .'

'The prince couldn't take his eyes off her!'

'How they danced!'

'How they talked!'

'She just left—not ten minutes ago!'

'Oh, Cap-of-Rushes, such an amazing evening!'

Cap-of-Rushes pulled her grassy cape closer around her. 'It must have been grand,' she said, but nothing more.

Next evening the music began again upstairs in the grand ballroom. All the servants changed into their best livery, but Cap-of-Rushes said she was too tired to do anything but sleep, and lay down in front of the stove.

As soon as they were gone, she changed her ugly cape and cap for a second dress—a black one sewn with diamonds like the night sky—and brushed her hair till it floated around her head as she ran upstairs.

Once again she danced all night with the prince and this time it was not so easy to slip away, for she could hardly bear to part from the prince, nor he from her. Even so, she was back in front of the stove before her friends burst excitedly into the room.

'Cap-of-Rushes! Oh, Cap-of-Rushes, you should have been there! That princess came again.'

'A black dress covered in diamonds!'

'The prince loves her for sure!'

Cap-of-Rushes pulled her grassy cape closer around her. 'It must have been grand,' she said, but nothing more.

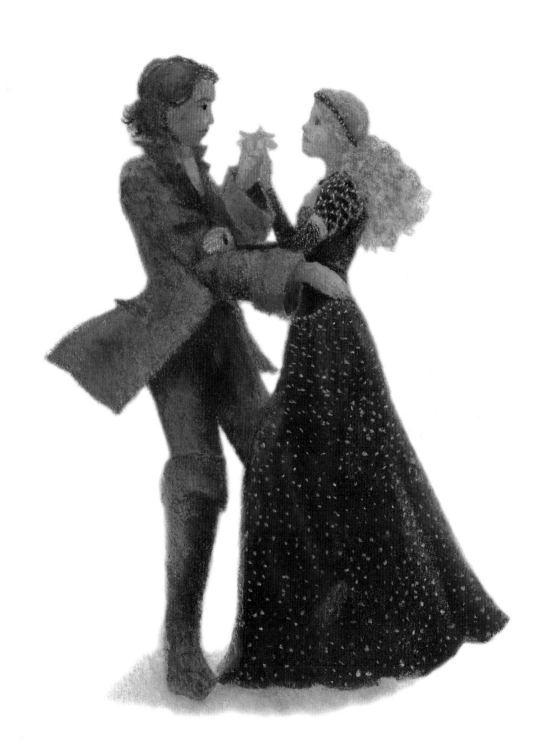

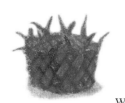 On the third evening, she again pretended she was too tired to go to the ball, and the others again went without her. As soon as they were gone, she put on her third dress—a red one sewn with rubies—and brushed her hair till it crackled with electricity. She could hardly wait to see the prince, for her love for him was big like a pain inside her.

As they danced, he asked to marry her—said he would die if he could not marry her—seized her hand and slipped his own ring of state on to her finger. But when Cap-of-Rushes looked into his eyes, she saw her own reflection and thought: what am I? A scullery maid, cast out by my father. When he finds out, the prince, too, will hate me. Wriggling free of his grasp, Cap-of-Rushes fled.

'Don't go!' cried the prince. 'Friends! Servants! Stop her for me, please! I mustn't lose her!'

Guests and guards, servants and maids scattered in every direction. Cooks and footmen tumbled down the back stairs into the kitchen, as fast as they could go . . . but found no one—only the little scullery maid asleep in front of the stove.

'Oh, Cap-of-Rushes! Cap-of-Rushes! Such a calamity! Wait till you hear!' wailed the head cook. (They did not realize that underneath that nasty cape of reeds rustled a gorgeous gown of red silk and rubies.)

Though riders galloped throughout the land, no trace could be found of the girl in the scarlet dress. And when it seemed she was gone forever, the prince cancelled all his royal engagements and stayed in his rooms, day after week after fortnight.

'Oh, Cap-of-Rushes! Cap-of-Rushes!' sobbed the cook, as she

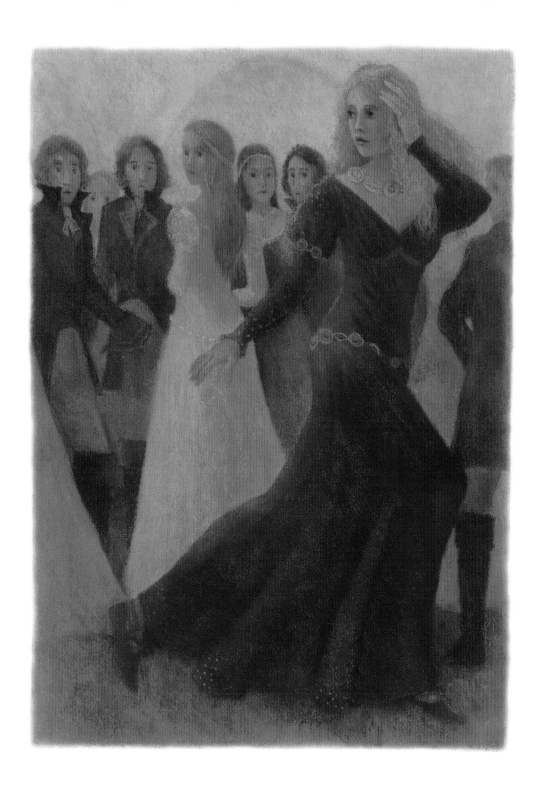

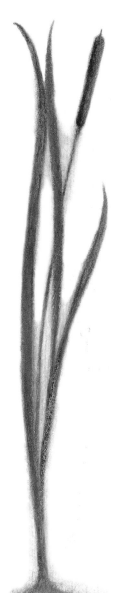

chopped onions one day. 'I'm afraid this is the last meal I shall ever cook for that poor young man!'

'What poor young man is that?' asked Cap-of-Rushes.

'I'm not supposed to say. It's a state secret,' said the cook, biting her lip. 'But the king sent for me this morning and told me to cook soup for the prince. Seems he won't eat, can't sleep. He's pining away with a broken heart.'

When Cap-of-Rushes heard that, she said, 'Let me make the soup. Please.' And as she prepared it, she slipped the ring of state into the serving dish.

The soup was sent up to the prince. At first he said he would not drink it, but at last the queen persuaded him to take one sip. And lo and behold! there in his spoon was the ring.

'LET THE COOK BE SENT FOR!'

The cry echoed down the back stairs. The cook quaked in her shoes. 'What have I done? Why me?' The footmen and maids gaped back at her and shrugged helplessly. So, wiping her trembling hands on her apron, the cook went to the prince's bedside and curtsied.

'Who cooked this soup?' the prince demanded to know, his face as pale as Death.

Thinking the soup was bad, and that poor little Cap-of-Rushes would get into trouble, the kind-hearted cook said, 'I did, your honour, if it please you, thank you kindly like.'

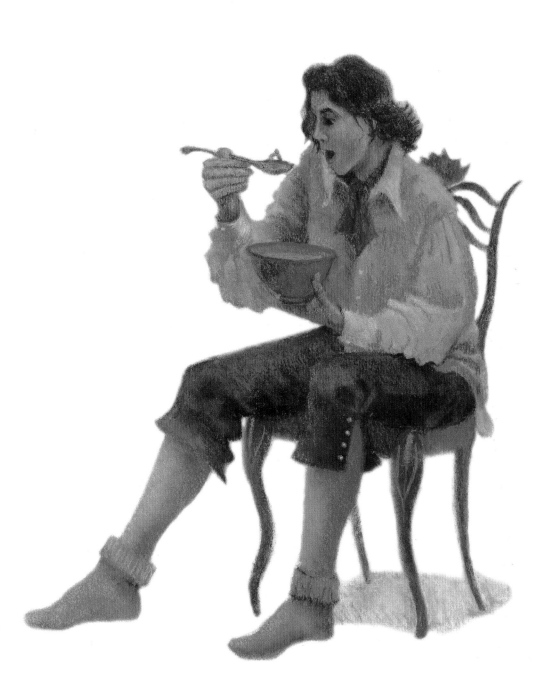

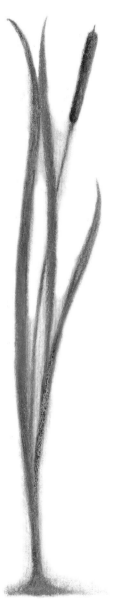

'No!' said the prince, bounding out of bed and advancing on the cook with the bowl outstretched in his hands. 'WHO COOKED THIS SOUP? TELL ME THE TRUTH.'

'Oh mercy!' cried the cook, putting her apron over her head. 'It was Cap-of-Rushes, your honour! But she's really such a good girl, if you just knew her!'

'Send her to me,' said the prince, and this time his voice was soft and gentle, because he knew he had found his missing princess.

When Cap-of-Rushes went to the prince's room it was not in her cape and cap of woven reeds. To the amazement of all the kitchen staff, she took that off and burned it on the stove, revealing a dress beneath of scarlet silk sewn with rubies. When the prince saw her, he knew he need not die; and when Cap-of-Rushes saw her prince, she suddenly knew how she could marry him after all and be happy evermore.

* * *

'Goneril! Regan! We are invited to a wedding in the kingdom next-door,' said the weary old king one morning. He had no wish to go—had rather lost his taste for parties and jollifications. But of course he could not refuse. So he and his daughters travelled to the wedding, and a very lavish affair it was, too.

The wedding feast covered seventeen trestle

tables—roast swan and quail and golden pheasant, roast beef and pork, lamb and venison, besides all the rolls and pâtés and pastries. More than a hundred guests stood up to toast the bride—(everyone said that behind that cloud of snowy veil she was a tremendous beauty). Then the serious business of eating began. Hands reached, forks glittered, teeth sank into the delectable fare. But ten minutes later everyone had lain down their forks.

The food was uneatable.

It tasted of nothing. The cooks had forgotten to use any salt!

It was embarrassing, yes. It was disappointing, true. Guests muttered between themselves that the head cook ought to be hanged. But even so! It was surely nothing to cry about! So why was the old retired king from the kingdom next-door sobbing as if his heart would break, face sunk in his hands, the tears running out between his fingers, dripping on to his uneaten meat? 'Whatever is the matter?' they asked him.

'I had . . . I had a daughter once,' wept the old man. 'I asked her how much she loved me and she said— oh, God forgive me!—she said, "As much as meat loves salt". I was so stupid that I threw her out into the stormy world to starve and die. It's only now—too late—I understand: she really loved me best of all!'

But before the other guests could burst into tears of sympathy, the bride clapped her hands. 'Footmen,

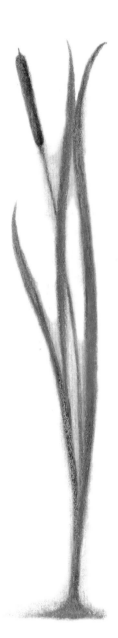

take this food away and feed it to the dogs!' she commanded. 'And, cook, fetch the other food—the dishes I told you to cook with salt.' Then she threw back her cloud-white veil, running the whole length of the table to kiss her father and show him her happy, shining face.

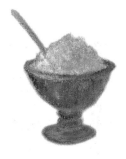

The Princess
and the Pea

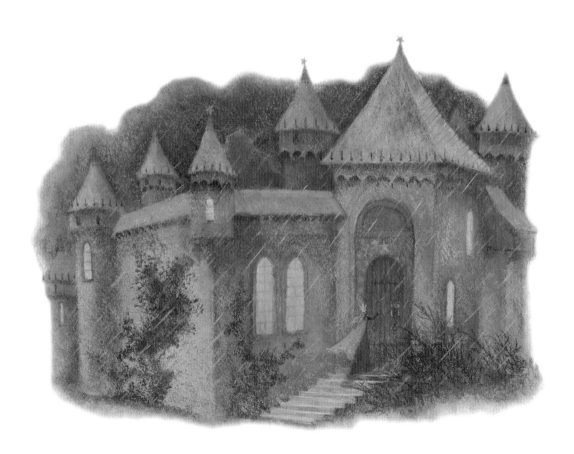

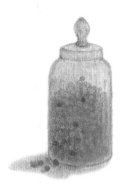

Some people are hard to please and some even harder. When it came to choosing a wife, Prince Particular was hardest of them all. 'Unless I can find a Real princess,' he said, 'I shall not marry at all.'

'A royal princess, don't you mean?' said his mother the queen.

'Not at all. A Real princess is what I said and a Real princess is what I meant. These days there are imitations everywhere—girls passing themselves off, girls giving themselves airs, girls stre-e-etching the truth.'

'But you would never marry such a one!' said the queen.

'Never!' agreed the prince, and went in search of his dream. He scoured the land. He placed advertisements in the newspapers:

WANTED:

a Real Princess with a view to marriage.
Genuine applicants only please.

He met countless girls and numberless women. He danced till his shoes and his conversation wore out. But though he met Princess Rose and Maharanee Myrtle, Infanta Flora, Sultana Sunflower, and Tsarina

Tulip—and all of them claimed to be Real—Prince Particular was not satisfied with any of them. Women smiled at him from behind veils, from behind fans, from behind masks. But Prince Particular did not smile back.

By the time he arrived home he was travel sick and sick of travel, heartsick and sick of seeking someone to whom he could give his heart. He abandoned all hope of marrying. It seemed there was not a Real princess left in the entire world. Like the dodo, they had all become extinct.

One stormy winter night, as draughts set all the castle doors banging and the tapestries riffled against the walls, and the rugs lifted along the floor, there came a knocking at the door.

'Who's there?' called the king through the grille.

'A traveller in need of shelter, sir! Princess Verity is my name. The storm frightened my horses and I fell from my carriage, and I am a stranger in these parts. I have walked many miles through this storm, and I am very cold and hungry!'

The king squinted through the grille. The girl outside did not look much like a princess. Her clothes were muddy and torn, her hair bedraggled and her face pinched with cold. But she was pretty and well spoken . . . and anyway the king would not have left a dog out on such a night. So he let her in to drip puddles on the hall floor.

'A princess, eh?' said Prince Particular with a smug, knowing look.

'A princess, eh?' said the queen. 'We shall see.'

The waif perched at the table and ate dinner in tiny morsels off the tip of her fork. She spoke of palaces and protocol, of archduke uncles and dowager aunts, of art and music and poetry. The prince's mouth fell wider and wider open as he watched the fork and the mouth into which it disappeared. He actually found himself wanting to believe. He found himself believing . . . Could this be? Could this storm-sodden urchin possibly be a Real princess?

The queen knew how to find out. 'We shall soon see,' she whispered to her son. 'There is one sure way of knowing.' To Verity she said, 'You must be tired out, child. I shall go and prepare a bed for you.'

The queen went upstairs and removed from the guest bed both eiderdown and mattress. On the base of the bed she laid a single dried pea. Then she put back the mattress, and the eiderdown too. On top she placed another mattress and another eiderdown. On top of that a third. In fact she went on piling mattresses and quilts on top of one another till the bed reached almost to the ceiling—a great sagging mountain of goose feathers. A ladder had to be

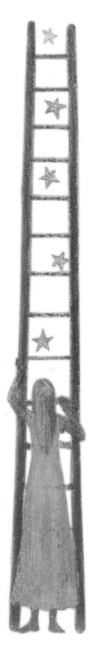

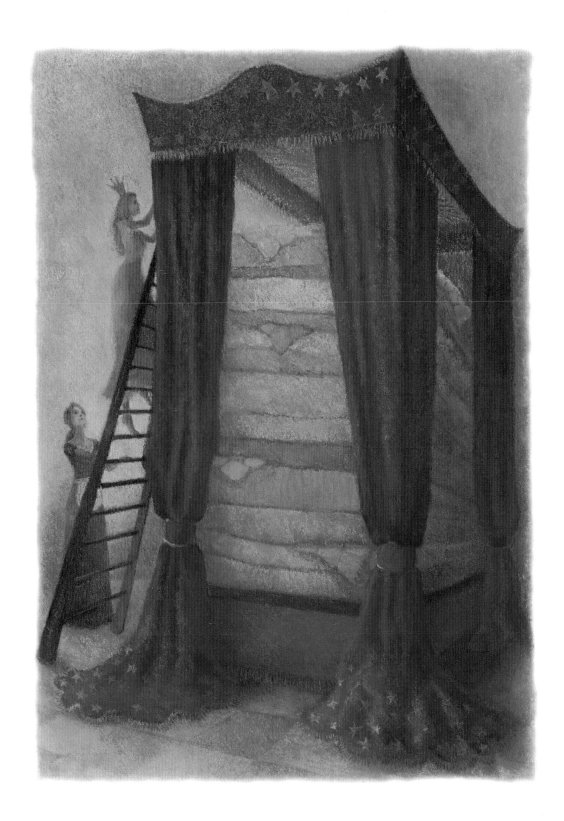

fetched before 'Princess' Verity could even climb into bed.

At breakfast next morning, Prince Particular found himself looking forward very much to seeing Verity again. He almost wished his mother had not set a test for her. He wished he knew what the test had been.

When Verity appeared, she had washed, and her hair was combed and she did not drip on the floor. But she looked almost as pale as she had the night before, with dark circles under her eyes and no colour in her cheeks.

'I hope you slept well, my dear?' asked the queen, inspecting the girl through a pair of spectacles on a stick.

Verity smiled wanly and curtsied, sitting down at table as if the seats were a little too hard. 'Thank you,' she said.

'Well, did you or didn't you?' asked the queen (rather rudely, Particular thought). 'Did you sleep well?'

Verity ducked her head. 'Quite well,' she said.

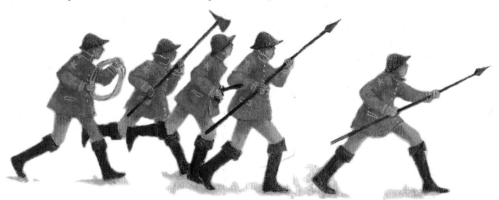

'Aha! I knew it!' exclaimed the queen, banging the table in a way that startled the footmen. 'Throw her out, the imposter!'

The footmen blinked, coughed awkwardly and shuffled their feet. The queen called out the guard. The soldiers came running with pikes and pistols and swords and cords. But as they laid hands on the poor girl, she cried, 'Oh, please don't grip me tightly, gentlemen. I am black and blue all over with bruises. Something in my bed . . .'

'Wait!' said the queen imperiously. 'Unhand her! What was that you said, girl?'

Verity blushed to the roots of her golden hair. 'Oh dear. You will think me dreadfully ungracious, after all your kindness. My dear mother the queen always taught me, a guest should never complain. It's just that in my bed . . .'

'Yes?'

'Last night . . .'

'Yes?'

'There seemed to be a . . .'

'Yes?'

'Something small and hard. I just couldn't sleep at all!'

Much to Verity's surprise, the queen whooped with joy and kissed the king. The king kissed the footman—and the prince kissed Verity.

'Only a princess is made of such delicate stuff that she can feel a pea through twenty mattresses!' cried the queen. 'My apologies, princess! But now I know that you are truly a Real princess!'

'That's just as well,' said Prince Particular under his breath. 'I was going to marry her anyway.'

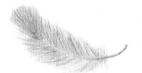